Diagnosis
of
Fungal
Infections

INFECTIOUS DISEASE AND THERAPY

Series Editor

Burke A. Cunha

*Winthrop-University Hospital Mineola, and
State University of New York School of Medicine
Stony Brook, New York*

Diagnosis
of
Fungal
Infections

Edited by

Johan A. Maertens
Universitaire Ziekenhuizen Leuven
Leuven, Belgium

Kieren A. Marr
Oregon Health and Science University
Portland, Oregon, USA

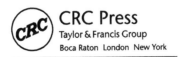

CRC Press
Taylor & Francis Group
Boca Raton London New York

CRC Press is an imprint of the
Taylor & Francis Group, an **Informa** business

First published 2007 by Informa Healthcare, Inc.

Published 2019 by CRC Press
Taylor & Francis Group
6000 Broken Sound Parkway NW, Suite 300
Boca Raton, FL 33487-2742

© 2007 by Taylor & Francis Group, LLC
CRC Press is an imprint of Taylor & Francis Group, an Informa business

First issued in paperback 2019

No claim to original U.S. Government works

ISBN 13: 978-0-367-45293-3 (pbk)
ISBN 13: 978-0-8247-2933-2 (hbk)

Visit the Taylor & Francis Web site at
http://www.taylorandfrancis.com

and the CRC Press Web site at
http://www.crcpress.com

Library of Congress Cataloging-in-Publication Data

Diagnosis of fungal infections / edited by Johan A. Maertens, Kieren A. Marr.
  p. ; cm. – (Infectious disease and therapy ; v. 47)
  Includes bibliographical references.
  ISBN-13: 978-0-8247-2933-2 (hardcover : alk. paper)
  ISBN-10: 0-8247-2933-1 (hardcover : alk. paper)
1. Mycoses–Diagnosis. I. Maertens, Johan A. II. Marr, Kieren A. III. Series.
  [DNLM: 1. Mycoses–diagnosis. W1 IN406HMN v.47 2007 / WC 450 D536 2007]

RC117.D47 2007
616.9'69075–dc22   2007023321

Preface

Fungal infections are a leading cause of death in multiple different patient populations; experience over the last few decades has been that these organisms are a leading cause of transplant-related mortality after stem cell transplantation, a frequent complication of organ transplantation, a leading cause of death in people with advanced human immunodeficiency virus disease, and a common cause of bloodstream infection among the hospitalized population. New studies are indicating that known fungi are involved as inciters in disease states not previously thought to be infectious (e.g., asthma and sinusitis), and "new" organisms are being discovered. Recognition of these organisms as important complications of the immunosuppressed state has generated much basic and clinical research since the 1980s and recent development of several new antifungal drugs. Despite these efforts and advancements, high mortality is at least in part resultant from difficulties in establishing confirmed diagnoses. Diagnostic difficulties have led to potentially inappropriate "empirical" antifungal administration strategies and over-utilization of antifungals and lack of appropriate therapy in the setting of established disease. Currently, appreciation of emerging resistance to several antifungal drugs complicates treatment decisions in the absence of microbial diagnoses. It appears that the field is largely at an impasse, awaiting development of new diagnostics.

Establishing the diagnosis of fungal infections is complicated, in part because these organisms are typically difficult to recover in the laboratory, either by laboratory culture, or by histopathological identification. Laboratory recovery of fungi has been improved in some settings; for instance, blood culture of *Candida* species has been facilitated with improvements in culture systems. However, other organisms remain elusive. For instance, filamentous organisms continue to be difficult to recover in culture, even in the presence of documented disease with visualized fungal fragments under the microscope. Recent observations suggest that there may be ways to improve laboratory cultivation of such organisms by adjusting growth conditions; however, optimized culture conditions appear to be relatively far from current practice. Other fungi, such as *Pneumocystis*, have never been cultivated in either clinical or basic research laboratories; we obviously have much to learn about fungal cultivation in the laboratory.

Given the complexities in obtaining diagnoses based on isolating organisms in the laboratory, efforts are now focused on developing diagnostics based on serologic tests, antigen identification, and advanced methods for detecting fungal nucleic acids. These tests have been in use for identifying endemic fungi, such as *Histoplasma*, for quite some time, and efforts have led towards relative optimization. However, other tests that detect *Candida* species and filamentous organisms are relatively younger in development and use, with differences in local and regional expertise guiding a great deal of variability in utilization. Other molecular tests that rely on polymerase chain reaction for identification of nucleic acids have become increasingly explored in research laboratories and are reaching some clinical microbiology laboratories. Much needs to be learned in order to most effectively use these types of tests for adjunctive diagnostics and for development of preventative strategies.

This book is focused on fungal diagnostics; it is timely in both the increasing toll of fungal infections worldwide, and in the heterogeneity of diagnostic practices. We have attempted to provide both a historical perspective and an update on state-of-the-art diagnostics, in both the general sense (Part I), and with considering the approach to specific infections (Part II).

In Part I, considerations of fungal diagnostics are discussed, with chapters that are focused on general methods. Establishing a clinical diagnosis with consideration of signs and symptoms is the first topic. Conventional diagnostics tools, including the roles of clinical microbiology and pathology laboratories, are discussed in the next chapter. Radiology, which is the staple for identification of fungal pneumonias, is addressed in one complete chapter. Following chapters deal with serodiagnostics, use of fungal metabolites, and molecular diagnostics; these chapters are not microbe-specific, but address multiple issues and tests across different pathogenic fungi.

Part II provides a more complete and detailed discussion of diagnostic methods for the most common superficial and invasive fungal infections. Specific chapters address superficial infections, mould infections, *Candida* and *Cryptococcus* infections, *Pneumocystis*, and endemic mycoses. These chapters all provide historical perspectives, as well as state-of-the-art approaches to diagnosing infectious complications in different hosts. Chapter 13 addresses the increasingly appreciated complication of fungal involvement in hypersensitivity and allergic conditions. The final chapter in the book raises perhaps the most "futuristic" issue concerning fungal diagnosis, which is molecular identification of emerging fungal pathogens, and our increasing understanding that as yet undiscovered organisms are the cause of disease states that have been historically considered to be non-infectious conditions. This topic is an apropos ending to summarize the general theme of the book, which is that we have learned a great deal, but we still have a great deal more to learn about fungal diagnostics.

This monograph is intended to offer both practical advice and to spur thoughts leading to new research. Our hope is that this will be found useful to laboratorians as well as clinicians of all varieties. The authors have provided both detailed reviews and thorough references. We acknowledge, at the onset, that there is much to be learned; with this in mind, we hope that this can be an effective platform from which gaps in knowledge can be identified and, subsequently, filled.

Johan A. Maertens, M.D.
Kieren A. Marr, M.D.

Contents

PART II: DIAGNOSTIC APPROACHES TO SPECIFIC FUNGAL INFECTIONS

PART III: MOVING FORWARD: "FUTURISTIC" ISSUES

Contributors

Gregory M. Anstead Division of Infectious Diseases, Department of Medicine, University of Texas Health Science Center, and Medical Service, South Texas Veterans Healthcare System, San Antonio, Texas, U.S.A.

Bethany Bergamo Department of Dermatology, University of Alabama at Birmingham, Birmingham, Alabama, U.S.A.

Methee Chayakulkeeree Division of Infectious Diseases, Department of Medicine, Duke University Medical Center, Durham, North Carolina, U.S.A., and Division of Infectious Diseases and Tropical Medicine, Department of Medicine, Siriraj Hospital, Mahidol University, Bangkok, Thailand

Hermann Einsele Department of Hematology and Oncology, Medizinische Klinik, Tübingen, Germany

David N. Fredricks Program in Infections Diseases at the Fred Hutchinson Cancer Research Center, and Division of Allergy and Infectious Diseases, Department of Medicine, University of Washington, Seattle, Washington, U.S.A.

John R. Graybill Division of Infectious Diseases, Department of Medicine, University of Texas Health Science Center, San Antonio, Texas, U.S.A.

Reginald Greene Department of Radiology, Massachusetts General Hospital and Harvard Medical School, Boston, Massachusetts, U.S.A.

Holger Hebart   Department of Hematology and Oncology, Medizinische Klinik, Tübingen, Germany

Carol A. Kauffman   Division of Infectious Diseases, Department of Internal Medicine, University of Michigan Medical School, and Veterans Affairs Ann Arbor Healthcare System, Ann Arbor, Michigan, U.S.A.

Juergen Loeffler   Department of Hematology and Oncology, Medizinische Klinik, Tübingen, Germany

Taruna Madan   Molecular Biochemistry and Diagnostics, Institute of Genomics and Integrative Biology, Delhi, India

Henry Masur   Critical Care Medicine Department, National Institutes of Health, Clinical Center, Bethesda, Maryland, U.S.A.

Christine J. Morrison   Office of the Chief Science Officer, Centers for Disease Control and Prevention, Atlanta, Georgia, U.S.A.

Marcio Nucci   Department of Internal Medicine, Hospital Universitário Clementino Fraga Filho, Universidade Federal do Rio de Janeiro, Rio de Janeiro, Brazil

Abigail Orenstein   Division of Pulmonary and Critical Care Medicine, Department of Medicine, University of Maryland School of Medicine, Baltimore, Maryland, U.S.A.

Luis Ostrosky-Zeichner   University of Texas Health Science Center at Houston, Houston, Texas, U.S.A.

Peter G. Pappas   Division of Infectious Diseases, University of Alabama at Birmingham, Birmingham, Alabama, U.S.A.

John R. Perfect   Division of Infectious Diseases, Department of Medicine and Department of Microbiology and Molecular Genetics, Duke University Medical Center, Durham, North Carolina, U.S.A.

Flavio Queiroz-Telles   Department of Communitarian Health, Hospital de Clínicas, Universidade Federal do Paraná, Curitiba, Paraná, Brazil

Anthonius J. M. M. Rijs   Department of Medical Microbiology, Radboud University Nijmegen Medical Center, Nijmegen University Center for Infectious Diseases, Nijmegen, The Netherlands

Fernanda P. Silveira   Division of Infectious Diseases, Department of Medicine, University of Pittsburgh, Pittsburgh, Pennsylvania, U.S.A.

Tania C. Sorrell   Centre for Infectious Diseases and Microbiology and Westmead Millennium Institute, University of Sydney, and Department of Infectious Diseases, Westmead Hospital, Westmead, New South Wales, Australia

Paul Stark   Department of Radiology, University of California, San Diego, California, U.S.A.

Henrich A. L. van der Lee   Department of Medical Microbiology, Radboud University Nijmegen Medical Center, Nijmegen University Center for Infectious Diseases, Nijmegen, The Netherlands

Paul E. Verweij   Department of Medical Microbiology, Radboud University Nijmegen Medical Center, Nijmegen University Center for Infectious Diseases, Nijmegen, The Netherlands

David W. Warnock   Division of Foodborne, Bacterial, and Mycotic Diseases, National Center for Zoonotic, Vector-Borne, and Enteric Diseases, Centers for Disease Control and Prevention, Atlanta, Georgia, U.S.A.

1

Pearls in Establishing a Clinical Diagnosis: Signs and Symptoms

Carol A. Kauffman

Division of Infectious Diseases, Department of Internal Medicine, University of Michigan Medical School, and Veterans Affairs Ann Arbor Healthcare System, Ann Arbor, Michigan, U.S.A.

INTRODUCTION

The symptoms and signs of fungal infection are protean. This is no surprise, given the variety of different types of fungi that are able to cause many different infections in humans. In some circumstances, the history and physical examination findings are so characteristic as to allow the diagnosis to be made at the bedside. In the majority of cases, however, the history and physical examination are suggestive of a possible fungal infection and will lead to more directed and definitive diagnostic tests. In a few situations, disease manifestations due to fungi clinically mimic those of bacterial infection so closely that the clinician is surprised when the laboratory identifies a fungus as the causative agent.

This chapter focuses on each of the components that physicians touch on as they obtain a history and perform a physical examination. As each of the areas of historical interest is explored, characteristics that point toward the diagnosis of a fungal infection, especially a specific fungal infection, are emphasized. With regard to the physical examination, abnormalities in those organ systems that are most frequently involved with fungal infections and in those that are readily seen on examination are emphasized.

HISTORY

Clues to the diagnosis of a fungal infection can be found by taking a thorough history. The specific elements of the history that are helpful include the obvious ones: history of the present illness, past medical and surgical history, and medications. Less immediately obvious, an in-depth social history that includes birthplace, travel, animal exposure (pets and others), occupation, leisure activities, and drug, cigarette, and alcohol use, provides valuable clues for the diagnosis of fungal infections. The review of systems occasionally may proffer a clue that helps with the diagnosis of a fungal infection, but this does not happen commonly. The history related to immunizations, allergies, and blood transfusions is less helpful.

History of Present Illness

The chief complaint and history of the present illness are obviously crucial elements in the history. All lines of questioning flow from these beginning historical points. General symptoms of infection, such as fever, chills, night sweats, fatigue, and anorexia are usually present, but obviously non-specific. Specific symptoms help focus on the affected organ systems, but those symptoms differ little from those due to bacterial infections. The context in which these symptoms occur, however, provides a much stronger impetus to include fungal infection in the differential diagnosis. For example, pleuritic chest pain and fever will cause great concern for fungal infection in a patient who has had an allogeneic stem cell transplant one year before and who has also been treated for severe chronic graft-versus-host disease in the preceding three months. However, non-fungal diagnoses will be entertained if the patient is an older adult who smokes and abuses alcohol or is a traveler who has just returned from a long overseas flight. As another example, a patient whose chief complaint is sudden development of a swollen painful eye with reduced vision will have fungal infection as the leading diagnosis, but only after the history of poorly controlled diabetes mellitus is obtained. Thus, although the history of the present illness sets the stage, ancillary material obtained from the rest of the history is even more important in directing the physician to consider fungal infections.

Past Medical and Surgical History

The past medical history reveals underlying illnesses that put the patient at risk for fungal infections, especially the opportunistic mycoses. For many patients, these underlying illnesses are central to the present illness and are already known to the physician. The most obvious are hematologic malignancies, transplants, or conditions for which immunosuppressive agents are given. Sometimes, a person who has received a transplant (usually heart or kidney) years before and has done well does not mention the transplant in the initial history because they are preoccupied with what they think is an unrelated symptom. Only in the past medical history does that important fact emerge.

Although the greatest risk for infections in general is in the immediate transplant period, certain patients remain at risk for fungal infections years after they receive a transplant. This includes solid organ transplant recipients who remain at risk for infection with endemic mycoses and cryptococcosis (1,2) and allogeneic stem cell transplant recipients who develop chronic graft-versus-host disease and who remain at risk for angioinvasive mold infections (3). On the other hand, patients with solid organ cancers do not appear to be at high risk for fungal infections unless they have received chemotherapy, which makes them neutropenic, or unless they are on corticosteroids (4).

Diabetes mellitus is clearly a risk factor for infections with the zygomycetes; the usual scenario is poorly controlled, insulin-dependent diabetes with episodes of ketoacidosis (5). Diabetes may also contribute to increased risk for recurrent vulvovaginal candidiasis (6). Underlying fibrotic lung disease, as seen with ankylosing spondylitis, sarcoidosis, and healed tuberculosis, predisposes to the development of pulmonary aspergilloma (7), and emphysema is always an underlying condition in patients with chronic cavitary pulmonary histoplasmosis (8). Many children and young adults with long-standing cystic fibrosis ultimately become colonized with *Aspergillus* species and develop allergic bronchopulmonary aspergillosis (7). Chronic granulomatous disease interferes with the ability of the host to defend against *Aspergillus*, as well as several other fungi; the presentation is usually one of a chronic pulmonary lesion or an osteoarticular infection with a draining sinus tract (9).

A history of HIV infection should be sought, as this infection places the patient at risk for several different fungal infections, including candidiasis, cryptococcosis, histoplasmosis, coccidioidomycosis, and aspergillosis (10–13). In fact, on many occasions, it is the diagnosis of a fungal infection that reveals a previously undiagnosed HIV infection.

Medications

Several types of medications play an important role in increasing the risk for fungal infections. Most, but not all, are immunosuppressive agents. Corticosteroids are especially important as a risk factor for invasive fungal infections (14). Cancer chemotherapeutic agents increase the risk for fungal infections, primarily because of the development of neutropenia, but their effects on gastrointestinal tract mucosa also allow opportunistic fungi, such as *Candida*, to gain access to the bloodstream (15). Calcineurin inhibitors, mycophenolate mofetil, and newer monoclonal anti-lymphocyte agents used in solid organ transplant recipients also increase the risk of opportunistic fungal infections (16). The expanded use of anti-tumor necrosis factor agents, infliximab, enteracept, and adalimumab, has led to an upsurge in fungal infections, both with opportunists, such as aspergillosis, and with the endemic mycoses, especially histoplasmosis and coccidioidomycosis (17–19).

Patients who have iron overload, and who are treated with the chelator deferoxamine, are at risk for development of invasive zygomycosis (20). *Rhizopus* is able to bind the chelator and use it as a siderophore capturing extra iron, a growth factor for enhancing fungal growth. Currently, this is more often noted in those with transfusion-dependent myelodysplastic syndromes than in dialysis patients compared with previous years. Localized mucocutaneous candidiasis, especially vulvovaginitis, is associated with the use of broad-spectrum antibiotic agents.

It is important to know if an immunocompromised patient is receiving an antifungal agent for prophylaxis. In this situation, a fungal infection that develops is most likely to be resistant to that agent. For example, if a patient on fluconazole prophylaxis develops fungemia, the most likely organisms will be *Candida glabrata* or *Candida krusei*, and not *Candida albicans* (21). A patient who is on voriconazole prophylaxis and who develops a nodular pulmonary infiltrate is more likely to have a zygomycete infection rather than a voriconazole-susceptible fungal infection (22–24).

Social History

Endemic Mycoses

For the endemic mycoses, the patient's history related to birthplace, travel, occupation, and leisure activities is extremely important. For example, a person who spent his or her childhood in the Mississippi or Ohio River drainage basins is likely to have been exposed to *Histoplasma capsulatum*. Years later, when presenting with a constellation of symptoms in New York City or Seattle, a perplexed physician cannot make a diagnosis of histoplasmosis until the question is asked as to where the patient's childhood was spent.

Recent travel that occurred just prior to the current illness for which the patient is seeking consultation is most helpful in establishing a diagnosis of an endemic mycosis. However, distant travel may also be relevant, especially when the patient is an immunosuppressed host whose current illness could reflect reactivation of distant infection, especially histoplasmosis or coccidioidomycosis. Travel while in the armed services also should be queried. A tour of duty that included southeastern Asia may have exposed the patient to *Penicillium marneffei*, a dimorphic fungus endemic to Thailand and several other areas in southeast Asia, but not found on other continents (25). Although less exotic, assignment to boot camp at a base in the southwestern or mid-western United States could have allowed exposure to the endemic fungi in those regions (26). For most travelers who are from other continents and who indulge in typical tourist activities in the United States, the risks of exposure to *H. capsulatum* or *Coccidioides immitis* are exceedingly low. However, exposure to *C. immitis* is possible if their tour takes them into the desert or they find themselves in the midst of a dust storm blowing from the desert (27).

Many people do things in their leisure time that are not expected, may seem out of character, and remain unknown to the physician unless specifically sought. It is mostly outdoor leisure activities that have been associated with exposure to the endemic fungi. The most straightforward is the association of gardening, especially rose gardening, with sporotrichosis (28). Another less obvious exposure that should be sought when a patient presents with skin lesions in a lympocutaneous distribution is playing in prairie hay (29,30). The leisure activity that is most often associated with the development of histoplasmosis is spelunking (31). Many caves in Central America and east of the Mississippi in the United States have large bat populations and luxurious growth of *H. capsulatum* in their guano, from which the conidia can be aerosolized when disturbed (32). Hunters and, interestingly, their dogs appear to have an increased risk of developing blastomycosis, presumably because of exposure to both as they rustle through wooded areas (33).

Participation in archeological digs in certain areas of Central America and the western United States puts those involved, many of whom do this as an eco-tour vacation, at risk for exposure to *C. immitis* (34). Almost any activity that disturbs the soil in the endemic area can lead to exposure to *C. immitis* arthroconidia. A dramatic recent event was the World Championship of Model Airplane Flying that was held in Kern County, California in which many individuals became infected when dust billowed into the air as the small planes took off (35). Well-meaning individuals who participated in building houses or churches in Central America have been infected with *C. immitis* when the soil was disturbed with construction activities (36).

Certain occupations place persons at risk for specific fungal infections. Landscapers and forestry workers are at risk for sporotrichosis (37–39). Bridge workers acquire histoplasmosis as they clean off the accumulated guano from birds and bats (40). Construction workers and those operating earth-moving equipment are also at risk for histoplasmosis (41), as are workers in the logging and wood pulp production industry (42). Less well known, however, is the risk of acquiring coccidioidomycosis by long-haul truck drivers whose routes go through the desert southwest (27). Veterinarians are at risk for acquiring sporotrichosis from infected cats, which often have ulcerated lesions that contain an enormous burden of *Sporothrix schenckii* (43).

With both leisure and occupational activities, obtaining a history of whether others have been similarly affected can be very helpful. Although a few bacteria, such as *Legionella* species, are associated with point source outbreaks, acute pneumonia in multiple persons indulging in the same outdoor activity is frequently a tip-off to an endemic mycosis (31).

With few exceptions, such as that noted above and a few others, fungal infections are not transmitted directly from animals. Scratches from cats, squirrels, and armadillos that are either colonized or live in burrows that are contaminated can transmit *S. schenckii* (44–47). Obviously, one asks about armadillo scratches only in patients who live in certain areas of

South America, such as Uruguay in which the animals are endemic and are used as food. The association of blastomycosis in hunters and their dogs is generally thought to be because they share the same exposure as they hunt (33); however, transmission from a dog bite has been noted (48). The *P. marneffei* life cycle involves bamboo rats, but generally there is no known direct exposure of humans to rats (25).

The use of alcohol, cigarettes, and illicit drugs puts the patient at risk for development of certain types of endemic mycotic infections. For example, alcoholism (for unknown reasons) is a risk factor present in most cases of pulmonary, osteoarticular, or relapsing lymphocutaneous sporotrichosis (37). Chronic cavitary pulmonary histoplasmosis occurs only in those with underlying chronic obstructive pulmonary disease related to cigarette smoking (8), and pulmonary sporotrichosis has this same condition as a risk factor, in addition to the frequent history of alcohol abuse (37).

Opportunistic Mycoses

For the opportunistic fungal infections, travel, occupation, leisure activities, and animal exposure are less important than they are for the endemic mycoses. Classically, cryptococcal infection has been associated with pigeons. Although a few cases have been described with exposure to pigeon excreta prior to development of cryptococcosis, most patients have no history of any direct contact with pigeons. Pigeon breeders have increased antibody titers against *Cryptococcus neoformans*, but no increased rate of infection (49). Cryptococcosis on the Australian continent is frequently due to *C. neoformans*, var *gattii*, an organism whose life cycle is intimately tied to the eucalyptus tree and the koalas that inhabit these trees. However, there appears to be no direct link between koalas and humans in terms of transmission of *Cryptococcus* (50).

An important clue to the occurrence of opportunistic fungal infections in a seemingly otherwise healthy person is a history of illicit drug use. Intravenous drug users are at risk for brain abscesses due to the zygomycetes (51), endophthalmitis due to both *Aspergillus* and *Candida* (52,53), and fungal endocarditis (54). A triad of endophthalmitis, sternoclavicular septic arthritis, and folliculitis due to *C. albicans* and involving the face and upper trunk has been described in intravenous users of brown heroin (55). In this particular syndrome, the rather insoluble brown heroin is cut with lemon juice, which has been found to be the source of *C. albicans* (56). Marijuana use puts patients, especially those with immunosuppression, at risk for pulmonary aspergillosis since the plant is heavily contaminated with the conidia of *Aspergillus* (57).

PHYSICAL EXAMINATION

There are clues that can be gleaned from the physical examination that make one think of certain fungal infections. Most helpful is examination of those organs that are readily accessible, notably the skin, eyes, nose, and throat.

General

General signs of infection, such as fever, tachycardia, and acutely toxic or chronically ill appearance, are non-specific and usually do not help point the clinician toward fungal infection as a diagnosis. Patients with disseminated candidiasis can appear quite toxic, as can individuals who have had a huge environmental exposure to an endemic mycosis and present with acute respiratory distress syndrome, but these findings are indistinguishable from those seen with bacterial infections. At the other end of the spectrum, AIDS patients with cryptococcal meningitis may have no fever and no physical findings suggesting meningitis; only a mild headache will prompt the astute clinician to perform a lumbar puncture. Orthostatic hypotension is a valuable hint to look for chronic progressive disseminated histoplasmosis with adrenal involvement causing Addison's disease (58).

Skin

Skin lesions are quite helpful in the diagnosis of both yeast and mold infections. Not only are some distinctive in appearance, but biopsy is simple, quick, and relatively painless. Daily examination of the skin in an at-risk patient can provide an early clue before cultures yield fungi. If the lesions are pustular, a smear and Gram stain can sometimes demonstrate yeasts. Although it takes longer to obtain the answer, a punch biopsy and silver staining of the tissue is more sensitive for finding organisms, especially filamentous fungi, and is much more specific in defining the endemic mycoses.

The angioinvasive molds, such as the zygomycetes, *Aspergillus*, *Fusarium*, and *Scedosporium*, cause a variety of skin lesions (59–62). The hallmark is necrosis, which is related to invasion of blood vessels and subsequent tissue infarction. The lesions begin as papules or nodules on an erythematous base; they gradually enlarge, become pustular, and develop central necrosis (Fig. 1). *Fusarium* generally causes painful lesions while the lesions of *Aspergillus* and *Scedosporium* are usually not painful. Disseminated *Fusarium* infection may arise from onychomycosis or from a paronychia; cellulitis develops around the nail and hematogenous dissemination occurs rapidly.

Disseminated candidiasis is associated with the appearance of pustular lesions on an erythematous base (Figs. 2 and 3) (63). In profoundly neutropenic patients, the lesions may remain macular. As the lesions progress, they can develop a central eschar, but they rarely cause necrosis as seen with the angioinvasive fungi. They can appear over any area of the body.

Although cryptococcosis causes primarily meningitis, skin lesions are commonly seen in those patients who have disseminated infection. Ulcerations, papules, nodules, and cellulitis have all been described (Fig. 4) (64). Multiple molluscum-like lesions are the most common skin manifestation in AIDS patients (65).

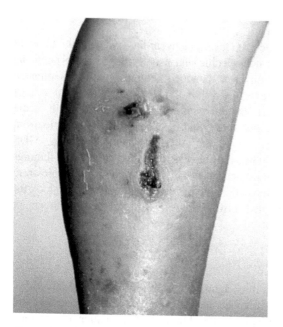

Figure 1 *Rhizopus* infection in an elderly man with myelodysplastic syndrome on deferoxamine chelation therapy.

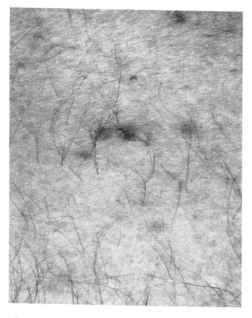

Figure 2 Skin lesions associated with candidemia on the back of a patient who had chronic lymphocytic leukemia and who was neutropenic.

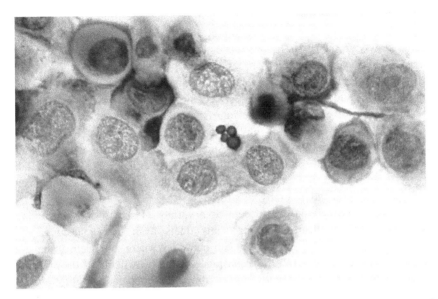

Figure 3　Wright's stain of smear from a lesion shown in Figure 2, showing a cluster of budding yeast.

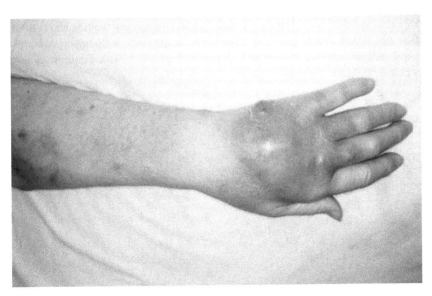

Figure 4　Cellulitis due to *Cryptococcus neoformans* in a patient who had renal failure and was on dialysis.

The endemic mycoses all can cause skin lesions, some of which are distinctive and lead directly to the correct diagnosis. Blastomycosis classically causes slowly growing, painless verrucous lesions with well-defined borders and a central area containing microabscesses with purulent exudate (Fig. 5) (66). Sporotrichosis is characterized by an initial nodular lesion that ulcerates and the subsequent development of similar lesions along the lymphatics draining the lesion (37). However, classic skin lesions are not always present. Blastomycosis can cause an acute eruption of multiple papules, and fixed cutaneous sporotrichosis, more commonly seen in South America, is manifested by a single, non-healing cutaneous ulceration (67). Conversely, a variety of mycobacterial, bacterial, and even drug-induced skin lesions can mimic the classic lesions seen with sporotrichosis and blastomycosis (68).

Coccidioidomycosis can present as a variety of skin lesions, including nodules, cellulitis, ulcers, draining sinus tracts from deeper lesions, and verrucous, non-painful lesions. They can occur anywhere, but seem to have a predilection for the face (69). Histoplasmosis is the least likely of the endemic mycoses to cause skin lesions, but in the AIDS population, eruptions of molluscum-like lesions, papules, folliculitis, and nodules containing *H. capsulatum* yeasts are not uncommon (70).

Head, Eyes, Ears, Nose, and Throat

The most obvious fungal infection involving the head and neck is oropharyngeal candidiasis, which presents as white plaques on the buccal and gingival mucosa, the palate, and the tongue. Isolated tongue involvement is uncommon and is more often not thrush but some other condition. In patients with upper dentures, plaques are uncommon, and painful palatal erythema is the sole manifestation of so-called "denture stomatitis" due to *Candida* (71).

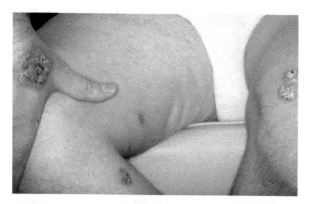

Figure 5 Multiple verrucous lesions due to *Blastomyces dermatitidis* in a farmer.

Disseminated histoplasmosis frequently presents with mucocutaneous lesions involving the palate, the tongue, the buccal or gingival mucosa, or the nasolabial area (58). Frequently these ulcers are painful, but firm, non-painful nodular lesions can also occur. Blastomycosis occasionally causes mass-like lesions in the oropharynx and larynx (72).

Swelling of the face, tenderness over the sinuses, and purulent nasal discharge are all signs associated with fungal sinusitis (73–76). The initial sign is usually facial pain and it is often out of proportion to other physical signs. This finding alone in an immunocompromised patient is enough to precipitate a work-up for invasive fungal sinusitis. A black eschar on the nasal mucosa or the palate indicates tissue necrosis associated with angioinvasive mold infections. However, before the mucosa of the palate or nose turns black, it may appear gray and demonstrate hypesthesia and the absence of bleeding when lightly brushed. Drainage from the nares can be purulent or dark and bloody. Rapidity of progression and involvement of the cavernous sinus and intracerebral vessels is characteristic of the zygomycetes (75); the rhinocerebral form of the disease occurs more often in diabetics in ketoacidosis than in those with hematologic malignancies or neutropenia.

Orbital apex syndrome (ophthalmoplegia, ptosis, and loss of vision) is seen with chronic invasive fungal sinusitis (76). This subacute to chronic infection is usually due to *Aspergillus* species, and appears to occur more often in elderly individuals who are not overtly immunosuppressed. The initial diagnosis is often malignancy until the biopsy reveals hyphal elements and granulomatous inflammation.

Examination of the retina can reveal the discrete white lesions associated with *Candida* chorioretinitis or more advanced infection with extension of fungal growth into the vitreous. The latter occurs with both *Aspergillus* and *Candida* endophthalmitis (53). Signs of intracranial pressure seen with fungal meningitis and with mass-occupying lesions due to angioinvasive fungi also can be seen on retinal examination.

Pulmonary

Even though the lung is the primary target organ for many of the filamentous fungi as well as the endemic mycoses, physical examination of the lungs often is not very helpful in the diagnosis of fungal infection. Rales are non-specific, occurring with any type of pneumonitis; they also are not a sensitive sign, as they are frequently absent, even with extensive disease on chest radiograph. As a late sign, a pleural rub can be appreciated in patients who have an angioinvasive fungal infection, and patients with both angioinvasive infection as well as chronic pulmonary involvement with the endemic mycoses can have hemoptysis. Imaging procedures are much more sensitive than the physical examination for fungal pulmonary involvement.

Cardiovascular and Abdominal

The findings in patients with cardiac involvement due to fungi do not differ from those seen in patients with bacterial endocarditis or arteritis. Similarly, there are few findings on abdominal exam that imply fungal infection. Hepatosplenomegaly occurs with disseminated histoplasmosis. Patients with chronic disseminated or hepatosplenic candidiasis have right upper quadrant tenderness and may have mild hepatomegaly.

Genitourinary Tract

Several fungi, notably *Blastomyces dermatitidis* and *C. neoformans*, frequently localize in the prostate during the course of disseminated infection (66,77). Examination of the prostate might reveal a nodular mass or an enlarged boggy prostate. Although uncommon, histoplasmosis can infect the prostate, epididymis, and testicles, usually presenting as a mass-like lesion (78,79). The classic presentation of *Candida* vulvovaginitis is that of a curd-like, white exudate, but thin, watery discharge with only erythema on the vaginal walls can also occur.

Central Nervous System

Fungal infection of the central nervous system (CNS) can present either as meningitis or brain abscess. The angioinvasive fungi are more likely to produce abscesses, as they invade through blood vessel walls and produce necrosis (80). New-onset motor or sensory deficits should prompt a search for an abscess, as should new-onset seizure activity. A frontal lobe abscess may remain relatively silent and produce only subtle mental status changes.

Meningitis is the usual manifestation of CNS involvement with cryptococcosis, coccidioidomycosis, and histoplasmosis. Patients usually have headache, photophobia and other visual complaints, and mental status changes; fever may or may not be present. With increased intracranial pressure, nausea and vomiting become prominent, cranial nerve palsies occur, and retinal examination shows papilledema.

CONCLUSIONS

By taking a complete history and doing a careful physical examination, the physician can gain some clues as to whether a fungal infection is present. Clearly, radiographic and laboratory studies are likely to be more specific, but the history and physical findings can help focus on those laboratory and radiographic studies that should be ordered. Careful attention to the evolution of signs and symptoms over time is also invaluable, especially in the case of immunocompromised hosts, whose clinical situation can change rapidly.

REFERENCES

1. Pappas PG, Perfect JR, Cloud GA, et al. Cryptococcosis in patients without HIV infection: management in the era of effective azole therapy. Clin Infect Dis 2001; 33:690–9.
2. Kauffman CA. Endemic mycoses after hematopoietic stem cell or solid organ transplantation. In: Bowden RA, Ljungman P, Paya CV, eds. Transplant Infections. 2nd ed. Philadelphia, PA: Lippincott Williams & Wilkins, 2003:524–34.
3. Marr KA, Carter RA, Boeckh M, Martin P, Corey L. Invasive aspergillosis in allogeneic stem cell transplant recipients: changes in epidemiology and risk factors. Blood 2002; 100:4358–66.
4. Lionakis MS, Kontoyiannis DP. The significance of isolation of saprophytic molds from the lower respiratory tract in patients with cancer. Cancer 2004; 100:165–72.
5. Ibrahim AS, Edwards JE, Filler SG. Zygomycosis. In: Dismukes WE, Pappas PG, Sobel JD, eds. Medical Mycology. New York: Oxford Press, 2003:241–51.
6. Sobel JD. Pathogenesis of recurrent vulvovaginal candidiasis. Curr Infect Dis Rep 2002; 4:514–9.
7. Judson MA. Noninvasive *Aspergillus* pulmonary disease. Semin Respir Crit Care Med 2004; 25:203–19.
8. Kauffman CA. Pulmonary histoplasmosis. Curr Infect Dis Rep 2001; 3:279–85.
9. Gallin JI, Alling DW, Malech HL, et al. Itraconzole to prevent fungal infections in chronic granulomatous disease. N Engl J Med 2003; 348:2416–22.
10. Hajjeh RA, Conn LA, Stephens DS, et al. Cryptococcosis: population-based multistate active surveillance and risk factors in human immunodeficiency virus-infected persons. J Infect Dis 1999; 179:449–54.
11. Wheat J. Histoplasmosis in the acquired immunodeficiency syndrome. Curr Top Med Mycol 1996; 7:7–18.
12. Mylonakis E, Barlam TF, Flanigan T, Rich JD. Pulmonary aspergillosis and invasive disease in AIDS. Review of 342 cases. Chest 1998; 114:251–62.
13. Ampel NM. Coccidioidomycosis among persons with human immunodeficiency virus infection in the era of highly active antiretroviral therapy (HAART). Semin Respir Infect 2001; 16:257–62.
14. Lionakis MS, Kontoyiannis DP. Glucocorticoids and invasive fungal infections. Lancet 2003; 362:1828–38.
15. Bow EJ, Loewen R, Cheang MS, Schacter B. Invasive fungal disease in adults undergoing remission-induction therapy for acute myeloid leukemia: the pathogenetic role of the antileukemic regimen. Clin Infect Dis 1995; 21:361–9.
16. Conti F, Morelon E, Calmus Y. Immunosuppressive therapy in liver transplantation. J Hepatology 2003; 39:664–78.
17. Bergstrom L, Yocum DE, Amperl NM, et al. Increased risk of coccidioidomycosis in patients treated with tumor necrosis factor-alpha antagonists. Arthritis Rheum 2004; 50:1959–66.
18. Wood KL, Hage CA, Knox KS, et al. Histoplasmosis after treatment with anti-tumor necrosis factor-alpha therapy. Am J Respir Crit Care Med 2003; 167:1279–82.

19. De Rosa FG, Shaz D, Campagna AC, Dellaripa PF, Khettry U, Craven DE. Invasive pulmonary aspergillosis soon after therapy with infliximab, a tumor necrosis factor-alpha-neutralizing antibody: a possible healthcare-associated case? Infect Control Hosp Epidemiol 2003; 24:477–82.

20. Daly AL, Velazquez LA, Bradley SF, Kauffman CA. Mucormycosis: association with deferoxamine therapy. Am J Med 1989; 87:468–71.

21. Wingard JR, Merz WG, Rinaldi MG, Johnson TR, Karp JE, Saral R. Increase in *Candida krusei* infection among patients with bone marrow transplantation and neutropenia treated prophylactically with fluconazole. N Engl J Med 1991; 325:1274–7.

22. Siwek GT, Dodgson KJ, de Magalhaes-Silverman M, et al. Invasive zygomycosis in hematopoietic stem-cell transplant patients receiving voriconazole prophylaxis. Clin Infect Dis 2004; 39:584–7.

23. Marty FM, Cosimi LA, Baden LR. Breakthrough zygomycosis after voriconazole treatment in recipients of hematopoietic stem-cell transplants. N Engl J Med 2004; 350:950–2.

24. Imhof A, Balajee SA, Fredricks DN, Englund JA, Marr KA. Breakthrough fungal infections in stem cell transplant patients receiving voriconazole. Clin Infect Dis 2004; 39:743–6.

25. Duong TA. Infection due to *Penicillium marneffei*, an emerging pathogen: review of 155 reported cases. Clin Infect Dis 1996; 23:125–30.

26. Crum N, Lamb C, Utz G, Amundson D, Wallace M. Coccidioidomycosis outbreak among United States navy SEALS training in a *Coccidioides immitis*-endemic area-Coalinga, California. J Infect Dis 2002; 186:865–8.

27. Kirkland TN, Fierer J. Coccidioidomycosis: a reemerging infectious disease. Emerg Infect Dis 1996; 2:192–9.

28. Kedes LH, Siemienski J, Braude AI. The syndrome of the alcoholic rose gardener. Sporotrichosis of the radial tendon sheath. Ann Intern Med 1964; 61:1139–41.

29. Dooley DP, Bostic PS, Beckius ML. Spook house sporotrichosis. A point-source outbreak of cutaneous sporotrichosis from hay bale props in a Halloween haunted-house. Arch Intern Med 1997; 157:1885–7.

30. Laur WE, Posey RE, Waller JD. A familial epidemic of cutaneous sporotrichosis occurring in north Texas. Cutis 1979; 23:205–8.

31. Cano M, Hajjeh RA. The epidemiology of histoplasmosis: a review. Semin Respir Infect 2001; 16:109–18.

32. Weinberg M, Weeks J, Lance-Parker S, et al. Severe histoplasmosis in travelers to Nicaragua. Emerg Infect Dis 2003; 9:1322–5.

33. Armstrong CW, Jenkins SR, Kaufman L, Kerkering TM, Rouse BS, Miller GB. Common-source outbreak of blastomycosis in hunters and their dogs. J Infect Dis 1987; 155:568–670.

34. Mardo D, Christensen RA, Nielson N, et al. Coccidioidomycosis in workers at an archeological site—Dinosaur National Monument, Utah, June–July 2001. Morbid Mortal Weekly Rep 2001; 50:1005–8.

35. Nicoll A, Evans B, Asgari N, et al. Coccidioidomycosis among persons attending the world championship of model airplane flying—Kern County, California, October 2001. Morbid Mortal Weekly Rep 2001; 50:1106–7.

36. Cairns L, Blythe D, Kao A, et al. Outbreak of coccidioidomycosis in Washington state residents returning from Mexico. Clin Infect Dis 2000; 30:61–4.

37. Kauffman CA. Sporotrichosis, state-of-the-art. Clin Infect Dis 1999; 29:231–7.

38. Hajjeh R, McDonnell S, Reef S, et al. Outbreak of sporotrichosis among tree nursery workers. J Infect Dis 1997; 176:499–4.

39. Dixon DM, Salkin IF, Duncan RA, et al. Isolation and characterization of *Sporothrix schenckii* from clinical and environmental sources associated with the largest U.S. epidemic of sporotrichosis. J Clin Microbiol 1991; 29:1106–13.

40. Jones TF, Swinger GL, Craig AS, McNeil MM, Kaufman L, Schaffner W. Acute pulmonary histoplasmosis in bridge workers: a persistent problem. Am J Med 1999; 106:480–2.

41. D'Allesio DJ, Heeren RH, Hendricks SL, Ogilvie P, Furcolow ML. Starling roost as source of urban epidemic histoplasmosis in area of low incidence. Am Rev Respir Dis 1965; 9:725–31.

42. Stobierski MG, Hospedales CJ, Hall WN, Robinson-Dunn B, Hoch D, Sheill DA. Outbreak of histoplasmosis among employees in a paper factory-Michigan 1993. J Clin Microbiol 1996; 34:1220–3.

43. Reed KD, Moore FM, Geiger GE, Stemper ME. Zoonotic transmission of sporotrichosis: case report and review. Clin Infect Dis 1993; 16:384–7.

44. Conti Diaz IA. Epidemiology of sporotrichosis in Latin America. Mycopathologia 1989; 108:113–6.

45. Frean JA, Isaacson M, Miller GB, Mistry BD, Heney C. Sporotrichosis following a rodent bite. A case report. Mycopathologia 1991; 116:5–8.

46. Saravanakumar PS, Eslami P, Zar FA. Lymphocutaneous sporotrichosis associated with a squirrel bite: case report and review. Clin Infect Dis 1996; 23:647–8.

47. Barros MBL, Schubach AO, Valle ACF, et al. Cat-transmitted sporotrichosis epidemic in Rio de Janeiro, Brazil: description of a series of cases. Clin Infect Dis 2004; 38:529–35.

48. Gnann JW, Bressler GS, Bodet CA, Avent CK. Human blastomycosis after a dog bite. Ann Intern Med 1983; 98:48–9.

49. Casadevall A, Perfect JR. Ecology of *Cryptococcus neoformans*. In: *Cryptococcus neoformans*. Washington, DC: ASM Press, 1998:41–70.

50. Sorrell TC. *Cryptococcus neoformans* variety *gattii*. Med Mycol 2001; 39:155–68.

51. Hopkins RJ, Rothman M, Fiore A, Gildblum SE. Cerebral mucormycosis associated with intravenous drug use: three case reports and review. Clin Infect Dis 1994; 19:1133–7.

52. Elliott JH, O'Day DM, Gutow GS, Podgorski SF, Akrabawi P. Mycotic endophthalmitis in drug abusers. Am J Ophthalmol 1979; 88:66–72.

53. Riddell J, McNeil SM, Johnson TM, Bradley SF, Kazanjian PH, Kauffman CA. Endogenous *Aspergillus* endophthalmitis: report of three cases and review of the literature. Medicine 2002; 81:311–20.

54. Ellis M. Fungal endocarditis. J Infect 1997; 35:99–103.

55. Bisbe J, Miro JM, Latorre X, et al. Disseminated candidiasis in addicts who use brown heroin: report of 83 cases and review. Clin Infect Dis 1992; 15:910–23.

56. Shankland GS, Richardson MD, Dutton GN. Source of infection in *Candida* endophthalmitis in drug addicts. Br Med J 1986; 292:297–308.

57. Levitz SM, Diamond RD. Aspergillosis and marijuana. Ann Intern Med 1991; 115:578–9.

58. Wheat LJ, Kauffman CA. Histoplasmosis. Infect Dis Clin North Am 2003; 17:1–19.

59. Boutati EI, Anaissie EJ. *Fusarium*, a significant emerging pathogen in patients with hematologic malignany: ten years experience at a cancer center and implications for management. Blood 1997; 90:999–1008.

60. Nucci M, Anaissie E. Cutaneous infection by *Fusarium* species in healthy and immunocompromised hosts: implications for diagnosis and management. Clin Infect Dis 2002; 35:909–20.

61. Castiglioni B, Sutton DA, Rinaldi MG, Fung J, Kusne S. *Pseudallescheria boydii* (anamorph *Scedosporium apiospermum*) infection in solid organ transplant recipients in a tertiary medical center and review of the literature. Medicine (Baltimore) 2002; 81:333–48.

62. Kontoyiannis DP, Wessel VC, Bodey GP, et al. Zygomycosis in the 1990s in a tertiary-care cancer center. Clin Infect Dis 2000; 30:851–6.

63. Sable CA, Donowitz GR. Infections in bone marrow transplant recipients. Clin Infect Dis 1994; 18:273–81.

64. Pema K, Diaz J, Guerra LG, Nabhan D, Verghese A. Disseminated cryptococcosis: comparison of clinical manifestations in the pre-AIDS and the AIDS era. Arch Intern Med 1994; 154:1032–4.

65. Cockerell CJ. Human immunodeficiency virus infection and the skin: a crucial interface. Arch Intern Med 1991; 151:1295–303.

66. Pappas PG. Blastomycosis. Semin Respir Crit Care Med 2004; 25:113–22.

67. Pappas PG, Tellez I, Deep AE, Nolasco D, Holgado W, Bustamante B. Sporotrichosis in Peru: description of an area of hyperendemicity. Clin Infect Dis 2000; 30:65–70.

68. Kostman JR, DiNubile MJ. Nodular lymphangitis: a distinctive but often unrecognized syndrome. Ann Intern Med 1993; 118:883–8.

69. Kim A, Parker SS. Coccidioidomycosis: case report and update on diagnosis and management. J Am Acad Dermatol 2002; 46:743–7.

70. Cohen PR, Bank DE, Silvers DN, Grossman ME. Cutaneous lesions of disseminated histoplasmosis in human immunodeficiency virus-infected patients. J Am Acad Dermatol 1990; 23:422–8.

71. Shay K, Truhlar MR, Renner RP. Oropharyngeal candidosis in the older patient. J Am Geriatr Soc 1997; 45:863–70.

72. Hanson JM, Spector G, El-Mofty SK. Laryngeal blastomycosis: a commonly missed diagnosis. Report of two cases and review of the literature. Ann Otol Rhinol Laryngol 2001; 109:281–6.

73. Gillespie MB, O'Malley BW, Francis HW. An approach to fulminant invasive fungal rhinosinusitis in the immunocompromised host. Arch Otolaryngol Head Neck Surg 1998; 124:520–6.

74. Iwen PC, Rupp ME, Hinrichs SH. Invasive mold sinusitis: 17 cases in immunocompromised patients and review of the literature. Clin Infect Dis 1997; 24:1178–84.

75. Ferguson BJ. Mucormycosis of the nose and paranasal sinuses. Otolaryngol Clin North Am 2000; 33:349–65.

76. deShazo RD, Chapin K, Swain RE. Fungal sinusitis. N Engl J Med 1997; 337:254–9.

77. Larsen RA, Bozette S, McCutchan JA, Chiu J, Leal MA, Richman DD. Persistent *Cryptococcus neoformans* infection of the prostate after successful treatment of meningitis. Ann Intern Med 1989; 111:125–8.

78. Mawhorter SD, Curley GV, Kursh ED, Farver CE. Prostatic and central nervous system histoplasmosis in an immunocompetent host: case report and review of the prostatic histoplasmosis literature. Clin Infect Dis 2000; 30:595–8.

79. Schuster TG, Hollenbeck BK, Kauffman CA, Chensue SW, Wei JT. Testicular histoplasmosis. J Urol 2000; 164:1652.

80. Walsh TJ, Hier DB, Caplan LR. Fungal infections of the central nervous system: comparative analysis of risk factors and clinical signs in 57 patients. Neurology 1985; 35:1654–7.

2

The Role of Conventional Diagnostic Tools

Paul E. Verweij, Henrich A. L. van der Lee, and Anthonius J. M. M. Rijs

Department of Medical Microbiology, Radboud University Nijmegen Medical Center, Nijmegen University Center for Infectious Diseases, Nijmegen, The Netherlands

INTRODUCTION

Many medical microbiology laboratories supporting the diagnosis of infectious diseases in humans culture fungi from clinical specimens. Fungi can be found by microscopic examination of clinical specimens or in cultures. As with other microbial diseases, the significance of these findings relies on the combination of the laboratory investigation with results of other tests or procedures and clinical observations. Within medical mycology, the availability of new diagnostic tools has had significant impact on the management of patients at risk for invasive fungal infection, as well as on the speed that results are available. New techniques include the detection of fungal antigens, such as cryptococcal antigen, mannan, galactomannan, and (1-3)-β-D-glucan, which were found to circulate in blood of patients with invasive fungal disease (1,2). Besides these biomarkers, the detection of genomic fungal DNA has been intensively investigated, and commercial formats are becoming available that help to diagnose invasive fungal infection early in the course of disease (3,4).

The development of these new techniques has been driven by the drawbacks of the conventional methods such as fungal culture. These drawbacks include, most notably, a low sensitivity and considerable delay in turn-around time due to slow growth of the fungus in culture and the time needed for its identification. The question is: Do conventional diagnostic methods, such as microscopy and culture, remain useful for the management of patients with invasive fungal infection?

IMPORTANCE OF CONVENTIONAL TOOLS FOR FUNGAL DIAGNOSIS

Given the increased complexity of patient populations subject to infection and the increasing variety of fungi that might cause infection, the necessity to identify the fungus causing disease to the species level has increased. Current guidelines recommend identifying all fungi (yeasts and molds) to the species level when cultured from sterile sites including blood, continuous ambulatory peritoneal dialysis (CAPD), and intravenous-line tips (5). Bronchoalveolar lavage (BAL) fluid is considered sterile, requiring all fungi, except *Candida*, to be fully identified (5). Adding to this is the increase of the number of antifungal compounds that are currently available to treat patients with invasive fungal infection, which differ in their antifungal spectrum. Both species identification and, to a lesser extent, in vitro susceptibility testing provide essential information to treat the patient with appropriate antifungal drugs. Species identification cannot be achieved with the systems that detect fungal antigens or metabolites, which at best enable a genus-specific diagnosis. The CT scan has become an essential tool to detect pulmonary lesions in neutropenic patients (6), but the lesions are not specific for a certain fungus. With these diagnostic tools, patients that require antifungal therapy can be identified early, but culture remains essential to confirm the diagnosis or to obtain etiologic identification.

In addition, routine culture of patients provides important information on the epidemiology. Systematic microbiological surveillance provides insights in trends of incidence of fungal pathogens and/or its resistance. It has been shown that the epidemiology can vary considerably between medical centers (7), and even within a single center the species distribution can vary between departments (8). Epidemic spread of certain strains can be detected using culture and further investigated by genotypic characterization of isolates (9). Finally, fungal isolates can be used for in vitro susceptibility testing to help guide antifungal therapy, as well as for monitoring changes of resistance. In vitro susceptibility testing of yeasts is common practice in most routine microbiology laboratories (10,11), but this is not the case for molds such as *Aspergillus*. The recently reported emergence of multiple-triazole resistance in *Aspergillus fumigatus* might change this practice and necessitate routine minimal inhibitory concentration (MIC) testing of clinically relevant mold isolates (12).

Although cultures typically take one or several days to become positive, direct examination of appropriate clinical specimens may provide significant diagnostic information very rapidly. This opportunity should be used in patients at high risk of invasive fungal disease.

DIRECT EXAMINATION AND STAINS

Direct examination is a rapid and cost-effective means of diagnosing fungal infection (13). Staining of clinical samples can be performed within minutes of receipt of the specimen and results are available within less than an hour, compared to one or several days for culture. Specific stains are available to aid the detection of fungi in wet preparations of the specimen and help to examine specific morphologic features that give direction to the etiologic agent. Furthermore, microscopy will be useful to interpret culture results, for instance in BAL fluid, which might yield a positive culture due to contamination with spores from the oral cavity. Specimens may be examined as a wet mount preparation with or without the addition of 10% potassium hydroxide, which aids in the visualization of hyphal elements through the partial digestion and clearing of proteinaceous material while leaving the fungal cell wall intact (14).

In many clinical microbiology laboratories the Gram stain is used as routine stain to identify microorganisms (primarily bacteria) in clinical specimens. Although this stain is useful for detection of bacteria, it is not optimal for detection of fungi. Nevertheless most fungi will be detected using the Gram stain, although some stain poorly like *Cryptococcus* spp. Most fungi are Gram positive (Fig. 1), but hyphal fragments may not stain and consequently be difficult to detect (Fig. 2). Fluorescent dyes such as Blankophor P, Calcofluor White, or Uvitex 2B are non-toxic dyes that bind to specific cell wall components, usually polysaccharides, cellulose, or chitin of fungi, and give intense fluorescence when examined through a fluorescence microscope. The probability of detecting fungal elements in clinical materials including tissue samples is higher than with the Gram stain, and morphological clues to which fungus is present can be detected that are easily overlooked when using only a Gram stain only (Fig. 3). If fungal elements are seen in the Gram stain, a new

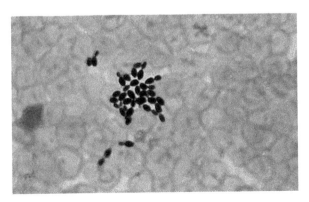

Figure 1 Gram stain of *Candida glabrata* in a blood culture. The yeast-cells are stained Gram positive.

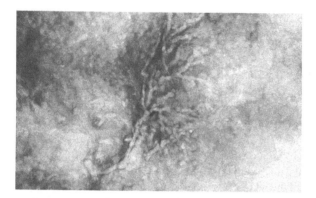

Figure 2 Gram stain of sputum with *Aspergillus fumigatus*. The hyphae do not take in the dyes and give a negative staining, which can easily be missed, especially when the smear is examined at high magnification.

wet preparation can be made to stain with the fluorescent dyes, but if such material is no longer available, the Gram-stained preparation can be used to stain with the fluorescent dye. Other stains commonly used for fungi are the India Ink which is used to detect encapsulated yeasts, such as *Cryptococcus* and the Giemsa stain, which is useful for detection of *Histoplasma capsulatum* in bone marrow and *Pneumocystis jiroveci* in respiratory secretions. A number of different stains commonly used in medical mycology are listed in Table 1 (15).

The microscopic morphology of fungi usually cannot be used to obtain a species identification of the etiologic fungus. At best, the difference between yeast and mold can be made as well as the distinction between *Aspergillus*-like

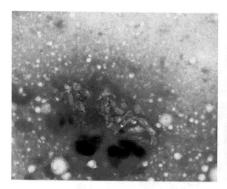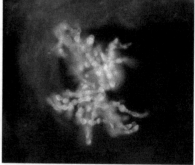

Figure 3 Gram stain of a liver biopsy (*left*) and Blankophor P stain (*right*) showing yeast-like structures. Cultures remained negative, but polymerase chain reaction identification was positive for *Candida albicans*.

Table 1 Some Commonly Used Methods for Direct Examination of Clinical Specimens for Fungi

Method	Use	Comments
Gram-stain	Detection of bacteria	Fungi commonly stain Gram positive
Calcofluor White, Blankophor P, Uvitex 2B	Detection of fungi, including *Pneumocystis jiroveci*	Fungi give bright green or blue fluorescence when examined with a fluorescence microscope. Can be mixed with 10% potassium hydroxide
Giemsa	Detection of fungi including *Histoplasma* spp., yeast cells, and trophozoites (not cysts) of *P. jiroveci*	Combines methylene blue and eosin
India Ink	Detection of *Cryptococcus neoformans*	The polysaccharide capsule of encapsulated organisms (e.g., *C. neoformans*) excludes the ink particles. Often used for CSF, sometimes difficult to distinguish yeast cells from leukocytes
Lactophenol cotton blue	Stain is recommended for mounting and staining yeast and molds	Organisms suspended in the stain are killed due to the presence of phenol
Potassium hydroxide (KOH) solution	Improves detection of fungi in keratinous material	Blue ink can be added as contrasting agent to improve detection of fungi

Abbreviation: CSF, cerebrospinal fluid.
Source: From Ref. 15.

hyphae and zygomycetes. Zygomycetes typically show broad, thin-walled hyphae with infrequent or absent septation, 5 to 25 μm wide, and branching sometimes occurs at strait 90° angles (Figs. 4 and 5). Zygomycetes involved in human disease typically involve *Rhizopus* spp., *Rhizomucor* spp., *Mucor* spp., *Absidia corymbifera*, *Apophysomyces elegans*, and *Cunninghamella bertholetiae* (17). The microscopic morphology of *Aspergillus* is quite different, consisting of septate hyphae, a uniform width of 3 to 6 μm, and dichotomous branching (Figs. 6 and 7). This morphology is not specific for *Aspergillus* and there are numerous molds that show similar features in tissue, including *Fusarium*, *Penicillium*, and *Scedosporium*. In general, it is difficult for an inexperienced practitioner to recognize these subtle microscopic differences. Also during treatment, the morphology might be atypical due to the growth conditions in tissue or exposure to antifungal agents (Fig. 8) (18). There are, however, some fungi that can be identified based on their characteristic morphology, including

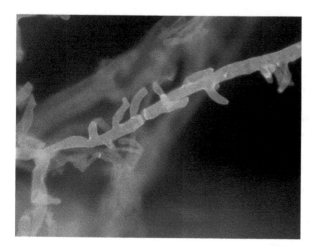

Figure 4   Blankophor P stain of lung specimen obtained at autopsy showing large, non-septate hyphae with branching at 90°. This morphology is consistent with a zygomycete and cultures were positive with *Rhizomucor pusillus*. *Source*: From Ref. 16.

Penicillium marneffei, H. capsulatum, Paracoccioides brasiliensis, Blastomyces dermatitidis, Coccidioides immitis, and *P. jiroveci.*

In the routine microbiology laboratory, the probability of fungi in for instance blood culture bottles is relatively low, and technicians might not be aware of fungi in the microscopy or may misidentify the fungus. Figure 9A shows a Gram stain of a blood culture of a hematology patient that was reported as being positive for yeasts. The microscopy showed both yeast-like elements as well as

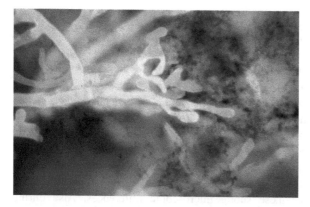

Figure 5   Calcofluor White stain of a lung specimen showing broad hyphae without septa, consistent with zygomycetes. Culture was negative, possibly due to previous antifungal treatment of the patient.

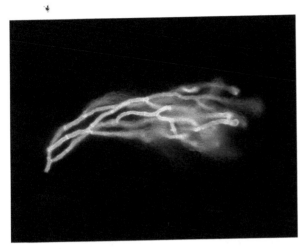

Figure 6 Blankophor P stain of a tissue biopsy of the skin of a patient with a necrotic lesion that had emerged during occlusion with a plaster. The morphology shows regular septate hyphae with dichotomous branching. The culture was positive with *Aspergillus flavus*.

hyphae, which is commonly seen in blood cultures than are positive with *Candida*. In this patient, however, a Blankophor P stain of the blood culture showed septate hyphae with monophialides bearing microconidia that were consistent with *Fusarium* (Fig. 9B). The culture was positive for *Fusarium oxysporum*. One should consider the possibility that yeast-like structures are not yeasts but actually spores from molds that are capable of producing spores in tissue. Although the probability that yeasts that are recovered in blood culture are members of the genus *Candida* is high, other possibilities need to be considered, such as *Cryptococcus* spp., *Malassezia* spp., and *Geotrichum* spp. Besides misinterpretation of the morphology, direct examination can be false-positive or false-negative.

Microscopy also helps to select culture media that will increase the probability of recovering the fungus in culture. For instance, a Sabouraud's dextrose agar could be added to blood agar plates in the case of detection of *Candida* in a blood culture bottle, or specific agars such as malt agar or bread agar can be used when the morphology is consistent with zygomycetes.

CULTURE

Since direct examination of clinical specimens does not allow identification to the species level, cultures should always be performed in addition to microscopy. Most clinically relevant yeast and molds grow readily on media routinely used in bacteriology.

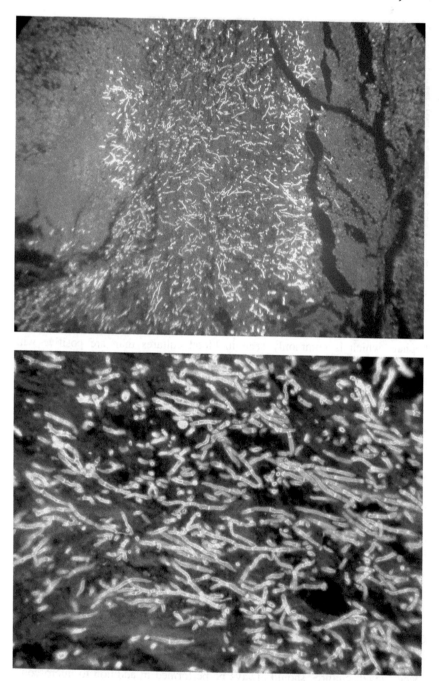

Figure 7   Blankophor P stain of a biopsy of a lesion in the oropharynx. The culture was positive with *Aspergillus fumigatus*. (*Top*, ×100; *bottom*, ×400.)

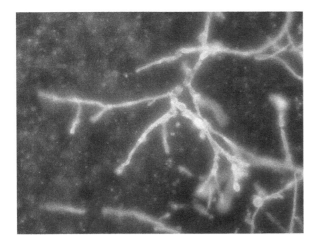

Figure 8 Blankophor P stain of a liver biopsy from a patient with primary hepatic invasive aspergillosis. The procedure was performed after several weeks of antifungal therapy. The morphology shows dichotomous branching of septate hyphae (suggestive for *Aspergillus*) but also yeast-like features (more in line with yeast). Culture was positive for *Aspergillus fumigatus* and there was no evidence for *Candida* species with negative culture and polymerase chain reaction. *Source*: From Ref. 17.

Blood culture remains an important means to diagnose invasive fungal infections, especially those caused by yeasts, as most molds, such as *Aspergillus*, fail to grow in blood cultures. When *Aspergillus* is recovered from the blood this is often caused by contamination of the blood culture bottle, although aspergillemia has been observed (19,20). Genuine aspergillemia was most often

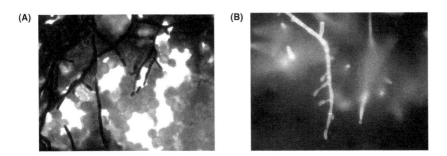

Figure 9 (**A**) Gram stain showing hyphal elements and yeast-like structures. These were interpreted and reported as consistent with a yeast, probably *Candida*. (**B**) Blankophor P stain of the same blood culture vial, as shown in (**A**), showing septate hyphae with monophialides bearing microconidia, consistent with *Fusarium*. The blood culture was positive with *Fusarium oxysporum*.

observed in cardiac patients or those with neutropenia. Pseudo-aspergillemia was characterized by negative results of repeat cultures (19,20). Only *Aspergillus terreus*, with its ability to produce yeast-like forms in tissue, was a common cause of true aspergillemia (21). Other angioinvasive molds, which have the ability to discharge a steady series of unicellular spores into the bloodstream during invasive infection in tissue, can readily be cultured from blood cultures, including *Fusarium* spp. (22), *Paecilomyces lilacinus*, *Acremonium* spp., and *Scedosporium prolificans* (23). This ability to sporulate in tissue and blood has been termed "adventitious sporulation" (24).

The sensitivity of automated blood culture systems with bottles that contain standard bacteriological medium for *Candida* is variable for different species, with *C. glabrata* showing very poor growth (Table 2) (25). For this species and *C. parapsilosis*, bottles containing Mycosis IC/F medium were significantly more sensitive (25). The mean time to detection in bottles containing standard bacteriological medium was over 18 hours for all *Candida* spp., with *C. glabrata* showing the longest time to detection (Table 2). The use of Mycosis IC/F was more effective, and it was advised to draw Mycosis IC/F vials in addition to standard bacteriological vials in patients with a high suspicion of fungemia (25). Also, other fungi, including *C. guillermondi*, *M. furfur*, *C. neoformans*, and *Fusarium* were detected more effectively when blood was cultured in the Mycosis IC/F vials (26,27). Delay in initiation of antifungal therapy has been shown to have significant impact on the survival of patients with candidemia. For patients that received at least one dose of empiric appropriate antifungal treatment prior to notification of a positive *Candida* blood culture result, the hospital mortality rate was lower, but not statistically significantly different, from those receiving appropriate antifungal treatment after notification of a positive blood culture result (28). However, overall, a multivariate analysis showed that delay of antifungal therapy was an independent risk factor for hospital mortality

Table 2 Positivity of Mycosis IC/F and Plus Aerobic/F Vials on Paired Blood Cultures According to Species and Time to Detection in Plus Aerobic/F Vials

Species	Mycologic IC/F (%)	Standard (plus aerobic/F) (%)	Mean detection time (hours ± standard deviation)
Candida albicans	82	78.1	39.9 ± 23.7
Candida parapsilosis	96.9	80	24.4 ± 14.5
Candida glabrata	95.3	37.5	61.5 ± 31.4
Candida tropicalis	91.1	83.9	18.5 ± 11.7
Candida krusei	89.7	89.7	26.7 ± 10.3

Source: From Ref. 25.

(28). This observation was confirmed by other investigators (29) and underscores the need to reduce the turn-around time for diagnostic tests of fungal infection.

Although most opportunistic fungi grow well on standard microbiological media, such as blood agar, chocolate agar, and brain heart infusion broth, medium that specifically supports the growth of fungi or inhibits the growth of other microorganisms is commonly used. Most commonly used are Sabouraud's dextrose agar and potato dextrose agar, which should be included in the work-up when mycological culture is specifically requested or when microscopy is positive for yeasts or hyphae. The yield of this agar is superior to standard bacteriologic medium (30). Antibacterial agents are commonly added in order to suppress the growth of bacteria, especially when material is obtained from a semi-sterile site (BAL fluid) or non-sterile sites. Antibiotics commonly used include chloramphenicol, gentamicin, penicillin, streptomycin, or ciprofloxacin (31). Another compound that is frequently incorporated into fungal culture media is the eukaryotic protein synthesis inhibitor cycloheximide. The addition of this compound is aimed at inhibiting the growth of saprobic molds that are clinically not relevant. However, clinically significant molds can also be inhibited, including *S. apiospermum*, *C. neoformans*, most zygomycetes, and some species of *Candida* and *Aspergillus* (31). In specific cases, plates with and without cycloheximide can be inoculated and incubated. Nutrient agars supplemented with other compounds can be used for the culture of specific fungi, such as dermatophytes (actidione), *Malassezia* spp. (oxe-bile and tween 40, Dixon agar), or *Cryptococcus* spp. (Guizotia abyssinia seeds, birdseed agar). As sporulation of molds is required to enable morphologic identification, media are used with reduced availability of nutrients in order to facilitate this process. Conventional Sabouraud's dextrose agar can be diluted (Takashio), or in some cases even water-based agar can be required to induce sporulation (32).

RECOVERY OF YEASTS

Invasive infections with *Candida* remain to be associated with significant morbidity and mortality (33). The importance of prompt treatment has been shown, and culture is one of the means by which a diagnosis can be established. *Candida* spp. commonly encountered in human disease include *C. albicans*, *C. glabrata*, *C. tropicalis*, and *C. parapsilosis*. These and other species readily grow within 24 to 48 hours on standard bacteriologic medium as well as mycological medium such as Sabouraud's dextrose agar (Fig. 10). When processing clinical specimens in the laboratory, and especially when yeasts are encountered, it is important to realize that some yeasts can be highly infectious, such as *C. immitis*, or that others might require specific nutrient requirements, such as *Malassezia* spp.

A rapid and simple test to achieve a presumptive identification of *C. albicans* is the germ-tube test. The test involves inoculation of several colonies of yeast into a substrate, usually fetal calf serum, and incubation at 37°C for three

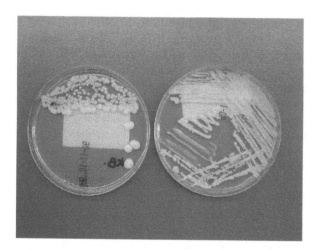

Figure 10 Growth of *Candida* species on Sabouraud's dextrose agar.

to four hours. *C. albicans* is characterized by the formation of germ-tubes, while other species usually do not produce germ-tubes within that time period. In approximately 5% of cases, *C. albicans* isolates fail to produce a germ-tube under these conditions. *C. dubliniensis* also produces germ-tubes in the germ-tube test, and additional phenotypic features need to be determined in order to differentiate it from *C. albicans* (Table 3; Fig. 11). Usually *Candida* colonies growing on blood agar or Sabouraud's dextrose plates after 24 hours of incubation are used to perform the germ-tube test. Some investigators have found that the test can be performed directly from positive blood culture vials (35).

Many commercial tests have become available over the past 10 years, including species-specific direct enzymatic color tests, differential chromogenic isolation plates, direct immunological tests, and enhanced manual and automated biochemical and enzymatic panels (36–39). Chromogenic isolation media demonstrate better detection rates of yeasts in mixed cultures than traditional

Table 3 Phenotypic Features that Help to Differentiate between *Candida albicans* and *Candida dubliniensis*

Test	*C. albicans*	*C. dubliniensis*
Growth at 37°C	+	+
Growth at 45°C	+/−	−
Assimilation of xylose	+	−
Production of chlamydospores[a]	+ (after 2 days)	+ + (after 1 day)

[a] See Figure 10.
Source: From Ref. 34.

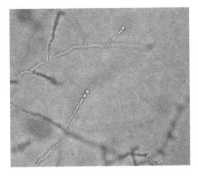 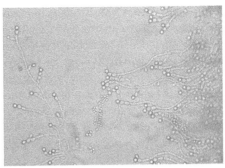

Figure 11 Microscopic morphology of chlamydospore formation of *Candida albicans* (*left*) and *Candida dubliniensis* (*right*) when grown on rice-cream agar.

media, and allow the direct identification of *C. albicans* by means of colony color. Comparative evaluation of rapid methods for *C. albicans* identification, including the germ-tube test, shows that chromogenic media may be economically advantageous (40). A rapid presumptive identification can also be obtained by the use of chromogenic agar plates (36). With the use of these rapid tests, however, it remains essential to take into account the morphological characteristics (both colony morphology and microscopic morphology) in order to support the biochemical result. Some commercial systems include the morphology as a feature that needs to be scored as part of the identification algorithm (37). Also, the proportion of isolates that are identified incorrectly and those reported as non-identification is important when deciding which system to use (37).

RECOVERY OF MOLDS

Most opportunistic fungi are ubiquitous, and their ability to cause invasive disease in humans is associated with their ability to grow at or near the human body temperature. When molds are recovered from clinical specimens, the main question is the significance of the culture. Since most opportunistic fungi are saprophytic fungi and produce spores that are airborne, the source of a positive culture could be variable, with possible contamination taking place at sample collection, specimen transportation, or handling of the sample in the microbiology laboratory. There are several options that can be followed in the clinical microbiology laboratory to interpret the significance of a mold cultured from a clinical specimen. These include the presence of fungal hyphae on direct microscopic examination of the same specimen, morphologically consistent with the culture result; the presence of the same fungus on multiple plates derived from the same specimen or isolated from repeat specimens; growth of the fungal colony in association with the sample or streaks made on the agar plate; and confirmation of the ability of the fungus to growth at body temperature. Of course, quality control measures should be in place in order to ensure that agar media are not contaminated with fungi. In addition to the general protocols for good laboratory practice in medical microbiology, for molds one should also avoid the use of natural materials, as these can be infested with fungi and can be a vehicle for transmission. Members of the zygomycetes are particularly associated with natural materials. In patients, infestation of wooden tongue depressors that were used as construct splints for intravenous and arterial cannulation sites was shown to be the cause of a cluster of invasive zygomycosis in neonates (41). In the laboratory, we have previously reported a pseudo-outbreak of zygomycosis due to the presence of *R. microsporus*, with positive cultures of clinical specimens from two departments (42). The pseudo-outbreak was caused by the use of wooden sticks in the laboratory, and the fungus grew from the sticks when incubated in broth (Fig. 12).

The significance of a fungal culture greatly depends on the sample from which it is cultured and, more importantly, from the host. Therefore, close communication between the microbiologist/mycologist and the treating physician is required. For invasive aspergillosis, several studies have demonstrated that the predictive value depends on the underlying disease or condition of the patient, with high significance when cultured from a patient with neutropenia or following stem cell transplantation and a low significance in HIV + individuals (30,43,44).

Isolation of zygomycetes from patients with cancer who have no risk factors or clinically evident infection probably represents colonization. The pretest probability of a culture positive for zygomycetes was high for patients with leukemia, since only 12% of these patients were deemed to be only colonized by zygomycetes (45). Nevertheless, the sensitivity of cultures for saprophytic molds such as *Aspergillus* and zygomycetes is low. A positive concordance for culture and histologic-cytologic examination was found to be

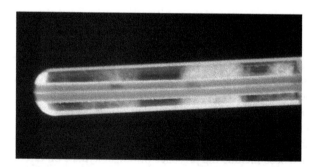

Figure 12 Infestation of wooden sticks that were used in the laboratory to suspend stool samples for culture. The wooden sticks were directly incubated in Sabouraud's broth showing growth of a fungus identified as the zygomycete *Rhizopus microsporus* var. *rhizopodiformis*. This infestation was the cause of a pseudo-outbreak of suspected infection. *Source*: From Ref. 42.

only 23% for *Aspergillus* (46). Cultures of lower respiratory specimens were negative for zygomycosis in 75% of the cases of histopathologically proven pulmonary zygomycosis (47). The positive predictive value of cultures that yield a less common pathogen such as *Scedosporium* appears to be higher (47).

The recovery of molds from clinical specimens in microbiological laboratories is influenced by many factors. Besides the incubation temperature, the available nutrients and the atmospheric conditions have significant impact on the ability of molds to grow in culture. Fungal cultures are commonly incubated in the presence of ambient air, while the conditions in vivo, typically necrotic and hypoxic tissue, are quite different. Adaptation to these very different conditions could be impossible to overcome by a eukaryotic organism, suggesting that matching of the in vivo and in vitro growth conditions could enhance the recovery of molds. This was found to be the case for *Aspergillus*, where temperature and microaerophilic incubation increased the overall recovery of this fungus with 31% (48). Also the recovery of zygomycetes was found to be significantly better when incubated at 37°C as compared to 25°C, both in an experimental setting and with clinical specimens (49). Finally, the ability for fungi to withstand freezing/thawing or chilling through refrigerating differs for the various pathogens, although limited data are available. In one study, clinical specimens were spiked with fungal pathogens, showing that *H. capsulatum* was killed by freezing as opposed to *A. fumigatus* and *C. immitis* (50). *Mucorales* are particularly susceptible to chilling in the refrigerator, and the potential yield may fall with temporary storage of the sample (5).

In tissue samples that show hyphae consistent with *Aspergillus*, 78% of cultures were positive with *Aspergillus*, while in samples with hyphae with a microscopic morphology consistent with zygomycetes, this was confirmed by culture in only 33% of samples (3). Recovery of zygomycetes from tissue is negatively influenced by the grinding of the tissue samples (51), since this might reduce the viability of the hyphae. However, culture positivity was also found to be dependent on the duration of exposure of the patient to antifungal agents, with a higher culture positivity in those patients with a short history of antifungal treatment (3). The sensitivity of polymerase chain reaction (PCR) analysis of tissue that revealed a mold was not affected by previous treatment and was higher than that of culture (sensitivity of culture was 63% compared to 96% for PCR, $P = 0.006$) (3).

STRAIN IDENTIFICATION

The necessity to identify clinically relevant fungi to the species level has been discussed previously. Many laboratories use commercial systems to identify (germ-tube negative) yeasts. The identification of filamentous fungi largely relies on the microscopic morphology, which can be easily examined when the fungi are cultured on slants (Fig. 13) and through examination of slides. Recently, the identification of zygomycetes was shown to be possible using carbon assimilation profiles that are available in commercial systems (52), which might prove useful as an addition to the microscopic identification. Clinical microbiology laboratories may identify frequently encountered molds, such as *Aspergillus* spp., within their own laboratory, and should rely on experienced reference laboratories for other less common fungi. However, limitations of morphological identification of filamentous fungi are increasingly being recognized. Within many taxa, new species are being recognized that are closely related to commonly known species within the clinical setting. *C. dubliniensis*, predominantly found in the oral cavity of HIV+ individuals, was first described in 1995. The yeast was closely related to *C. albicans*, also producing germ-tubes when incubated in fetal calf serum (53). The initial observation that this new species might be less susceptible to azoles was not confirmed (54). More recently, *A. lentulus* was described as new species, closely related to *A. fumigatus* within the section *Fumigati*, characterized by slow sporulation (55). The new species was shown to exhibit reduced susceptibility against multiple antifungal agents. As a consequence, the correct identification is not only of interest to taxonomists, but also has clinical significance. Further studies by these authors showed that a collection of slowly sporulating strains previously identified as *A. fumigatus* contained both *A. lentulus* and *A. udagawae*, further illustrating the limited accuracy of morphologic identification (56). The application of molecular tools has lead to the description of an increasing number of species within the *A.* section *Fumigati* (57), leading taxonomists to discussion how to define new species. A polyphasic approach will probably be followed that includes macro- and micro-morphology, growth temperature regimes, extrolite patterns, and DNA analyses including gene sequences such as beta-tubulin, calmodulin, and actin (58). Similar taxonomic changes are taking place with other molds and raise the question as to how clinical isolates should be reported, given the limitations of morphologic identification. At a recent workshop on *Aspergillus* systematics (59), it was recommended that *A. fumigatus*, *A. flavus*, *A. terreus*, and *A. niger* be reported as *A. fumigatus* complex, *A. flavus* complex, *A. terreus* complex, and *A. niger* complex, respectively, unless speciation is performed through molecular methods.

Another issue of debate is the preferred nomenclature of molds that are cultured in the clinical setting, i.e., should the anamorphic name be reported to the clinician or the teleomorphic name? For those who are not mycologists this can be very confusing. Examples of molds that are reported by both names are *Pseudoallescheria boydii* and *S. apiospermum*, or *A. nidulans* and *Emericella nidulans*. Since the anamorph state of the fungus is usually associated with invasive fungal disease, it might be preferable to agree to use only the anamorph nomenclature in clinical mycology. Alternatively, if an *A. nidulans* is cultured from a clinical specimen, and the isolate produces ascospores in culture, it can be advocated to report what is actually found in culture, in this case, the teleomorph name. However, the production of the sexual state depends on many factors, including the medium used to culture the fungus. Consensus on this topic should

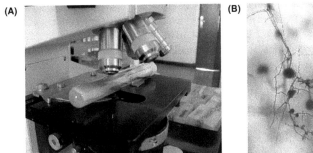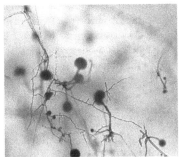

Figure 13 Slants with positive cultures can be examined directly under the microscope allowing morphologic identification. (**A**) Direct microscopic examination of the slant. (**B**) Image of the morphologic morphology with rhizoides, unbranched sporangiophores, and the sporangia consistent with *Rhizopus* spp.

be sought in order to reduce confusion in those treating the patient and in the literature.

CONCLUSION

The number of immunocompromised patients and subsequent invasive fungal infections continues to rise. Diagnosing invasive fungal infection and the correct identification of clinically relevant isolates has become more complex. The variety of isolates that might cause invasive fungal disease has increased, with patients emerging that are infected by multiple fungi (45). The necessity to identify the infecting fungus/fungi to the species level has increased due to several reasons, most notably the broadening arsenal of antifungal agents available for treatment that differ in spectrum of activity. Furthermore, developments in taxonomy lead to the description of new species, some of which are relevant clinically due to reduced susceptibility to antifungal drugs and the re-classification of existing fungal species. The conventional methods used to diagnose invasive fungal disease and to obtain the isolates that cause the infection remain essential in combination with other diagnostic tests and procedures. These developments contrast with surveys that indicate that the number of laboratory professionals in the field of medical mycology is declining (60). Effective recruitment, retention, and training of personnel are essential and must be concurrent with advances in technology (60,61).

REFERENCES

1. Mennink-Kersten MA, Donnelly JP, Verweij PE. Detection of circulating galacto-mannan for the diagnosis and management of invasive aspergillosis. Lancet Infect Dis 2004; 4:349–57.
2. Mennink-Kersten MA, Verweij PE. Non-culture-based diagnostics for opportunistic fungi. Infect Dis Clin North Am 2006; 20:711–27.

3. Rickerts V, Mousset S, Lambrecht E, et al. Comparison of histopathological analysis, culture, and polymerase chain reaction assays to detect invasive mold infections from biopsy specimens. Clin Infect Dis 2007; 44:1078–83.

4. Wheat LJ. Antigen detection, serology, and molecular diagnosis of invasive mycoses in the immunocompromised host. Transpl Infect Dis 2006; 8:128–39.

5. Denning DW, Kibbler CC, Barnes RA. British Society for Medical Mycology. British Society for Medical Mycology proposed standards of care for patients with invasive fungal infections. Lancet Infect Dis 2003; 3:230–40.

6. Greene RE, Schlamm HT, Oestmann JW, et al. Imaging findings in acute invasive pulmonary aspergillosis: clinical significance of the halo sign. Clin Infect Dis 2007; 44:373–9.

7. Morgan J, Wannemuehler KA, Marr KA, et al. Incidence of invasive aspergillosis following hematopoietic stem cell and solid organ transplantation: interim results of a prospective multicenter surveillance program. Med Mycol 2005; 43(Suppl. 1):S49–58.

8. Martin D, Persat F, Piens MA, Picot S. *Candida* species distribution in bloodstream cultures in Lyon, France, 1998–2001. Eur J Clin Microbiol Infect Dis 2005; 24:329–33.

9. Vos MC, Endtz HP, Horst-Kreft D, et al. *Candida krusei* transmission among hematology patients resolved by adapted antifungal prophylaxis and infection control measures. J Clin Microbiol 2006; 44:1111–4.

10. Rex JH, Pfaller MA. Has antifungal susceptibility testing come of age? Clin Infect Dis 2002; 35:982–9.

11. Bille J. When should *Candida* isolates be tested for susceptibility to azole antifungal agents? Eur J Clin Microbiol Infect Dis 1997; 16:281–2.

12. Verweij PE, Mellado E, Melchers WJ. Multiple-triazole-resistant aspergillosis. N Engl J Med 2007; 356:1481–3.

13. Yuen KY, Woo PC, Ip MS, et al. Stage-specific manifestations of mold infections in bone marrow transplant recipients: risk factors and clinical significance of positive concentrated smears. Clin Infect Dis 1997; 25:37–42.

14. Hope WW, Walsh TJ, Denning DW. Laboratory diagnosis of invasive aspergillosis. Lancet Infect Dis 2005; 5:609–22.

15. Merz WG, Roberts GD. Algorithms for detection and identification of fungi. In: Murray PR, Baron EJ, Jorgensen JH, Pfaller MA, Yolken RH, eds. Manual of Clinical Microbiology. 8th ed. Washington, DC: ASM Press, 2003:1668–85.

16. Verweij PE, van der Velden WJ, Donnelly JP, Blijlevens NMA, Warris A. Invasieve zygomycose, een opkomende infectieziekte. Ned Tijdschr Geneesk 2007 (in press).

17. Roden MM, Zaoutis TE, Buchanan WL, et al. Epidemiology and outcome of zygomycosis: a review of 929 reported cases. Clin Infect Dis 2005; 41:634–53.

18. van der Velden WJ, Blijlevens NM, Klont RR, Donnelly JP, Verweij PE. Primary hepatic invasive aspergillosis with progression after rituximab therapy for a post transplantation lymphoproliferative disorder. Ann Hematol 2006; 85:621–3.

19. Duthie R, Denning DW. *Aspergillus* fungemia: report of two cases and review. Clin Infect Dis 1995; 20:598–605.

20. Simoneau E, Kelly M, Labbe AC, Roy J, Laverdiere M. What is the clinical significance of positive blood cultures with *Aspergillus* sp. in hematopoietic stem cell transplant recipients? A 23 year experience Bone Marrow Transplant 2005; 35:303–6.

21. Kontoyiannis DP, Sumoza D, Tarrand J, Bodey GP, Storey R, Raad II. Significance of aspergillemia in patients with cancer: a 10-year study. Clin Infect Dis 2000; 31:188–9.

22. Nucci M, Marr KA, Queiroz-Telles F, et al. *Fusarium* infection in hematopoietic stem cell transplant recipients. Clin Infect Dis 2004; 38:1237–42.

23. Maertens J, Lagrou K, Deweerdt H, et al. Disseminated infection by *Scedosporium prolificans*: an emerging fatality among haematology patients. Case report and review. Ann Hematol 2000; 79:340–4.

24. Schell WA. New aspects of emerging fungal pathogens: a multifaceted challenge. Clin Lab Med 1995; 15:365–87.

25. Meyer MH, Letscher-Bru V, Jaulhac B, Waller J, Candolfi E. Comparison of mycosis IC/F and plus aerobic/F media for diagnosis of fungemia by the Bactec 9240 System. J Clin Microbiol 2004; 42:773–7.

26. Fricker-Hidalgo H, Chazot F, Lebeau B, Pelloux H, Ambroise-Thomas P, Grillot R. Use of simulated blood cultures to compare a specific fungal medium with a standard microorganism medium for yeast detection. Eur J Clin Microbiol Infect Dis 1998; 17:113–6.

27. Hennequin C, Ranaivoarimalala C, Chouaki T, et al. Comparison of aerobic standard medium with specific fungal medium for detecting *Fusarium* spp. in blood cultures. Eur J Clin Microbiol Infect Dis 2002; 21:748–50.

28. Morrell M, Fraser VJ, Kollef MH. Delaying the empiric treatment of *Candida* bloodstream infection until positive blood culture results are obtained: a potential risk factor for hospital mortality. Antimicrob Agents Chemother 2005; 49:3640–5.

29. Garey KW, Rege M, Pai MP, et al. Time to initiation of fluconazole therapy impacts mortality in patients with candidemia: a multi-institutional study. Clin Infect Dis 2006; 43:25–31.

30. Horvath JA, Dummer S. The use of respiratory-tract cultures in the diagnosis of invasive pulmonary aspergillosis. Am J Med 1996; 100:171–8.

31. Sutton DA. Specimen collection, transport, and processing: mycology. In: Murray PR, Baron EJ, Jorgensen JH, Pfaller MA, Yolken RH, eds. Manual of Clinical Microbiology. 8th ed. Washington, DC: ASM Press, 2003:1659–67.

32. Meis JF, Kullberg BJ, Pruszczynski M, Veth RP. Severe osteomyelitis due to the zygomycete *Apophysomyces elegans*. J Clin Microbiol 1994; 32:3078–81.

33. Pfaller MA, Diekema DJ. Epidemiology of invasive candidiasis: a persistent public health problem. Clin Microbiol Rev 2007; 20:133–63.

34. Larone DH. Medically Important Fungi. 4th ed. Washington, DC: ASM Press, 2002.

35. Terlecka JA, du Cros PA, Orla Morrissey C, Spelman D. Rapid differentiation of *Candida albicans* from non-albicans species by germ tube test directly from BacTAlert blood culture bottles. Mycoses 2007; 50:48–51.

36. Freydiere AM, Guinet R, Boiron P. Yeast identification in the clinical microbiology laboratory: phenotypical methods. Med Mycol. 2001; 39:9–33.

37. Verweij PE, Breuker IM, Rijs AJ, Meis JF. Comparative study of seven commercial yeast identification systems. J Clin Pathol 1999; 52:271–3.

38. Sanguinetti M, Porta R, Sali M, et al. Evaluation of VITEK 2 and RapID yeast plus systems for yeast species identification: experience at a large clinical microbiology laboratory. J Clin Microbiol 2007; 45:1343–6.

39. Freydiere AM, Perry JD, Faure O, et al. Routine use of a commercial test, GLABRATA RTT, for rapid identification of *Candida glabrata* in six laboratories. J Clin Microbiol 2004; 42:4870–2.

40. Ainscough S, Kibbler CC. An evaluation of the cost-effectiveness of using CHROMagar for yeast identification in a routine microbiology laboratory. J Med Microbiol 1998; 47:623–8.

41. Mitchell SJ, Gray J, Morgan ME, Hocking MD, Durbin GM. Nosocomial infection with *Rhizopus microsporus* in preterm infants: association with wooden tongue depressors. Lancet 1996; 348:441–3.

42. Verweij PE, Voss A, Donnelly JP, de Pauw BE, Meis JF. Wooden sticks as the source of a pseudoepidemic of infection with *Rhizopus microsporus* var. *rhizopodiformis* among immunocompromised patients. J Clin Microbiol 1997; 35:2422–3.

43. Yu VL, Muder RR, Poorsattar A. Significance of isolation of *Aspergillus* from the respiratory tract in diagnosis of invasive pulmonary aspergillosis. Am J Med 1986; 81:249–54.

44. Perfect JR, Cox GM, Lee JY, et al. Mycoses Study Group. The impact of culture isolation of *Aspergillus* species: a hospital-based survey of aspergillosis. Clin Infect Dis 2001; 33:1824–33.

45. Kontoyiannis DP, Wessel VC, Bodey GP, Rolston KV. Zygomycosis in the 1990s in a tertiary-care cancer center. Clin Infect Dis 2000; 30:851–6.

46. Tarrand JJ, Lichterfeld M, Warraich I, et al. Diagnosis of invasive septate mold infections. A correlation of microbiological culture and histologic or cytologic examination. Am J Clin Pathol 2003; 119:854–8.

47. Lionakis MS, Kontoyiannis DP. The significance of isolation of saprophytic molds from the lower respiratory tract in patients with cancer. Cancer 2004; 100:165–72.

48. Tarrand JJ, Han XY, Kontoyiannis DP, May GS. *Aspergillus hyphae* in infected tissue: evidence of physiologic adaptation and effect on culture recovery. J Clin Microbiol 2005; 43:382–6.

49. Kontoyiannis DP, Chamilos G, Hassan SA, Lewis RE, Albert ND, Tarrand JJ. Increased culture recovery of Zygomycetes under physiologic temperature conditions. Am J Clin Pathol 2007; 127:208–12.

50. Thompson DW, Kaplan W, Phillips BJ. The effect of freezing and the influence of isolation medium on the recovery of pathogenic fungi from sputum. Mycopathologia 1977; 61:105–9.

51. Spellberg B, Edwards J, Jr., Ibrahim A. Novel perspectives on mucormycosis: pathophysiology, presentation, and management. Clin Microbiol Rev 2005; 18:556–69.

52. Schwarz P, Lortholary O, Dromer F, Dannaoui E. Carbon assimilation profiles as a tool for identification of zygomycetes. J Clin Microbiol 2007; 45:1433–9.

53. Sullivan DJ, Westerneng TJ, Haynes KA, Bennett DE, Coleman DC. *Candida dubliniensis* spp. nov.: phenotypic and molecular characterization of a novel species associated with oral candidosis in HIV-infected individuals. Microbiology 1995; 141:1507–21.

54. Pinjon E, Moran GP, Coleman DC, Sullivan DJ. Azole susceptibility and resistance in *Candida dubliniensis*. Biochem Soc Trans 2005; 33:1210–4.

55. Balajee SA, Gribskov JL, Hanley E, Nickle D, Marr KA. *Aspergillus lentulus* spp. nov., a new sibling species of *A. fumigatus*. Eukaryot Cell 2005; 4:625–32.

56. Balajee SA, Nickle D, Varga J, Marr KA. Molecular studies reveal frequent misidentification of *Aspergillus fumigatus* by morphotyping. Eukaryot Cell 2006; 5:1705–12.
57. Yaguchi T, Horie Y, Tanaka R, Matsuzawa T, Ito J, Nishimura K. Molecular phylogenetics of multiple genes on *Aspergillus* section *Fumigati* isolated from clinical specimens in Japan. Nippon Ishinkin Gakkai Zasshi 2007; 48:37–46.
58. Hong SB, Go SJ, Shin HD, Frisvad JC, Samson RA. Polyphasic taxonomy of *Aspergillus fumigatus* and related species. Mycologia 2005; 97:1316–29.
59. www.aspergilluspenicillium.org
60. McClenny N. Laboratory detection and identification of *Aspergillus* species by microscopic observation and culture: the traditional approach. Med Mycol 2005; 43(Suppl. 1):S125–8.
61. Steinbach WJ, Mitchell TG, Schell WA, et al. Status of medical mycology education. Med Mycol 2003; 41:457–67.

3

The Role of Radiology in the Diagnosis of Fungal Infections

Reginald Greene

Department of Radiology, Massachusetts General Hospital and Harvard Medical School, Boston, Massachusetts, U.S.A.

Paul Stark

Department of Radiology, University of California, San Diego, California, U.S.A.

IMAGING MODALITIES

Imaging plays a central role in the management of patients with suspected invasive fungal infection, especially in immunocompromised patients. Computed tomography (CT) and plain chest radiography (CXR) provide essential tools for detecting disease at an early stage, narrowing differential diagnosis, providing clues for the start of early-targeted treatment, and assessing response to therapy. To a lesser extent, other modalities, like positron emission tomography (PET), magnetic resonance imaging (MRI), and ultrasound (US), also can contribute to special aspects of problem solving. When conditions permit, imaging can also serve as a guide for percutaneous tissue sampling, which, in immunocompromised patients, can be expected to identify etiologic organisms about 80% of the time (1). This chapter naturally focuses on chest imaging because the lung is the most common portal of entry for suspected invasive fungal infection.

Modern, state-of-the-art, multi-detector CT scanning is the acknowledged gold-standard for clinical imaging of the lung, pleura, and mediastinum. The technique provides high-speed image acquisition that can minimize breathing artifacts, improve image quality, and allow high quality multi-planar reconstructed images. Various technical maneuvers can also be used to optimize imaging and reduce radiation exposure (2). Few critical clinical management decisions with respect to invasive fungal infection can be made without reference to chest CT findings. Although initial imaging findings of invasive fungal infection may be nonspecific, when they are interpreted in an appropriate clinical context, they can help narrow the differential diagnostic possibilities, identify important noninfectious disease, and, at times, justify pre-emptive specific therapy.

CXR continues to be the mainstay day-to-day survey tool for detecting new chest disease and monitoring its evolution. The technique has the advantages over CT of more ready availability, low cost, and much lower radiation exposure. Over the past two decades, new digital technology has increased the dynamic range, optimization of imaging quality, and repeatability of optical density of sequential radiographic images (3). Radiography has the advantage of being suitable for bedside chest imaging for seriously ill patients, but the diagnostic accuracy of such bedside imaging is much lower than radiography performed in an imaging department. In general, positive radiographic findings should be corroborated by a follow-up CT. When the risk of invasive fungal infection is very high, chest CT scan should probably follow a negative CXR, particularly if the CXR has been done at the bedside. On CXR, diffuse miliary lesions and ground glass opacities are frequently undetected, and large areas of the chest are not visible at all or are poorly seen, especially in bedside studies.

MRI of the chest has only been used sporadically to assess immune compromised patients with invasive fungal infection infections (4,5). In general, chest MRI does not now match the overall utility of CT in assessing these patients. In febrile neutropenic patients, nodules less than 10 mm are detected less well with MRI than with CT (5). Motion and breathing artifacts, especially in older and otherwise severely ill patients, tend to selectively degrade MRIs, particularly for small lesions (5). In a recent study, no significant difference could be detected between MRI and CT in lesion-location and distribution of pulmonary nodules, ground-glass opacity areas, and consolidation, but MRI was not as capable of evaluating the internal characteristics of lesions, such as cavitations. In the abdomen, central nervous system (CNS), paranasal sinuses, and bones and joints, MRI and CT both have important recognized roles.

US of the chest is useful in detecting pleural effusions, and for controlling percutaneous interventions, each of which can be performed at the bedside. US has the advantage of not producing ionizing radiation, and not requiring the use of iodinated intravenous contrast medium. CT, as compared with either US or MRI, provides the best global assessment of the entire abdominopelvic compartment.

PET imaging with F-18 fluorodeoxyglucose (FDG) is now widely used as a sensitive method of detecting metabolically active tumors. The technique still does not have an established role in clinical evaluation of inflammation and pneumonia. It has been used infrequently to detect invasive fungal infection, partly because there is crossover activity with malignant tumors (6) and other noninfectious inflammations, e.g., drug-induced pulmonary toxicity (7).

Anecdotal studies have identified a wide spectrum of FDG-avid lung lesions in patients with chronic and acute inflammatory lesions and infections.

ASPERGILLOSIS

Invasive Pulmonary Aspergillosis

Invasive pulmonary aspergillosis (IPA) is the main example of a ubiquitous opportunistic mold that rarely causes invasive infection in the immunocompetent host, but frequently causes life-threatening primary invasive fungal pneumonia in the immunocompromised patient. Immunocompromised patients at highest risk are hematopoietic stem cell transplant (HSCT) recipients and those with hematologic conditions, especially those with prolonged neutropenia. Since the lung is the most common portal of entry, it is not surprising that invasive aspergillosis involves the lung in about 90% of such infections (8). In the HSCT recipient there are two peak periods of *Aspergillus* infection: during the first 30 days following transplantation (the pre-engraftment period when neutropenia may be severe), and later, after the first 90 days post-transplantation, during the late post-engraftment period, when prolonged high levels of immunosuppression for graft versus host disease lead to functional neutropenia. Thus, a large fraction of IPA develop in the HSCT recipients as outpatients following hospital discharge (9). In other immunocompromised groups, such as solid organ transplant recipients, high-dose corticosteroid recipients, and patients with AIDS who suffer predominantly from T-cell dysfunction, IPA occurs more sporadically and at a lower incidence than in the two high risk groups mentioned above. Angio-invasive pathogenesis in the peripheral lung airways and airspaces is by far the most common sequence, and likely accounts for (>90%) of instances of IPA (8,10). IPA develops in patients with previously normal lungs, wherein immunodeficiency allows germination of *Aspergillus* spores inhaled into the distal lung airways and airspaces where angio-invasive mycelial penetration develops a hemorrhagic nodule of infection and coagulation necrosis. The much less common invasive mold infection (IMI) caused by Zygomycetes tends to follow the same angio-invasive pathogenetic sequence. As a result, the clinical backgrounds and imaging findings of these two IMIs are essentially identical, but the treatment is different.

Imaging

The two most common initial CT findings of IPA in patients at the highest risk of IMI are the pulmonary macronodule and the halo sign (10).

At the time of detection, the pulmonary macronodule is by far the most frequent initial finding IPA; it can be identified in >90% of patients (10). The macronodule is defined as a localized space-occupying, ovoid nodular opacity ≥1 cm diameter that displaces rather than conforms to the shape of the pre-existing aerated lung, and completely obscures the background bronchovasculature. By convention, a nodule is called a "mass" when it is greater than 3 cm diameter. The macronodule is such a common feature on initial CT that its absence argues against the diagnosis of angio-invasive aspergillosis (10). The differential diagnosis of the macronodule is wide, and includes many other infectious processes, such as other fungal infections, nocardiosis, tuberculosis, and lung abscess. Common noninfectious causes associated with macronodules include bland pulmonary infarcts, lung cancer, lung metastases, lymphoproli-ferative disorders, and vasculitis.

The halo sign is found on initial imaging in a significant fraction of patients depending on how early CT is employed in such patients. In a large series of patients with IPA, it was identified in about 60% of patients (10). The halo sign consists of a macronodule that possesses a perimeter of ground-glass opacity, i.e., intermediate increased lung density between solid and air density through which vasculature is still visible (Fig. 1). The halo corresponds to coagulation necrosis, infection and oozing hemorrhage that develops at the perimeter of the macronodule of infarction (11). The halo sign is highly transient. In one longitudinal CT study, 72% of patients with IPA had a halo sign on initial CT, but only 22% of these patients still had a halo sign hemorrhage after the first 10 days (4). In another study, the frequency of the halo sign rapidly decreased to about one fifth of its initial frequency 7–10 days following an initial CT scan (12). Some data suggest that there may even be a significant fall-off in the frequency of the halo sign during the first three days following the initial CT scan (12). The ground glass perimeter of the halo sign should be substantial enough to permit clear visualization of background vasculature through it (10). The nodule with a halo sign needs to be differentiated from the nodule with un-sharp edges due to irregularity of nodule outline, and to partial volume effect

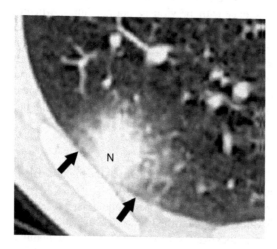

Figure 1 Halo sign. Computed tomography scan of a neutropenic patient with a subpleural macronodule (N) surrounded by a halo of ground-glass opacification (*arrows*).

caused by thick CT sections or respiratory motion. The halo sign can be caused by uncommon angio-invasive fungi, such as Zygomycetes, and other rare, normally saprophytic, angio-invasive fungi, such as *Trichosporon* spp., (13), *Penicillium* spp., (14) and *Fusarium* spp., (15). These rare angio-invasive fungi can also produce nodular metastatic nodules in the liver and spleen similar to those formed in chronic candidiasis.

The halo sign has been reported in infections due to *Coccidioides immitis* and *Candida* spp., *Nocardia* spp., *Mycobacterium tuberculosis, cytomegalovirus,* and herpes simplex virus, and angio-invasive bacterial infections, such as those caused by *Pseudomonas aeruginosa* (16). Noninfectious causes of the halo sign include bronchiolo-alveolar cell carcinoma, lymphoproliferative disorders, metastatic angiosarcoma, Kaposi sarcoma, Wegener granulomatosis, eosinophilic lung disease, and organizing pneumonia (17–19).

Pre-Emptive Therapy Based on the Halo Sign

Because the halo sign is regarded as a specific indicator of IPA in patients with a compatible illness who are at very high risk of IMI, it has been used to justify pre-emptive specific antifungal therapy (8,20–25). The rationale for pre-emptive treatment of patients at high risk of IMI based on finding a halo sign is supported by outcome findings in a subgroup analysis of 235 patients with IPA who had an initial CT (8). Of 222 patients who presented with at least one macronodule, 143 presented with a halo sign, versus 79 who presented with nodules lacking a halo sign. At 12 weeks, the halo sign group had a significantly higher satisfactory response rate irrespective of treatment arm (52% vs. 29%), and better survival rates than the other group (71% vs. 53%). These findings corroborated those of smaller prior studies (24). The difference in treatment response held true irrespective not only for treatment arm, but also for underlying condition, namely hematological conditions or non-hematological conditions, baseline neutropenia or no baseline neutropenia, and allogeneic HSCT. Since the improved outcome in the halo sign group in the above study is arguably related to the earlier stage of infection in those with halo signs, early performance of CT scanning should take a high priority in patients with compatible illnesses who are at high risk of developing an IMI. The evanescent nature of the halo signs emphasizes the urgency of obtaining a CT at the earliest opportunity.

The air crescent sign is a cavitary lesion in which a semilunar pocket of gas surmounts a partially detached nodule of devitalized lung (Fig. 2) (22,26). It is identified at presentation in only about 10% of patients with IPA, and is a sign of late IPA that usually occurs after recovery of neutrophil function. In those who are at the highest risk of developing IPA, the air crescent sign as well as the halo sign are considered specific indicators of IPA in patients with a compatible illness (8,10,20,22,23,27,28). In the period of 4–10 days following initial chest CT when halo signs rapidly become less frequent, air crescent signs become more prevalent (4,12). Thick-walled and thin-walled cavities without air crescents can be found in a small minority of initial CT studies of patients with IPA, but

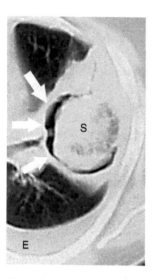

Figure 2 Air crescent sign. Computed tomography scan demonstrates an air crescent sign due to angio-invasive pulmonary zygomycosis in an immunocompromised patient with an underlying hematological malignancy. The finding is indistinguishable from an air crescent sign caused by angio-invasive pulmonary aspergillosis. A crescent of air (*arrows*) surrounds a soft tissue mound of sequestrum (S) due to vitalized lung. This is a sign of late angio-invasive mold infection. There is also a dependent left pleural effusion (E) along the dorsal surface of the left chest wall.

these findings do not seem to have the same diagnostic predictive value as the air crescent sign, from which they should be differentiated (29). In limited experience with invasive aspergillosis, MR studies have demonstrated necrotic target lesions with a rim with T-2 weighted hyperintensity, and gadolinium rim enhancement (4). The differential diagnosis of the air crescent sign is broad, but like the halo sign, invasive aspergillosis is the most common cause of the air crescent sign when it is found in patients at high risk of IMI. The sign is also found in many conditions other than invasive aspergillosis, e.g., nocardiosis, tuberculosis, bacterial lung abscess, cavitary hematoma, and cavitary lung cancer (30,31). The sequestrum of devitalized lung in the air crescent sign needs to be differentiated from the fungus ball of saprophytic aspergillosis, which is often mobile. The sign also needs to be differentiated from thin and thick-walled cavities that lack air crescents.

    Initial imaging findings less common than the macronodule include consolidations and consolidative infarcts with or without air bronchograms that can be found in about one-third of patients, and small airway opacities that occur in about a tenth of patients with IPA (10). In addition to IPA, the common differential diagnostic considerations for localized lung consolidation includes any a wide range of fungal and bacterial as well as noninfectious conditions, such as aspiration, bland infarction, hemorrhage, partial atelectasis, lymphoproliferative disorders, and radiation injury. Centrilobular opacities include sub-centimeter nodular opacities located in the center of secondary lobules, and are often found in conjunction with opacified segments of small branching bronchi and bronchioli, i.e., tree-in-bud opacities, and/or patches of peribronchial consolidation. These findings, identified either separately or in combination, are taken as general indicators of bronchiolitis or bronchopneumonia that results from spread of infection along the airways (32). While small airways findings are uncommon in angio-invasive aspergillosis, they are the rule in airway-invasive aspergillosis, a less common pathogenetic sequence in IPA that tends to occur in previously injured lungs, such as in the lung transplant patient where the invasion is dominated by airway imaging findings rather than by macronodules (33). These findings can be found in a wide variety of bronchopneumonias, such as those caused by cryptococcal, mycobacterial, common bacterial, and viral infection. A chronic form of airway invasive aspergillosis, i.e., chronic tracheobronchial aspergillus infection that spreads along the airways, results in bronchial wall thickening and nodularity, bronchostenosis, and bronchiectasis that can lead to peribronchial consolidation and atelectasis, especially in HSCT and lung transplant recipients, and in AIDS patients (33). Ancillary findings, such as pleural effusion, pericardial effusion, and hilar or mediastinal lymphadenopathy, are identified in small fraction of patients with IPA ($\sim 10\%$).

MRI images in patients with IPA have identified nodular and segmental non-nodular lung lesions and demonstrated target-like T1-weighted central high signal, and rim-enhancement after intravenous gadolinium injection (25). Hyperintensity on T-l weighted imaging correlates with sub-acute hemorrhage induced by angio-invasive aspergillus infection (25). A CT/MRI comparative study found that the CT halo sign was much more specific than the analogous MRI halo sign in identifying patients with invasive aspergillosis (25).

Extra-pulmonary intrathoracic invasion by IPA, such as into the great vessels, pleura and pericardium, hila, and mediastinum, occur infrequently (10) but are capable of disastrous consequences. Occasionally, hyphal elements invade adjacent large vessels to cause thrombosis, pseudo aneurysm, and the risk of rupture and exsanguination. Blood-borne dissemination into the lungs may result in disseminated lung nodules or diffuse or multi-focal consolidation.

Cerebral aspergillosis occurs by direct extension from sino-nasal aspergillosis or from systemic hematogenous dissemination. Initial brain lesions are similar in appearance to those in the lung; usually well-defined, macronodular, low-attenuation lesions or large vessel infarcts surrounded by edema on CT. On MRI, cerebral lesions are t2w hyperintense surrounded by edema, and exhibit t1w enhancement after intravenous gadolinium (34). In later stages, central necrosis and rim enhancement are the primary findings (35). Sino-nasal aspergillosis may demonstrate soft tissue masses or abscesses in the nasal cavities or paranasal sinuses from which there may be extension to the brain or orbit via the cribriform plate, sometimes associated with bone destruction or cavernous sinus

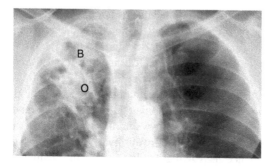

Figure 3 Chronic pulmonary aspergillosis. Chest radiograph shows apical bullous disease in a patient with bullous emphysema (B), progressive paracystic lung opacity (O), and pleural thickening in the right upper lobe.

thrombosis (36). Visceral dissemination into the abdomen is associated with solid nodular masses, abscesses, or infarcts in the liver, spleen, and kidneys.

Chronic aspergillosis tends to occur in elderly, often debilitated patients who usually have pre-existing chronic cystic lung disease such as bullous emphysema, apical cystic tuberculosis and end-stage sarcoidosis (37). The further enlargement of lung cysts, the development of new lung cysts, the appearance of para cystic lung opacities, and progression of local pleural thickening in association with progressive constitutional symptoms are all signs of chronic aspergillosis. There are pathologic signs of tissue invasion, but dissemination does not usually occur. The findings may simulate post primary tuberculosis (Fig. 3). Long-term anti-aspergillus therapy is the rule. About half of these patients develop aspergillomas in the lung cysts.

ZYGOMYCOSIS

Pulmonary zygomycosis (PZ) is an uncommon invasive fungal infection relative to IPA, but its frequency has recently been reported to be increasing, especially among patients with hematological malignancy and in HSCT recipients (38). In general, zygomycosis is indistinguishable from angio-invasive aspergillosis in clinical presentation, pathogenetic sequence, pathology, and imaging findings (Fig. 2) (39–41). Angio-invasive zygomycosis differs from angio-invasive aspergillosis primarily in its rarity (42) in the high at-risk groups for IMI and in its resistance to standard anti-aspergillus therapy. It has been reported as a breakthrough infection in patients treated for IPA with voriconazole (43). Several factors lead to problems with differential diagnosis between IPA and PZ: among cancer patients, first, they both have similar risk factors for IMI, second, they usually present with primary pulmonary infection, and third, they both have similar angio-invasive pathogenesis that results in similar imaging features. The problem has serious therapeutic implications because effective treatment for one is not adequate for the other. In an attempt to help differentiate between

PZ and IPA, a relatively small retrospective review of 45 consecutive patients with either isolated IPA or isolated PZ, and similar risk factors for IMI, found that nodular lesions were the predominant finding in patients with either PZ or IPA (about 80% of patients), but, that there was a higher number of patients with ≥ 10 nodules in PZ versus IPA (64% vs. 18%); $p < 0.02$ (38). The presence of ≥ 10 nodules independently correlated with PZ. Even though the imaging findings are not usually distinguishable from one another, the detection of a halo sign on presentation is much more likely attributable to IPA than to PZ because Zygomycetes are so much less common causes of angio-IMI than Aspergillus in those at high risk of IMI. Thus, lesions attributed to Aspergillus without confirmatory mycology based on the halo sign should always be regarded as potential PZ infections, particularly if the response to standard anti-aspergillus therapy is unsatisfactory. In such cases of zygomycosis, surgical resection is often utilized when possible. As mentioned above, rare angio-invasive fungi other than Zygomycetes can also produce imaging features similar to those of IPA.

CANDIDIASIS

Candida is the most important example of a ubiquitous opportunistic fungus that rarely causes primary invasive pneumonia, but commonly causes systemic dissemination to the lungs and solid organs. *Candida* infection is commonly associated with synchronous infection by other pathogenic and opportunistic microbes (44). Those at high risk are usually severely immunosuppressed, such as patients with leukemia, and often with neutropenia. *Candida* rarely causes primary invasive pneumonia, and most often causes secondary pneumonia, either as a result of hematogenous dissemination to the lung, or by super-infection of lung that has been previously damaged by a noninfectious process or by other contemporaneous infection. Because of the frequent multiplicity of co-infectious agents, imaging findings of pulmonary candidiasis tend to defy meaningful categorization. The fungus can be identified in lung tissue that shows no evidence of significant lung damage (45). In general, there is a lack of correlation between patient outcome and the detection of localized versus diffuse imaging findings, whether candidiasis is considered primary, i.e., due to airway aspiration, or secondary, i.e., due to hematogenous dissemination. The pulmonary imaging findings attributed to invasive candidiasis are often bilateral and diffuse as a result of systemic dissemination. Focal findings may also occur in areas of damaged lung that have become infected.

On CT, a wide variety of focal or diffuse imaging findings have been described, including nodules (46), a bronchiolitis-bronchopneumonia pattern (47), and diffuse miliary nodules (1–3 mm discrete nodules too numerous to count). Focal nodules detected in pulmonary candidiasis do not seem to have the same clinical relevance as early nodular lesions found in invasive aspergillosis, where early detection and treatment can impact patient outcome (46).

Contemporaneous initial abdominal CT studies may also demonstrate disseminated nodular lesions in the liver, spleen, or kidneys.

The differential diagnosis of diffuse lung opacification in the immunosuppressed patient is broad and mainly dependent on the particular type of lung lesions that make up the diffuse opacification. In general, in the severely immune-deficient patient, diffuse lung opacification may be found in candidiasis, *Pneumocystis carinii* (*jirovecii*) pneumonia (PCP), viral pneumonia, toxoplasmosis, and disseminated endemic or opportunistic mycoses. It can also be found in pulmonary edema, Kaposi sarcoma, ARDS, capillary leak syndromes, pulmonary hemorrhage, alveolar proteinosis, transfusion reactions, drug toxicity, idiopathic interstitial pneumonias, and metastatic cancer.

Extra-pulmonary candidiasis results from variable portals of entry, e.g., transcutaneous infusion lines and aspiration. The infection is usually disseminated in multiple organs at the time of the initial CT study. CT studies may demonstrate pulmonary lesions alone or in combination with extra pulmonary infection. Chronic hepatosplenic candidiasis often occurs in acute leukemia after remission-induced chemotherapy during recovery from prolonged neutropenia (48) when the patient has improved neutrophil function and the capability to form focal granuloma formation (49). In hepatosplenic candidiasis, CT, MRI, and US characteristically demonstrate multiple, 5–15 mm, well-defined, solid nodules in the liver, spleen, and/or kidneys (Fig. 4). In acute

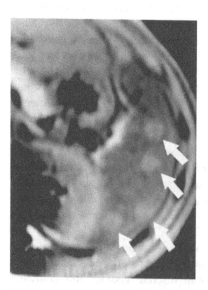

Figure 4 Chronic hepatosplenic *Candidiasis*. T1-weighted magnetic resonance imaging demonstrates four 10–15 mm high signal nodules (*arrows*) in the spleen in a severely immunosuppressed patient with disseminated *candidiasis*.

hepatosplenic candidiasis, before neutrophil function has recovered, these same nodules consist of liquefied or partially liquefied abscesses, rather than solid lesions. Patients suspected of chronic disseminated candidiasis are best studied with contrast-enhanced CT, but upper abdominal US may also be useful because lesions that are not visible on CT may be apparent with US (50). The converse is also true. Disseminated granulomatous infection in the liver, spleen, or kidneys can be found even when chest radiographic studies are normal (51). US studies may demonstrate well-defined hypoechoic nodules, often with a "wheels within wheels" appearance, consisting of a hypoechoic outer rim, hyperechoic inner rim, and hypoechoic infectious-necrotic core. Sometimes the hypoechoic nodules have hyperechoic cores called "Bull's eye" lesions (52,53). MRI of deep visceral candidiasis appears as well-defined, T-2 hyperintense nodules (52). Similar, multiple, sub-acute or chronic macroscopic hepatosplenic nodules (hypoechoic on US and hypo attenuating on CT) can be found in immunosuppressed patients with other disseminated fungal, mycobacterial, and suppurative infections caused by aspergillosis and fusaria, tuberculosis, atypical mycobacteria, and multiple bacterial abscesses. Even after satisfactory clinical response to treatment, hepatosplenic nodules tend to persist for long periods (52,54,55).

CRYPTOCOCCOSIS

Cryptococcus neoformans is the most common ubiquitous pathogenic fungus that causes clinical progressive primary lung infection in immune-competent patients (53). Most infections occur in immune-deficient patients with very low CD4 counts in whom the fungus commonly causes life-threatening disseminated infection. Other patients at high risk of infection are those immuno-suppressed from steroid use, malignant disease, and organ transplantation. The infection results from new primary pulmonary infection, or activation of a dormant focus.

The most commonly presenting chest findings in both immune-competent and immune-deficient patients is the pulmonary nodule or mass that ranges in size from 0.5–5 cm diameter (Fig. 5) (56,57). The nodule is often subpleural and may be cavitated (56). The differential diagnosis of cavitary pulmonary nodules in AIDS patients includes invasive aspergillosis, PCP, lung cancer, and lung abscess, among others (58). Some nodules have been reported to have ground-glass halos (59). Nodules are often detected in the asymptomatic patient. Since dormant infections may leave no residue, the pulmonary nodule may be the only chest finding. In AIDS patients, *Cryptococcus* is the most common cause of fungal pneumonia.

Regional spread may develop from a subpleural nodule, resulting in peribronchial lung parenchymal opacification. There may be associated local lymphatic spread to bronchopulmonary and hilar lymph nodes and to the pleural space, causing an effusion. Hematogenous dissemination from pulmonary cryptococcosis can result in a miliary pattern of 1–3 mm nodules diameter

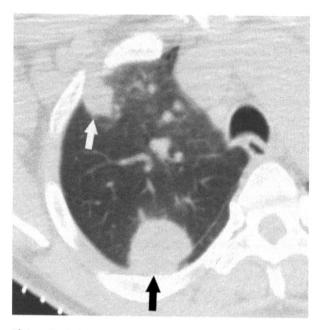

Figure 5 Pulmonary cryptococcosis. Two subpleural nodules (*arrows*) in an AIDS patient with low CD4 count and meningeal involvement with cryptococcosis.

nodules that are too numerous to count. The differential diagnosis of diffuse miliary findings includes all other hematogenously disseminated infections, especially endemic mycoses and non-fungal infectious etiologies, such as disseminated mycobacterial infection, *Pneumocystis jirovecii* pneumonia, and viral pneumonia, such as cytomegalovirus pneumonia. Differential diagnoses also include hypersensitivity pneumonitis, cryptogenic organizing pneumonia, lymphoid interstitial pneumonia, Kaposi sarcoma, hematogenous metastases, drug-induced disease, diffuse alveolar damage, acute interstitial pneumonia, stage I sarcoidosis, silicosis, and hematogenous metastases to the lung.

Cerebral cryptococcosis is the most common invasive fungal infection of the CNS. Both on CT and on MRI, it can be occult, or demonstrate non-enhancing solid lesions or enhancing basal ganglia lesions, pseudo cysts, meningitis, or meningoencephalitis with gyral enhancement with or without hydrocephalus (58). The differential diagnosis of CNS cryptococcosis in AIDS patients with very low CD4 counts includes toxoplasmosis. In the majority of patients with lung lesions, there is concurrent, often asymptomatic, CNS infection (60). About a quarter of AIDS patients who present with CNS cryptococcosis will be found to have clinically silent pulmonary lesions. Abdominal cryptococcosis may demonstrate disseminated low attenuation nodules in the liver similar to those encountered in other disseminated fungal infections.

ENDEMIC MYCOSES

North American endemic mycoses include *Histoplasma capsulatum, C. immitis,* and *Blastomyces dermatididis*. In immune-competent hosts, respiratory infection is generally sub clinical and followed by spontaneous resolution. In the immunosuppressed patient, respiratory infection generally results in disseminated life-threatening infection. At the time of initial assessment, dissemination has usually already occurred. The main risk factor for infection is severe impairment in T-cell immunity, such as in AIDS patients with low CD4 counts (58,61). The lung is the main portal of entry for these infections. They usually arise from activation of a dormant focus, or acquisition of a new primary infection. In either case, rapid dissemination occurs within the lungs and/or spreads to extra-pulmonary sites or to the lungs via hematogenous dissemination. Sites of extra-pulmonary dissemination include the brain, meninges, solid abdominal viscera, gastrointestinal tract, and bones. Alternative initial sites of infection include the paranasal sinuses and skin.

CXR is initially negative in about half of affected patients, even when dissemination has occurred. Positive initial chest findings are varied (62) but tend to follow three overall patterns: focal or multi-focal lung lesions, such as nodules or consolidations that represent a reactivated dormant focus, or a progressive primary infection; diffuse lung opacities that indicate hematogenous dissemination from progressive primary pulmonary infection or from secondary sites of extra-pulmonary infection; and from extra-pulmonary dissemination to the CNS, intra-abdominal organs, or lymph nodes. The diffuse lung lesions of the second pattern may be discrete miliary nodules (1–3 mm diameter), larger nodules, macronodules (≥ 1 cm diameter), or consolidation. On chest radiographs, the miliary lesions of CT may appear as vague, nonspecific, irregular opacities. When the miliary nodules of hematogenous dissemination are present, nodules or consolidations of the previously dormant focus or the new site of progressive primary infection may also be visible. The underlying immunodeficiency that make these patients susceptible to endemic mycoses also put them at increased risk of infection from bacteria, viruses, protozoa, and other fungi. These infections include mycobacteria, *Nocardia asteroides, Legionella* spp., varicella-zoster virus, herpes simplex virus, cytomegalovirus, Epstein–Barr virus, *P. carinii,* and *T. gondii*. (63,64). Hilar, mediastinal, and intra-abdominal lymph adenopathy is a common feature of endemic mycoses, and needs to be differentiated from similar findings in disseminated infection due to tuberculosis, atypical mycobacteria and other fungi, and to metastatic tumor and lymphoma.

H. capsulatum causes endemic infection primarily in the Mississippi valley region of central United States. Like other endemic fungal infections, histoplasmosis generally produces a mild, self-limited infection in the lung in immunocompetent patients: histoplasmosis only rarely causes progressive or disseminated infection because normal patients are protected by the ability to develop tuberculoid granulomas that can calcify and become dormant (65).

In immunocompromised patients, histoplasmosis is uncommon, even in endemic areas (66). When it does occur, infection is often disseminated on first discovery. In the lung, a diffuse radiographic abnormality reflecting hematogenous dissemination is identified in about half of the patients (67). The diffuse lung lesions consist of miliary nodules, some of which calcify after recovery (Fig. 6). Diffuse disease may also be manifest as diffuse macronodules, vague reticulonodular opacities, or consolidations. Focal radiographic lung opacities are identified in only a small fraction of patients (68). Enlarged hilar and mediastinal lymph nodes, calcified granulomas, and cavitated granulomas are also identifiable (Figs. 7 and 8) (68). Increased focal opacity and/or cavitation within the diffuse lung disease may indicate the site of an activated dormant focus. Even when imaging does identify findings consistent with disseminated histoplasmosis, concurrent tuberculosis must be considered, especially in the AIDS patient with a low CD4 count. Miliary nodules caused by systemic disseminated histoplasmosis are indistinguishable from those caused by *Cryptococcus*, other endemic fungi, mycobacteria, or metastatic tumor (Figs. 6 and 8). Extra-pulmonary findings include hepatosplenomegaly, lymphadenopathy, and solid organ enlargement. Disseminated extra-pulmonary histoplasmosis is an important diagnostic consideration in the immunocompromised patient from an endemic area who develops a febrile illness associated with pneumonic consolidation, paratracheal mediastinal and intra-abdominal lymphadenopathy, superior vena cava syndrome, and in the patient with calcified or non-calcified miliary lesions in the lung, lymph nodes, spleen, or adrenal glands.

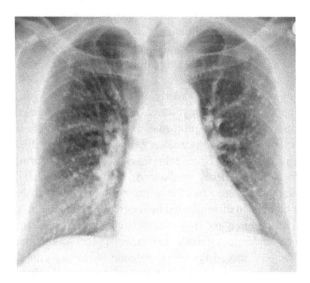

Figure 6   Calcified residua of miliary histoplasmosis. Chest radiograph shows numerous bilateral pulmonary calcifications in a non–immune-compromised patient with a prior episode of miliary histoplasmosis.

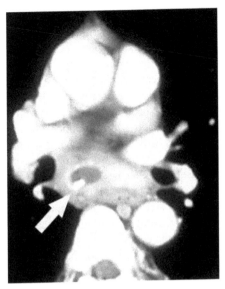

Figure 7 *Histoplasma* lymphadenopathy. Computed tomography scan demonstrates mediastinal lymphadenopathy with calcified granuloma and low-density abscess (*arrow*) in a non–immune-compromised patient.

C. immitis, is a cause of endemic mycosis in the southwestern United States. The lung is the primary portal of entry. In the immunodeficient patient, systemic infection rapidly disseminates, often manifested by miliary lung nodules (Fig. 8A,B). In the immunocompetent person, T-cell immunity helps confine coccidoidomycosis to the lungs and intrathoracic lymph nodes, during

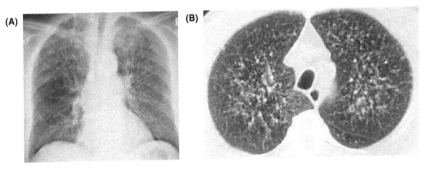

Figure 8 Disseminated coccidoidomycosis. (**A**) Chest radiograph demonstrates numerous 2–4 mm nodular lung opacities in an immune-compromised host with AIDS and low CD4 count. (**B**) Computed tomography scan demonstrates numerous bilateral 2–4 mm randomly distributed pulmonary nodules due to disseminated coccidoidomycosis in the same patient.

which time the disease is usually self-limited and influenza-like. A small fraction of symptomatic immunocompetent patients exhibit imaging evidence of pneumonia. When present, imaging findings may show segmental or lobar airspace opacities, sometimes with hilar adenopathy and/or pleural effusion. Residue of these infections consist of nodules or cavities that my progress, or slowly resolve or evolve, into thin-walled cysts over a number of months (69). In immunocompromised patients dissemination carries a high risk of mortality. Hematogenous dissemination to the lungs often causes diffuse micronodules (miliary) (68) or diffuse reticulonodular opacities, often with hilar lymphadenopathy and pleural effusions (Fig. 8) (70,71). In about one-fourth of patients with disseminated disease, localized lung disease can also be found. Pericardial involvement may lead to pericardial effusion, cardiac tamponade, or constrictive pericarditis. Extra-pulmonary coccidoidomycosis to the brain may show meningitis, i.e., marked thickening of basal meninges and intense contrast enhancement, communicating hydrocephalus in the cervical subarachnoid space and cisterns (basilar, sylvian, and inter-hemispheric) on CT and MRI (36,72). Focal parenchymal MRI abnormalities may suggest ischemia or infarction, brain abscess, or granulomas (73). Extra-pulmonary dissemination can produce bone abscesses, synovitis, abscesses, or granulomas in the liver and other infra-abdominal organs in CT or MRI.

  B. dermatididis is a soil fungus co-endemic with *H. capsulatum* in the south-central and mid-western United States. It is an uncommon cause of invasive mycosis in the severely immunocompromised HIV patient. The two main portals of entry are the lung and the skin. Cell-mediated immunity appears to be less important for protection against blastomycosis than it is for protection against other endemic mycoses. In immunocompetent patients with acute blastomycosis,

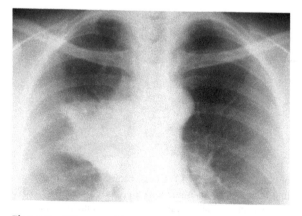

Figure 9 Pulmonary blastomycosis. Chest radiograph shows a consolidative mass in the right upper lobe of an immune-competent host with pulmonary blastomycosis.

imaging findings demonstrate airspace disease (often with air bronchograms), or mass-like opacities in more than half of patients (Fig. 9) (74–76). Mass lesions usually indicate chronic disease (76). In a small minority of patients, presentations consist of nodules, cavities, and interstitial lung findings. Miliary lesions and diffuse alveolar damage are rare in the immunocompetent patient (76). In the immunosuppressed patient, imaging findings often consist of consolidations and mass lesions that are often extensive and progressive (77). Superimposition of disseminated miliary lung lesions or an ARDS-like pattern may be identified in disseminated disease (78). Cavitation and pleural abnormalities occur in a minority of patients. Extra-pulmonary dissemination may involve the liver, spleen, bone marrow, pancreas, brain, meninges, and endocrine glands, especially in the AIDS patient with very low CD4 count. CNS involvement typically demonstrates meningitis or cerebral abscess.

PNEUMOCYSTIS CARINII (JIROVECII) PNEUMONIA

In the immunocompromised patient, PCP presents with sub acute fever, shortness of breath, dyspnea on exertion, nonproductive cough, and hypoxemia. A diagnosis of PCP is corroborated when sputum, bronchoalveolar lavage, or lung biopsy stains are positive for *Pneumocystis jirovecii*. In such a patient, for example an AIDS patient with a CD4+T lymphocyte count <200/L, PCP is suspected when there is a hazy diffuse lung opacification on a chest radiograph. A significant number of these patients will have normal or only very minimal visible lung opacification on CXR.

CT will identify virtually all patients symptomatic with PCP. In these patients, there are three common diffuse patterns of lung findings: (*i*) in about 1/4, there is a diffuse homogeneous pattern that consists of more or less symmetric involvement of the lungs involved by ground-glass opacity and airspace consolidation with delicate air bronchograms; the latter is likely due to airspace disease caused by acute outpouring of fluid into the alveolar airspaces; (*ii*) in the largest group, about 1/2 of all patients with PCP, there is a patchwork mosaic pattern that consists of a combination of ground glass opacity, consolidation, and interstitial lesions, with multiple spared secondary lobules; and (*iii*) in the smallest fraction of patients, about 1/6 of the total, there is primarily an interstitial pattern consisting of interstitial reticular opacities with septal and bronchial wall thickening.

Pneumocystis carinii Pneumonia: Spectrum of Parenchymal CT Findings

These diffuse CT findings (Fig. 10A,B) (79) may have a preferential distribution in the lung periphery (cortex), the lung center (medulla), the upper or lower lung, or in a single part of the lung. PCP may cause isolated ground-glass opacification (80), isolated consolidation, or isolated nodules. Although PCP may present

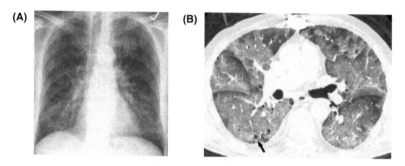

Figure 10 *Pneumocystis carinii (jirovecii)* pneumonia. (**A**) Chest radiograph shows diffuse, predominantly peri-hilar, hazy opacities in a patient with AIDS and a low CD4 count. (**B**) CT scan in the same patient demonstrates diffuse ground-glass opacities with patchy subpleural sparing. A few small cysts are visible in the right lower lobe (*arrow*).

atypically as a cavitated or non-cavitated nodular opacity, this appearance, when found in association with diffuse lung disease caused by PCP, should suggest the possibility of a second infectious, neoplastic, or leukemic process (81).

Other potential findings that are common include air cysts of ≥1 cm diameter that tend to occur in the lung apices (Fig. 10A,B) (82). The latter structural abnormality, which is often thin-walled, may lead to spontaneous pneumothorax (83). Other potential findings include mediastinal lymphadenopathy that may calcify, pleural effusions, and bronlchiectasis. In AIDS patients, high-resolution CT can help distinguish the most characteristic patterns of PCP from the dense localized consolidation, or tree-in-bud opacities, that are more characteristic of non–PCP-related lung infection (84). After clinical recovery, residual ground glass or airspace consolidation, often with recognizable septal thickening, are often still visible, especially in the lung periphery. Air cysts may clear after several months, but persistence is common.

In an appropriate clinical setting, empiric treatment of PCP may be initiated in the patient who also has characteristic radiographic findings. In addition to continued efforts to establish a specific diagnosis, chest CT is strongly recommended to substantiate the plain film findings because similar diffuse radiographic appearances can be found in disseminated mycobacterial infection (both typical and atypical), disseminated fungal infection, Kaposi sarcoma, drug-induced disease, and lymphomatoid disorders, such as lymphocytic interstitial pneumonitis and disseminated lymphoma (85,86). Since clinical response while on empiric therapy does not establish a diagnosis, and chest CT obtained at some later time point is likely to be confounded by intervening therapies, a CT at the time of initiation of therapy makes more sense than waiting for lack of response to therapy. One potentially important confounder in interpreting later imaging findings is the paradoxical deepening of consolidation that may occur when corticosteroids are tapered or discontinued.

REFERENCES

1. Hwang SS, Kim HH, Park SH, Jung JI, Jang HS. The value of CT-guided percutaneous needle aspiration in immunocompromised patients with suspected pulmonary infection. AJR Am J Roentgenol 2000; 175:235–8.
2. Kalra MK, Maher MM, Toth TL, et al. Strategies for CT radiation dose optimization. Radiology 2004; 230:619–28.
3. McAdams HP, Samei E, Dobbins J, III, Tourassi GD, Ravin C. Recent advances in chest radiography. Radiology 2006; 241:663–83.
4. Blum U, Windfuhr M, Buitrago-Tellez C, et al. Invasive pulmonary aspergillosis. MRI, CT, and plain radiographic findings and their contribution for early diagnosis. Chest 1994; 106:1156–61.
5. Eibel R, Herzog P, Dietrich O, et al. Pulmonary abnormalities in immunocompromised patients: comparative detection with parallel acquisition MR imaging and thin-section helical CT. Radiology 2006; 241:880–91.
6. Filmont JE, Czernin J, Yap C, et al. Value of F-18 fluorodeoxyglucose positron emission tomography for predicting the clinical outcome of patients with aggressive lymphoma prior to and after autologous stem-cell transplantation. Chest 2003; 124:608–13.
7. Stumpe KD, Dazzi H, Schaffner A, von Schulthess GK. Infection imaging using wholebody FDG-PET. Eur J Nucl Med 2000; 27:822–32.
8. Herbrecht R, Denning DW, Patterson TF, et al. Voriconazole versus amphotericin B for primary therapy of invasive aspergillosis. N Engl J Med 2002; 347:408–15.
9. Patterson JE, Zidouh A, Miniter P, Andriole VT, Patterson TF. Hospital epidemiologic surveillance for invasive aspergillosis: patient demographics and the utility of antigen detection. Infect Control Hosp Epidemiol 1997; 18:104–8.
10. Greene RE, Schlamm HT, Oestmann JW, et al. Imaging findings in acute invasive pulmonary aspergillosis: clinical significance of the halo sign. Clin Infect Dis 2007; 44:373–9.
11. Shibuya K, Paris S, Ando T, Nakayama H, Hatori T, Latge J-P. Catalases of *Aspergillus fumigatus* and inflammation in aspergillosis. Jpn J Med Mycol 2006; 47:249–55.
12. Caillot D, Couaillier JF, Bernard A, et al. Increasing volume and changing characteristics of invasive pulmonary aspergillosis on sequential thoracic computed tomography scans in patients with neutropenia. J Clin Oncol 2001; 19:253–9.
13. Saul SH, Khachatoorian T, Poorsattar A, et al. Opportunistic Trichosporon pneumonia. Association with invasive aspergillosis. Arch Pathol Lab Med 1981; 105:456–9.
14. Huang SN, Harris LS. Acute disseminated penicilliosis: report of a case and review of pertinent literature. Am J Clin Pathol 1963; 39:167–74.
15. Young NA, Kwon-Chung KJ, Kubota TT, Jennings AE, Fisher RI. Disseminated infection by *Fusarium moniliforme* during treatment for malignant lymphoma. J Clin Microbiol 1978; 7:589–94.
16. Armstrong D, Young LS, Meyer RD, Blevins AH. Infectious complications of neoplastic disease. Med Clin North Am 1971; 55:729–45.
17. Primack SL, Hartman TE, Lee KS, Muller NL. Pulmonary nodules and the CT halo sign. Radiology 1994; 190:513–5.
18. Kim Y, Lee KS, Jung KJ, et al. Halo sign on high resolution CT: findings in spectrum of pulmonary diseases with pathologic correlation. J Comput Assist Tomogr 1999; 23:622–6.

19. Gaeta M, Blandino A, Scribano E, et al. Computed tomography halo sign in pulmonary nodules: frequency and diagnostic value. J Thorac Imaging 1999; 14:109–13.

20. Denning DW. Invasive aspergillosis. Clin Infect Dis 1998; 26:781–803.

21. Hruban RH, Meziane MA, Zerhouni EA, et al. Radiologic-pathologic correlation of the CT halo sign in invasive pulmonary aspergillosis. J Comput Assist Tomogr 1987; 11:534–6.

22. Orr DP, Myerowitz RL, Dubois PJ. Patho-radiologic correlation of invasive pulmonary aspergillosis in the compromised host. Cancer 1978; 41:2028–39.

23. Kuhlman JE, Fishman EK, Siegelman SS. Invasive pulmonary aspergillosis in acute leukemia: characteristic findings on CT, the CT halo sign, and the role of CT in early diagnosis. Radiology 1985; 157:611–4.

24. Caillot D, Casasnovas O, Bernard A, et al. Improved management of invasive pulmonary aspergillosis in neutropenic patients using early thoracic computed tomographic scan and surgery. J Clin Oncol 1997; 15:139–47.

25. Herold CJ, Kramer J, Sertl K, et al. Invasive pulmonary aspergillosis—evaluation with MR imaging. Radiology 1989; 173:717–21.

26. Curtis AM, Smith GJ, Ravin CE. Air crescent sign of invasive aspergillosis. Radiology 1979; 133:17–21.

27. Gefter WB, Albelda SM, Talbot GH, et al. Invasive pulmonary aspergillosis and acuteleukemia. Limitations in the diagnostic utility of the air crescent sign. Radiology 1985; 157:605–10.

28. Aquino SL, Kee ST, Warnock ML, Gamsu G. Pulmonary aspergillosis: imaging findings with pathologic correlation. AJR Am J Roentgenol 1994; 163:811–5.

29. Godwin JD, Webb WR, Savoca CJ, Gamsu G, Goodman PC. Multiple, thin-walled cystic lesions of the lung. AJR Am J Roentgenol 1980; 135:593–604.

30. Ryu JH, Swensen SJ. Cystic and cavitary lung diseases: focal and diffuse. Mayo Clin Proc 2003; 78:744–52.

31. Tuncel E. Pulmonary air meniscus sign. Respiration 1984; 46:139–44.

32. Logan PM, Primack SL, Miller RR, Muller NL. Invasive aspergillosis of the airways: radiographic, CT, and pathologic findings. Radiology 1994; 193:383–8.

33. Kramer MR, Denning DW, Marshall SE, et al. Ulcerative tracheobronchitis after lung transplantation. A new form of invasive aspergillosis. Am Rev Respir Dis 1991; 144:552–6.

34. Cox J, Murtagh FR, Wilfong A, Brenner J. Cerebral aspergillosis: MR imaging and histopathologic correlation. AJNR Am J Neuroradiol 1992; 13:1489–92.

35. Osborn AG. Diagnostic Neuroradiology. St. Louis: Mosby, 1994:706–9.

36. Bowen BC, Post MJD. Intracranial infection. In: Atlas SW, ed. Magnetic Resonance Imaging of the Brain and Spine. New York: Raven Press, 1991:501–38.

37. Denning DW, Riniotis K, Dobrashian R, Sambatakou H. Chronic cavitary and fibrosing pulmonary and pleural aspergillosis: case series, proposed nomenclature and review. Clin Infect Dis 2003; 37:S265–80.

38. Chamilos D, Marom EM, Lewis RE, Lionakis MS, Kontoyianis DP. Predictors of pulmonary zygomycosis versus invasive pulmonary aspergillosis in cancer patients. Clin Infect Dis 2005; 41:60–6.

39. Funada H, Misawa T, Nakao S, Saga T, Hattori KI. The air crescent sign of invasive pulmonary mucormycosis in acute leukemia. Cancer 1984; 53:2721–3.

40. Vogl TJ, Hinrichs T, Jacobi V, Bohme A, Hoelzer D. Computed tomographic appearance of pulmonary mucormycosis. Rofo Fortschr Geb Rontgenstr Neuen Bildgeb Verfahr 2000; 172:604–8.
41. Jamadar DA, Kazerooni EA, Daly BD, White CS, Gross BH. Pulmonary zygomycosis: CT appearance. J Comput Assist Tomogr 1995; 19:733–8.
42. Wheat LJ. Fungal infections in the immunocompromised host. In: Rubin RH, Young LS, eds. Clinical Approach to Infection in the Compromised Host. New York: Plenum, 1981:211–37.
43. Kontoyiannis DP, Lionakis MS, Lewis RE, et al. Zygomycosis in the era of Aspergillus-active antifungal therapy in a tertiary care cancer center: a case-control observational study of 27 recent cases. J Infect Dis 2005; 191:1350–60.
44. Dubois PJ, Myerowitz RL, Allen CM. Pathoradiologic correlation of pulmonary candidiasis in immunosuppressed patients. Cancer 1977; 40:1026–36.
45. Masur H, Rosen PP, Armstrong D. Pulmonary disease caused by *Candida* species. Am J Med 1977; 63:914–25.
46. Cairns MRI, Durack DT. Fungal pneumonia in the immunocompromised host. Semin Respir Infect 1986; 1:166–85.
47. Buff SJ, McLelland R, Gallis HA, Matthay R, Putman CE. *Candida albicans* pneumonia: radiographic appearance. AJR Am J Roentgenol 1982; 138:645–8.
48. Haron E, Feld R, Tuffnell P, et al. Hepatic candidiasis: an increasing problem in immunocompromised patients. Am J Med 1987; 83:17–26.
49. Haron E, Vartivarian S, Anaissie E, Dekmezian R, Bodey GP. Primary Candida pneumonia. Experience at a large cancer center and review of the literature. Medicine (Baltimore) 1993; 72:137–42.
50. Pastakia B, Shawker TH, Thaler M, O'Leary T, Pizzo PA. Hepatosplenic candidiasis: wheels within wheels. Radiology 1988; 166:417–21.
51. Thaler M, Pastakia B, Shawker TH, O'Leary T, Pizzo PA. Hepatic candidiasis in cancer patients: the evolving picture of the syndrome. Ann Intern Med 1988; 108:88–100.
52. Mudad R, Vredenburgh J, Paulson EK, et al. A radiologic syndrome after high dose chemotherapy and autologous bone marrow transplantation, with clinical and pathologic features of systemic candidiasis. Cancer 1994; 74:1360–6.
53. Fox DL, Müller NL. Pulmonary cryptococcosis in immunocompetent patients: CT findings in 12 patients. AJR 2005; 185:622–6.
54. Shirkhoda A. CT findings in hepatosplenic and renal candidiasis. J Comput Assist Tomogr 1987; 11:795–8.
55. Shirkhoda A, Lopez-Berestein G, Holbert JM, Luna MA. Hepatosplenic fungal infection: CT and pathologic evaluation after treatment with liposomal amphotericin B. Radiology 1986; 159:349–53.
56. Woodring JH, Ciporkin G, Lee C, Worm B, Woolley S. Pulmonary cryptococcosis. Semin Roentgenol 1996; 31:67–75.
57. Maroon B, Khoury MB, Godwin JD, et al. Thoracic cryptococcosis: immunologic competence and radiologic appearance. AJR 1984; 141:893–6.
58. Cornell SH, Jacoby CG. The varied computed tomographic appearance of intracranial cryptococcosis. Radiology 1982; 143:703–7.
59. Zinck SE, Leung AN, Frost M, Berry GJ, Muller NL. Pulmonary cryptococcosis: CT and pathologic findings. J Comput Assist Tomogr 2002; 26:330–4.

60. McGuinness G. Changing trends in the pulmonary manifestations of AIDS. Radiol Clin North Am 1997; 35:1029–82.
61. Connolly JE, Jr., McAdams HP, Erasmus JJ, Rosado-de-Christenson ML. Opportunistic fungal pneumonia. J Thorac Imaging 1999; 14:51–62.
62. Conces DJ, Jr. Endemic fungal pneumonia in immunocompromised patients. J Thorac Imaging 1999; 14:1–8.
63. Oh YW, Effmann EL, Godwin JD. Pulmonary infections in immunocompromised hosts: the importance of correlating the conventional radiologic appearance with the clinical setting. Radiology 2000; 217:647–56.
64. Greene R. Opportunistic pneumonias. Semin Roentgenol 1980; 15:50–72.
65. Wheat J. Histoplasmosis experience during outbreaks in Indianapolis and review of the literature. Medicine (Baltimore) 1997; 76:339–54.
66. Williams DM, Krick JA, Remington JS. Pulmonary infection in the compromised host. Am Rev Respir Dis 1976; 114(2): 359–94.
67. Vathesatogkit P, Goldenberg R, Parsey M. A 27-year-old HIV-infected woman with severe sepsis and pulmonary infiltrates Disseminated histoplasmosis with severe sepsis and acute respiratory failure. Chest 2003; 123:272–6.
68. Goldstein E. Miliary and disseminated coccidioidomycosis. Ann Intern Med 1978; 89:365–6.
69. Dublin AB, Phillips HE. Computed tomography of disseminated coccidiodomycosis. Radiology 1980; 135:361–8.
70. Batra P, Batra RS. Thoracic coccidioidomycosis. Semin Roentgenol 1996; 31:28–44.
71. Ampel NM, Dols CL, Galgiani JN. Coccidioidomycosis during human immuno-deficiency virus infection: results of a prospective study in a coccidioidal endemic area. Am J Med 1993; 94:235–40.
72. Wrobel CJ, Meyer S, Johnson RH, Hesselink JR. MR findings in acute and chronic coccidioidomycosis meningitis. AJNR Am J Neuroradiol 1992; 13:1241–5.
73. Erly WK, Bellon RJ, Seeger JF, Carmody RF. MR imaging of acute coccidioidal meningitis. AJNR Am J Neuroradiol 1999; 20:509–14.
74. Brown LR, Swensen SJ, Van Scoy RE, et al. Roentgenologic features of pulmonary blastomycosis. Mayo Clin Proc 1991; 66:29–38.
75. Halvorsen RA, Duncan JD, Merten DF, Gallis HA, Putman CE. Pulmonary blastomycosis: radiologic manifestations. Radiology 1984; 150:1–5.
76. Winer-Muram HT, Beals DH, Cole FH, Jr. Blastomycosis of the lung: CT features. Radiology 1992; 182:829–32.
77. Pappas PG, Pottage JC, Powderly WG, et al. Blastomycosis in patients with the acquired immunodeficiency syndrome. Ann Intern Med 1992; 116:847–53.
78. Evans ME, Haynes JB, Atkinson JB, Delvaux TC, Jr., Kaiser AB. Blastomyces dermatitidis and the adult respiratory distress syndrome. Case reports and review of the literature. Am Rev Respir Dis 1982; 126:1099–102.
79. Kuhlman JE, Kavuru M, Fishman EK, Siegelman SS. *Pneumocystis carinii* pneumonia: spectrum of parenchymal CT findings. Radiology 1990; 175:711–4.
80. Miller WT, Jr., Shah RM. Isolated diffuse ground-glass opacity in thoracic CT: causes and clinical presentations. Radiology 1990; 175:711–4.
81. Scott WW, Kuhlman JE. Focal pulmonary lesions in patients with AIDS: percutaneous transthoracic needle biopsy. Radiology 1991; 180:419–21.

82. Kuhlman JE, Knowles MC, Fishman EK, et al. Premature bullous pulmonary damage in AIDS: CT diagnosis. Radiology 1989; 173:22–6.
83. Sandhu JS, Goodman PC. Pulmonary cysts associated with *Pneumocystis carinii* pneumonia in patients with AIDS. Radiology 1989; 173:33–5.
84. Hidalgo A, Falco V, Mauleon S, et al. Accuracy of high-resolution CT in distinguishing between *Pneumocystis carinii* pneumonia and non-*Pneumocystis carinii* pneumonia in AIDS patients. Eur Radiol 2002; 13:1179–84.
85. McGuinness G, John V, Scholes JV, et al. Unusual lymphoproliferative disorders in nine adults with HIV or AIDS: CT and pathologic findings. Radiology 1995; 197:59–65.
86. Bazot M, Cadranel M, Benayoun S, Tassart M, Bigot JM, Carette MF. Primary pulmonary AIDS-related lymphoma: radiographic and CT findings. Chest 1999; 116:1282–6.

4

Serodiagnosis: Antibody and Antigen Detection

Christine J. Morrison

Office of the Chief Science Officer, Centers for Disease Control and Prevention, Atlanta, Georgia, U.S.A.

David W. Warnock

Division of Foodborne, Bacterial, and Mycotic Diseases, National Center for Zoonotic, Vector-Borne, and Enteric Diseases, Centers for Disease Control and Prevention, Atlanta, Georgia, U.S.A.

INTRODUCTION

The definitive diagnosis of invasive fungal infections is usually based upon the isolation and identification of a specific etiologic agent in culture, and/or on the microscopic demonstration of the etiologic agent in histopathologic or other clinical specimens. The management of invasive fungal infections is, however, often hampered by difficulties in obtaining good specimens for histopathologic or microbiologic investigation, and by the fact that fungal cultures sometimes become positive only late in the infection. In this situation, other methods are essential to allow early diagnosis and treatment. New procedures, based on the detection of fungal DNA in clinical material, are presently being developed (1,2) (see Chapter 6). These molecular tests offer great hope for the rapid detection and identification of difficult-to-culture organisms, and for rapid diagnosis directly from clinical samples. However, few DNA-based tests are currently available for routine clinical use.

Serologic tests provide rapid results compared with the length of time required for culture and identification of fungal pathogens, and consequently they are often used as a basis for decisions regarding management of patients with invasive fungal infections. The majority of tests are based on the detection of antibodies to specific fungal pathogens, although tests for fungal antigens are now becoming more widely available. At their best, individual serologic tests can be diagnostic, e.g., tests for antigenemia in cryptococcosis. In general, however, the results of these tests must be interpreted with caution and need to be considered alongside the results of other clinical and laboratory investigations.

ANTIBODY TESTING

Although serologic testing has long been used to establish the presumptive diagnosis of a number of fungal infections, the results of antibody detection tests are seldom helpful in immunocompromised individuals with opportunistic infections, such as invasive aspergillosis or candidiasis. Among the reasons for the poor sensitivity and specificity of antibody testing in these infections are that antibodies are sometimes present in colonized but uninfected persons, and that immunocompromised individuals are often incapable of mounting a detectable antibody response to infection. In other cases, the infection is so fulminant that there is insufficient time for a detectable response to occur. Antibody detection tests have proved more useful in the diagnosis of endemic fungal infections, such as histoplasmosis and coccidioidomycosis, which are sometimes difficult to diagnose by traditional methods such as culture.

Numerous methods are available for the detection of antibodies in persons with fungal diseases. Immunodiffusion (ID) is a simple and inexpensive method for qualitative detection of precipitating antibodies, but it is insensitive and this reduces its usefulness as a screening test. Counterimmunoelectrophoresis (CIE) is a more rapid and sensitive method for the detection of precipitins. Complement fixation (CF) is a sensitive, quantitative test, but more difficult to perform and interpret than ID. However, it remains an important method contributing to the diagnosis of a number of endemic fungal infections, including histoplasmosis and coccidioidomycosis.

Early tests for the detection of fungal antibodies relied on the use of unpurified or semipurified antigens and this resulted in major problems with cross-reactions due to the presence of determinants shared among pathogenic fungi. Many of these reactions are due to polysaccharide components within these preparations. Moreover, tests that depend on unpurified antigens may be impeded by difficulties in producing reproducible reagents. For this reason, recent investigations have focused on developing standardized antigens that are derived from the application of recombinant procedures.

ANTIGEN TESTING

Another approach to the diagnosis of invasive fungal infections is to use serologic tests to detect fungal antigens in body fluids. The latex agglutination (LA) test for *Cryptococcus neoformans* capsular antigen, introduced in the 1960s, remains one of the most useful of all serologic tests for fungal infection. Similar tests are currently being evaluated for the detection of fungal cell wall components, such as galactomannan and mannan, in patients with invasive aspergillosis or candidiasis, respectively. In contrast to cryptococcosis, the antigens released in patients with these infections are often cleared very rapidly from the circulation by receptor-mediated endocytosis in the liver (3,4). As a result, antigenemia is often sporadic rather than sustained. Unless serial samples are tested, the diagnosis will often be missed.

The LA test is a simple but insensitive method that nevertheless has proved highly successful for detection of the polysaccharide capsular antigens of *C. neoformans*, which are released in large amounts in most patients with cryptococcosis. LA has, however, proved much less useful for the early detection of fungal cell wall components, such as galactomannan and mannan, in patients with invasive aspergillosis or candidiasis, respectively. More sensitive antigen detection procedures, such as radioimmunoassay (RIA), have been developed for the diagnosis of these and a number of other fungal diseases, in particular, histoplasmosis. However, there are legal restrictions on the use and disposal of radioactive isotopes, making RIA-based tests less appealing for use in clinical microbiology laboratories. In contrast, enzyme-linked immunosorbent assay (ELISA) is more suitable for routine clinical use, and methods have been developed and evaluated for several diseases, including aspergillosis, candidiasis, coccidioidomycosis, histoplasmosis, paracoccidioidomycosis, and penicilliosis.

In general, antigen detection tests that use polyclonal antibodies raised against unpurified or semipurified fungal antigens have significant cross-reactions with other pathogenic fungi (5). Furthermore, assays that use polyclonal antibodies may be subject to variability among different lots of antisera. Monoclonal antibody-based antigen detection tests offer several advantages over polyclonal antibody-based procedures, including reduced batch-to-batch variability, and the ability to generate standardized reagents in almost unlimited quantities. However, monoclonal antibody-based antigen detection tests are sometimes less sensitive than otherwise identical methods that use polyclonal antibodies.

EVALUATING THE PERFORMANCE OF SERODIAGNOSTIC TESTS

In general, four measures are used to evaluate the usefulness of a diagnostic test, based on the number of patients with or without the disease who have a positive or negative test result. *Sensitivity* is defined as the proportion of individuals having the disease who have positive results, and *specificity* as the proportion of non-diseased individuals who have negative results. Estimates of sensitivity and specificity make the assumption that the diagnosis has already been established. The *positive predictive value* (PPV) of a test is defined as the proportion of individuals with a positive test result who have the disease, and the *negative predictive value* (NPV) is the proportion of individuals with a negative result who do not have the disease. These estimates assume that the test result has already been established and ask whether the test correctly predicted the diagnosis. Both kinds of analysis require that an intermediate or indeterminate result is either excluded or reclassified as positive or negative. Both analyses assume that the cut-off value separating these categories has already been selected. Often, however, the cut-off is not obvious and is decided as a compromise between sensitivity and specificity. A better approach is to prepare receiver operator characteristic (ROC) curves for each test method under evaluation: at each potential cut-off value, the sensitivity is plotted on the y axis and 1 minus the specificity is plotted on the x axis. The cut-off value plotted on the ROC curve that demonstrates maximum sensitivity and minimum (1—specificity) can then be selected as a suitable value to define test positivity.

Assessing the performance of a diagnostic test requires the use of standard case definitions of infection. Such definitions are essential to permit reliable categorization of the patients from whom samples are obtained. Uncertainty in disease diagnosis is one of the most important variables that influence comparisons among diagnostic tests. It also complicates analysis of different evaluations of the performance of the same test. Many invasive fungal infections are difficult to diagnose, and this is reflected in the large number of different case definitions and diagnostic criteria that have been employed (6). Thus, infection may be classed as definite, proven, probable, suspected, presumptive, or possible. These terms may take on a range of meanings, and there is often wide variation in their interpretation. As a result, even when a simple commercial test, such as the LA method for Aspergillus galactomannan antigen detection, was evaluated in different institutions, differences in disease diagnosis contributed to variations in test sensitivity that ranged from 27.5% to 95% (7,8). Consensus definitions have been developed for invasive fungal infections in patients with cancer and in hematopoietic stem cell transplant (HSCT) recipients (9) and these are now being applied to clinical trials of antifungal agents. Their application to evaluations of new serodiagnostics should lead to a clearer understanding of the merits and limitations of particular tests and reagents.

It should be borne in mind that the consensus definitions for invasive fungal infections (9) were developed for use in clinical trials and relied on conservative criteria to assure a correct diagnosis. One issue that arises when these definitions are used to analyze the performance of novel diagnostic tests is the insensitivity of current "gold standard" tests such as culture and/or histopathology. As a result, it can be difficult to interpret a positive antigen test result in the absence of a positive culture or histopathologically documented disease.

In addition to the use of consistent case definitions, evaluations of the performance of diagnostic tests should be carried out in defined patient populations appropriate for testing the question being asked (10). It is important that the patients from whom samples are obtained have a homogenous underlying condition and a high probability of having the fungal disease under investigation. In studies in which there is no assurance that homogenous populations are being evaluated, the selection of subjects may well be biased and, therefore, the findings cannot be used to make generalizations about the test being evaluated. It is well established that the kinetics of antibody and antigen production differ in different patient populations and therefore the performance of each new test and reagent needs to be evaluated in each group separately. Furthermore, the prevalence of the disease in the population under investigation is an important factor that greatly influences the positive and negative predictive values of the procedure, especially when disease prevalence is very low. In the case of the commercial sandwich ELISA for Aspergillus galactomannan antigen detection, the PPV of the test was 10% in a group of 211 HSCT recipients, 20 of whom had positive test results, but only two of who had aspergillosis (11). In contrast, the PPV was 95% in a second group of 297 oncohematologic patients with suspected lung infection, 42 of whom gave positive results, and 40 of whom had aspergillosis (11).

Another issue that creates difficulty when interpreting the results of diagnostic tests is how to evaluate multiple test results that are obtained from an individual patient. In most studies, subjects have been classified as "cases" (with infection) or "controls" (without infection). However, this does not allow for evaluation of test performance in the setting of clinical variables that change over time. These variables can impact test performance dramatically; examples include receipt of antifungal therapy, changes in neutrophil count, and time relative to culture-confirmed diagnosis. More recent studies have included per-test analyses to assess the impact of clinical variables that can change over time.

The diagnosis of most invasive fungal infections requires a combination of clinical, radiologic, microbiologic, and histopathologic investigations. With few exceptions, no single test is sufficient to diagnose these infections, and serologic tests require confirmation by clinical signs and symptoms, radiologic abnormalities, and/or culture. Although most new serologic tests have been evaluated in comparison with conventional diagnostic tests, comparisons between non-culture based methods are also of great interest. The most important issue remains the need for tests that allow early detection of disease or, equally important, provide reliable evidence for the absence of fungal infection.

SEROLOGIC DIAGNOSIS OF FUNGAL INFECTIONS

Aspergillosis

Antibody Detection

Tests for Aspergillus antibodies have been extensively evaluated and are of proven usefulness in the diagnosis of several clinical forms of aspergillosis, in particular allergic bronchopulmonary aspergillosis (ABPA) and aspergilloma (colonization of existing cavities in the lungs). Of the different serologic tests that have been developed, the most popular are those that detect precipitins, such as ID and CIE. Serologic tests have, however, proved less successful in immunocompromised patients with invasive aspergillosis, even when more sensitive procedures, such as ELISA, are used. Furthermore, it has been difficult to evaluate and compare the different methods, because the tests and antigen preparations have not been standardized, and patient populations studied have differed.

In studies conducted prior to the 1980s, unpurified mycelial or culture filtrate antigens of *Aspergillus fumigatus* were used to detect antibodies in the serum of patients with invasive aspergillosis. However, marked differences were noted in the composition of similar antigen preparations, depending on the strain(s) used in their production, the conditions of culture, and the method of extraction (12,13). In addition to cross-reactions due to determinants shared with other fungi, some unpurified *Aspergillus* antigens also showed cross-reactions with C-reactive protein, present in the serum of patients with a range of infectious and noninfectious diseases. In light of these problems, semipurified or purified standardized antigens began to be used in the 1980s. Antigenic preparations of *A. fumigatus* contain numerous protein and polysaccharide components, but the latter are responsible for most of the cross-reactions with other fungi. Most recent investigators have used the protein and glycoprotein antigens of *A. fumigatus* to detect antibodies in patients with aspergillosis (14–16).

Since 1990 much effort has been expended to isolate and characterize relevant antigens of *A. fumigatus* to the molecular level (17). Among these antigens are an 18 kDa ribonuclease (18), a 90 kDa catalase (19), and an 88 kDa dipeptidyl-peptidase (20). In addition, galactomannan, isolated from cell wall or culture filtrate preparations of *A. fumigatus* has been well characterized (21,22). Because of difficulties in producing large amounts of these antigens in pure form from traditional cultures, attention has turned to the use of molecular biological methods to produce pure recombinant protein antigens of *A. fumigatus*. Such antigens can be used as the basis for the development of quantitative methods, such as ELISA, for measurement of the antibody response.

In recent years, more than 20 recombinant *A. fumigatus* antigens have been identified and characterized, and a number of these have been extensively evaluated for their diagnostic performance in serologic studies of asthmatic individuals, and patients with cystic fibrosis with or without ABPA (23–26). Although the reactivity of these individual antigens shows considerable variation (25,27), some of these pure recombinant *A. fumigatus* antigens have been shown to be useful in differentiating ABPA from other *Aspergillus*-induced allergic disorders and in monitoring disease progression and response to treatment (23,24,28).

Tests for *Aspergillus* antibodies have been extensively evaluated for the rapid diagnosis of invasive aspergillosis, but their role remains uncertain. Using unpurified culture filtrate antigens, Holmberg et al. (29) detected *A. fumigatus* precipitins by CIE in serial serum specimens from seven of 10 oncohematologic patients with aspergillosis. In contrast, Young and Bennett (30) were unable to detect antibodies to culture filtrate antigens by ID in any of 15 patients with hematologic malignancies and confirmed invasive aspergillosis. The reported variations in the success of these tests may be due to differences in the composition of the antigen preparations used, or the timing of sample collection. Differences in the level of immunosuppression of patients studied could also be an important factor.

The role of antibody testing in the diagnosis of invasive aspergillosis in non-neutropenic high-risk groups has not been extensively evaluated. Several reports suggest that the detection of anti-Aspergillus antibodies might be useful in solid organ transplant recipients. Trull et al. (31) used an ELISA to measure anti-Aspergillus IgG levels in serial serum samples from 19 heart transplant recipients with proven invasive aspergillosis. Sixteen patients developed raised titers of antibodies to culture filtrate or somatic antigens of *A. fumigatus* at some time after transplantation. However, it was noted that, even though samples were tested with an ELISA, repeated testing was required for the detection of an antibody response. In addition, antibody levels often declined to within the normal range even during fulminant infection. Tommee et al. (32) noted a close correlation between anti-Aspergillus IgG levels and Aspergillus infection in four lung transplant recipients. Clearly, further evaluation is needed in order to establish the diagnostic value of Aspergillus antibody detection in solid organ transplant recipients and other groups of relatively immunocompetent patients at risk of invasive Aspergillus infection.

Yuen et al. (33) described the cloning and characterization of the *AFMP1* gene, which encodes an antigenic cell wall galactomannoprotein of *A. fumigatus*. In a more recent report, this group described the development of an ELISA for the serodiagnosis of *A. fumigatus* infections, based on purified recombinant galactomannoprotein antigen (34). This test proved 100% sensitive for patients with aspergilloma, and gave positive results in one third of patients with invasive aspergillosis. More recently, Sarfati et al. (26) tested eight recombinant protein antigens and showed that, although an 18 kDa ribonuclease, a 360 kDa catalase, and an 88 kDa dipeptidyl-peptidase were useful in the diagnosis of ABPA and aspergilloma, no changes in levels of antibody response to these antigens could be detected by ELISA in immunocompromised patients during invasive Aspergillus infection. Antibody detection may be useful as a means of establishing a diagnosis of aspergillosis in hosts who have undergone immunological reconstitution, or who have "allergic" forms of aspergillosis, but antigen detection tests may be a more appropriate diagnostic method for those who remain immunocompromised.

Antigen Detection

Isolation in culture of the organism, together with its histopathologic demonstration in tissue, remains the definitive method for diagnosis of invasive forms of aspergillosis in immunocompromised individuals (9). There are, however, problems associated with these approaches, and these relate both to the differentiation of Aspergillus colonization from infection and to the invasive nature of the methods required to obtain specimens. Aspergillus infection is often not recognized until a late stage and, as a consequence, the outcome is dismal. Because the prognosis can be improved if infection is detected promptly and if appropriate treatment is instigated, several non-culture-based methods of diagnosis have been the subject of extensive investigation. These include tests for the detection of Aspergillus antigens in blood and other body fluids, as well as methods to detect circulating Aspergillus DNA.

The choice of test procedure and reagents for Aspergillus antigen detection is important. The reagents should detect antigens from all of the major pathogenic *Aspergillus* species and the test procedure should be sensitive because the amount of antigen in clinical specimens is likely to be small. Among the methods that have been developed and evaluated are RIA (35,36), inhibition ELISA (37,38), LA (7), and sandwich ELISA (39). With these tests, Aspergillus antigens have been detected in serum, urine, and bronchoalveolar lavage fluid (BALF) of infected animals and humans with invasive aspergillosis. Several antigens have been studied as potential targets, but galactomannan, a major structural glycoprotein from the fungal cell wall, has received the most attention (17). Animal studies have shown that the concentration of circulating Aspergillus antigen correlates with the extent of infection, at least in neutropenic models (40–42).

Two tests to detect circulating Aspergillus galactomannan antigen are now commercially available in a number of countries. Both utilize the same rat monoclonal antibody, EB-A2, in either an LA or sandwich ELISA format. The LA test was the first to be developed (Pastorex Aspergillus, Bio-Rad Laboratories, Paris, France) and has been extensively evaluated using serum samples from HSCT recipients and patients with hematologic malignancies (7,8,43–47). However, despite its ease of use, the LA test is relatively insensitive (detection limit of 15–20 ng of galactomannan per mL) and detects galactomannan only during the late stages of the disease (46,47). In one report, the LA test was positive in only 12% of serum samples from patients with hematologic malignancies on the day that a diagnosis of invasive aspergillosis was made (48). The LA test cannot be used to detect Aspergillus antigen in urine. In one report, false-positive results were obtained with 42% of urine samples from control subjects (44).

More recently, a sandwich ELISA (Platelia Aspergillus, Bio-Rad Laboratories) has been developed that employs the same monoclonal antibody as the LA test. This test, which was recently approved by the U.S. Food and Drug Administration (FDA) for use with serum samples, is more sensitive because the monoclonal antibody functions both as a captor and a detector, thereby allowing the detection limit to be lowered 10-fold to 0.5 to 1.0 ng of galactomannan per mL (39). Initial clinical studies suggested that the ELISA had a sensitivity of

83% to 90% and a specificity of 81% to 84% (8,49). The test appeared able to detect galactomannan in serum at an earlier stage of infection than the LA procedure, before symptoms and clinical signs became apparent (39,49).

As clinical experience has increased, it has become clear that results obtained with the Platelia Aspergillus ELISA depend on a number of factors, including the prevalence of the disease among the population studied, the stage of the disease at the time of testing, and the age of the population studied. The latter factor is important because more false-positive results occur among children than adults (specificity 98% vs. 48%, respectively) (11). The use of azole prophylaxis is another factor to consider, because this has been shown to decrease test sensitivity (42,50). Published results have also depended on several test parameters, including the cut-off value used, and whether two consecutive positive test results were required for significance.

The Platelia Aspergillus ELISA results are reported as a ratio between the optical density of the patient's sample and that of a control with a low but detectable amount of galactomannan. The optimal cut-off value to maximize test sensitivity and specificity has been the subject of debate since this test first became available. The manufacturer initially considered a ratio of >1.5 to be positive, a ratio of 1.0 to 1.5 to be indeterminate (requiring the test to be repeated), and a ratio <1.0 to be negative. This cut-off value was used in many early studies, but has been progressively revised downwards. Several recent studies have indicated that the cut-off value could be reduced to 1.0 (51–53), or even to as low as 0.5 (42,54). A cut-off value of 0.5 is currently accepted by the FDA.

The diagnostic potential of the Platelia Aspergillus ELISA has been confirmed in several large-scale evaluations (11,42,52,53,55). However, direct comparisons between the results of these studies are difficult, due to differences in the populations studied and the test parameters selected. Using a positive cut-off value of 1.0, and a requirement for two consecutive positive test results, in a hematologic patient population with a high incidence of fatal aspergillosis, the galactomannan ELISA had a sensitivity of almost 93%, a specificity of 95%, a PPV of almost 93%, and a NPV of 95% (52). In contrast, in a study of autologous HSCT recipients with less definite and less fatal disease, a lower prevalence of aspergillosis, and requiring only a single positive test result with a cut-off value of 1.5, sensitivity was only 26%, specificity was 99%, PPV was 92%, and NPV was 83% (11). Pfeiffer et al. (56) have reported a meta-analysis of 27 studies in which consensus case definitions for aspergillosis were used (9). Overall, for proven cases of infection, the Platelia Aspergillus ELISA had a sensitivity of 71% and a specificity of 89%. For both proven and probable cases of infection, the test had a sensitivity of 61% and a specificity of 93%. For proven cases, the PPV was quite low, ranging from 25% to 62% as the prevalence of infection increased from 5% to 20%. In contrast, the NPV was high, ranging from 92% to 98% (56). These data suggest that the Platelia Aspergillus ELISA is good at ruling out the diagnosis of aspergillosis but less so at confirming the diagnosis. The performance of the test shows substantial variation depending on the population under investigation. It appears most useful for patient groups with a high pretest probability of having the disease.

It remains controversial whether invasive aspergillosis can be diagnosed by Platelia Aspergillus ELISA before any clinical or radiologic signs develop. Although one recent report suggests that galactomannan detection does not precede the presence of a halo sign on a thoracic CT scan (57), other prospective studies show that antigenemia can be detected before a diagnosis is made by clinical or radiologic means in approximately two-thirds of cases (median, 5–8 days earlier; range, 1–27 days) (52,53,55). Reducing the cut-off value for a positive result from 1.5 to 0.5 extends the time interval between the first positive antigen test and clinical onset of disease in HSCT recipients to about one to two weeks (42). These findings led the FDA to approve the assay to be used with a cut-off value of 0.5 so as to assist the early diagnosis of invasive aspergillosis in adult neutropenic patients and HSCT recipients.

The usefulness of serial galactomannan monitoring in the assessment of therapeutic response has been demonstrated in animal models of invasive aspergillosis. Antigen levels have been observed to increase in untreated animals (40–42), and fall in those treated with amphotericin B, posaconazole, or voriconazole (42,58,59). The course of the Aspergillus galactomannan antigen titer has also been shown to correlate with clinical outcome in allogeneic HSCT recipients with invasive aspergillosis. In several published studies, antigen levels increased in patients who died from infection despite receiving antifungal treatment, but remained unchanged or decreased in those who survived or died because of causes other than aspergillosis (42,55,60). These results suggest that serial determination of galactomannan levels might be a useful tool for assessing prognosis in some groups of high-risk patients. However, the usefulness of serial antigen testing may depend on the concomitant antifungal treatment given. Animal studies showed that during treatment with the echinocandin drug, caspofungin, antigen levels did not decrease despite clinical improvement (61). A paradoxical increase in circulating galactomannan levels has been observed during treatment with caspofungin in a patient with proven aspergillosis (62). In contrast, Maertens et al. (63) reported that four of five patients who responded to treatment with caspofungin had no detectable antigen by treatment end, while 10 of 12 patients who showed no improvement in antigen levels during treatment showed persistence or progression of their Aspergillus infection.

Although the Platelia Aspergillus ELISA is a promising tool for the early diagnosis of aspergillosis, false-positive results have been reported for 75% of pediatric HSCT recipients (11), for 20% of lung transplant recipients (64), and for 13% of liver transplant recipients (65). The causes of these false-positive results are unclear. However, the monoclonal antibody, EB-A2, used in the Platelia Aspergillus ELISA, has been reported to cross-react with a number of other organisms, including *Fusarium oxysporum*, *Trichophyton rubrum*, *Paecilomyces variotii*, *Penicillium chrysogenum*, and *Penicillium digitatum* (66–68). Other reported causes of false-positive results include infant milk formulas (69), gastrointestinal colonization with *Bifidobacterium bifidum* (70), and enteral feeding with a liquid nutrient that contained soybean protein (71).

Patients at risk for invasive aspergillosis are often receiving treatment with broad-spectrum antibiotics. Should these drugs cross-react with the Platelia Aspergillus ELISA, there is potential for an erroneous diagnosis and inappropriate treatment. Ansorg et al. (72) noted that piperacillin and amoxicillin cross-react in vitro with EB-A2. More recently, there have been numerous reports of the occurrence of false-positive results associated with piperacillin–tazobactam and other beta-lactam antibiotics, including ampicillin, amoxicillin and amoxicillin–clavulanic acid (73–78). Although false-positive results caused by these antibiotics disappear when the drug is discontinued, they may persist for up to five days (78–80). When tested for galactomannan, 12 of 15 batches of piperacillin–tazobactam gave positive results (75). Piperacillin and amoxicillin are semi-synthetic drugs derived natural compounds produced by moulds of the genus *Penicillium* that contain galactomannan in the cell wall. It remains to be established if the basis for the cross-reactivity with EB-A2 is a chemical reaction with the drug itself, or with another compound found in the pharmaceutical preparation, such as a galactomannan or galactofuranose.

Despite the fact that the Platelia Aspergillus ELISA has only been licensed for testing of serum samples, specimens of other body fluids have also been tested for detection of antigen. These include BALF (81–84) and cerebrospinal fluid (CSF) (85,86). Although the number of reports is limited, the evidence thus far suggests that galactomannan can be detected in each of these samples from patients with invasive aspergillosis with higher sensitivity than is the case with culture (87). Well-designed prospective studies with systematic sampling and use of consensus case definitions (9) are needed to compare the performance of antigen detection in samples other than serum specimens with that in serum samples.

In addition to antigen detection, a number of other approaches have been developed for the rapid diagnosis of invasive aspergillosis. As well as PCR-based assays, these include tests to detect (1-3)-β-ᴅ-glucan, a cell wall component of many fungi. The Fungitell assay (Associates of Cape Cod, Falmouth, Massachusetts) was approved by the FDA in 2004 for the diagnosis of invasive fungal infections, including aspergillosis. In a comparative assessment with the Platelia Aspergillus ELISA, Kawazu et al. (88) reported sensitivities of 100% and 55% for the galactomannan test and the (1-3)-β-ᴅ-glucan test, respectively. Pazos et al. (89) monitored neutropenic patients retrospectively for both galactomannan and (1-3)-β-ᴅ-glucan, and noted a sensitivity of 88%, a specificity of 90%, a PPV of 70%, and a NPV of 96% for both methods in the diagnosis of invasive aspergillosis. However, the experience to date is insufficient to conclude that the (1-3)-β-ᴅ-glucan test is as useful as the Platelia Aspergillus ELISA.

Although numerous investigators have reported good performance characteristics of their in-house molecular tests for the diagnosis of aspergillosis in comparison to conventional diagnostic methods, there have been fewer head-to-head comparisons of antigen and PCR-based DNA detection methods. However, several reports have indicated that antigen detection in serum is more sensitive than PCR (90,91). Musher et al. (84) compared the performance of the Platelia Aspergillus ELISA and a quantitative PCR in tests with BALF. The sensitivity of the ELISA was 61% with a cut-off value of 1.0 and 76% with a cut-off value of 1.5; the corresponding specificities were 98% and 94%, respectively. The PCR had a sensitivity of 67% and a specificity of 100%. Further direct comparisons between different methods are essential, not only to provide information about their comparative sensitivity and specificity, but also to help in the design of improved management strategies for invasive aspergillosis.

At present, it appears that maximum benefit can be obtained from the Platelia Aspergillus ELISA if it is used as a screening test, rather than a diagnostic test, in those patients who are at high risk to develop disease. Such individuals might include allogeneic HSCT recipients or neutropenic cancer patients with a new fever. Samples should be obtained from these patients at least twice a week, and should be tested prospectively during the period of high risk and if sampling is continued during antifungal therapy. If an individual is at high risk of having aspergillosis, obtaining two consecutive positive results appears to offer strong support for the diagnosis, provided the patient is not being treated with piperacillin or amoxicillin. It remains to be determined whether prospective screening is of benefit in terms of improved patient survival, or reduction in use of empiric antifungal agents. However, Maertens et al. (92) recently reported that the rate of empiric antifungal treatment for neutropenic fever in patients at high risk for aspergillosis was reduced from 35% to 8% by monitoring for galactomannan antigenemia. By withholding treatment from antigen-negative patients, liposomal amphotericin B usage was reduced by almost 80%.

Candidiasis

Antibody Detection

Tests for Candida antibodies have been extensively evaluated but remain of uncertain usefulness in the diagnosis of invasive forms of candidiasis. Numerous methods have been developed, but the most popular tests are those that detect agglutinins or precipitins, such as ID and CIE. However, these tests are complicated by false-positive results in patients with mucosal colonization or superficial infection, and by false-negative results in immunocompromised individuals. Since 1980, numerous attempts have been made to improve the specificity and sensitivity of antibody detection tests by selecting antigens that are associated with invasive infection rather than colonization, and by using more sensitive procedures, such as RIA and ELISA. However, published studies on different tests and antigens are difficult to compare because of differences in the patient populations, case definitions of infection, numbers of samples collected from individual patients, and the retrospective or prospective design employed.

All normal individuals possess antibodies to mannan, the major cell wall mannoprotein of *Candida* species, and its presence in antigen preparations made from unpurified culture filtrates or cell homogenates accounts for most of the false-positive precipitin test results seen in surgical patients without invasive candidiasis (93,94). Nevertheless, attempts have been made to develop more sensitive tests, such as RIA and ELISA, to detect antibodies to mannan and adapt them to the diagnosis of invasive candidiasis. Using an ELISA to measure levels of antimannan antibodies in sequential serum samples from neutropenic patients, Greenfield et al. (95) detected rising levels in five of 20 patients with invasive candidiasis compared with only one of 80 control subjects. However, other groups have reported that up to 20% of patients with no evidence of invasive candidiasis show significant rises in antibodies to mannan (96). An ELISA to detect circulating anti-*Candida albicans* mannan antibodies is now being marketed in a number of countries (Platelia Candida Antibody, Bio-Rad Laboratories). The test had a sensitivity of 53%, a specificity of 94%, a PPV of 85%, and a NPV of 84% in a recent retrospective evaluation of 162 serum samples from 43 patients with invasive candidiasis and 230 serum samples from 150 controls (97).

Cytoplasmic antigens, prepared from blastospore suspensions of *C. albicans*, were among the first to be used in ID and CIE tests on the assumption that the host is exposed to these only during invasive disease. However, because these antigens were prepared by cell disruption, the extracts became contaminated with mannan during this process. As a result, test specificity was poor, and did not improve until methods were developed to fractionate and identify the immunodominant components in these preparations. Greenfield and Jones (98) identified and purified a 54 kDa major cytoplasmic component of *C. albicans* antigen that was recognized by antibodies present in samples from patients with invasive candidiasis. Subsequently, Greenfield et al. (95) used this antigen to detect antibodies by ELISA in serial serum samples from neutropenic patients. Although the test had a specificity of 100%, sensitivity was only 21%. Other investigators noted significant rises in antibody levels to the 54 kDa antigen in 10% of individuals with no evidence of candidiasis (96).

Antigens with similar molecular masses to the 54 kDa antigen described by Greenfield and Jones (98) have been reported by other groups, including antigens of 44 to 52 kDa (99), 47 kDa (100), 45 kDa (101), and 43 kDa (102). Two of these antigens have been extensively characterized. The 47 kDa antigen of *C. albicans* has been shown to be a breakdown product of the heat shock protein (HSP) 90 (103), and the 44 to 52 kDa antigen has been identified as the glycolytic enzyme enolase (104,105). Antibodies to the 47 kDa antigen were detected by immunoblotting of serum samples from 71% to 74% of patients with invasive candidiasis, and from 38% of patients with superficial infection or colonization (100,106). However, these antibodies have also been found in 70% of critical-care patients without evidence of invasive candidiasis (107). Of particular interest is the fact that all patients who recovered from the infection produced strong antibody responses to the 47 kDa antigen, while those who died showed little or no response, leading the authors to suggest that tests designed to detect antibody to this antigen could have prognostic utility (100,106).

Antibodies to the 48 kDa enolase antigen of *C. albicans* were detected in seven of 10 serum samples from patients with invasive candidiasis (99). Moreover, these patients had significantly higher levels of antibody to this antigen than did patients with non-invasive forms of candidiasis, other fungal infections, or normal individuals. Using an ELISA to detect antibodies to enolase, van Deventer et al. (108) reported a sensitivity of 50% and a specificity of 86% in immunocompetent patients, and a sensitivity of 53% and a specificity of 78% in immunocompromised patients. Using immunoblotting to detect antibodies to enolase, Mitsutake et al. (109) noted a sensitivity of 93% and a specificity of 95% in immunocompetent patients.

In addition to enolase, a number of other Candida enzymes have been evaluated as potential targets for antibody detection. Staib et al. (110,111) showed that patients with invasive candidiasis and colonized individuals had antibodies that reacted with culture filtrates containing proteolytic enzymes of *C. albicans*. Macdonald and Odds (112,113) detected antibodies to a purified *C. albicans* proteinase by CIE, and noted that patients with invasive disease had higher levels than individuals without candidiasis. However, using an ELISA and a purified *C. albicans* proteinase, Ruchel et al. (114) reported that serial monitoring of antibody levels alone was not useful in the diagnosis of invasive candidiasis. More recently, Na and Song (115) noted that an ELISA for detection of antibodies against *C. albicans*-secreted aspartyl proteinase had a sensitivity of 70% and a specificity of 76% in a retrospective evaluation of 33 patients with invasive candidiasis. Using an ELISA to detect antibodies against a 52 kDa metallopeptidase antigen of *C. albicans*, El Moudni et al. (116) reported a sensitivity of 83%, a specificity of 97%, a PPV of 97%, and a NPV of 82% in a retrospective evaluation of 40 patients with invasive candidiasis.

Evans et al. (117) were the first to suggest that the use of mycelial-form-specific antigens of *C. albicans* might provide a more reliable indication of invasive disease, since this morphologic form of the fungus is more common during infection. Several groups have since reported finding antigens on the surface of germ tubes of *C. albicans* that are either absent from, or found in insignificant amounts, on blastospores (118–120). Among the mannoproteins found in the Candida cell wall, Ponton and Jones (121) identified a 230 to 250 kDa component from the germ tube cell wall surface that was recognized by serum from patients with invasive candidiasis. Quindos et al. (122) developed an indirect immunofluorescence (IF) test to detect antibodies against this antigen, and have subsequently reported the method to be useful in several groups of individuals with invasive candidiasis, including hematologic and intensive care patients (122–124). Overall, the IF test showed a sensitivity of 77% to 89% and a specificity of 91% to 100%.

Although substantial progress has been made in improving antibody detection tests for the diagnosis of invasive candidiasis, there is a general belief that these methods are both insensitive and nonspecific (2). This is especially problematic when only a single serum sample is tested. By testing serial samples and combining the results of a commercial ELISA for detection of antimannan antibodies (Platelia Candida Antibody, Bio-Rad Laboratories) with those of an ELISA for detection of circulating *C. albicans* mannan antigen (Platelia Candida Antigen, Bio-Rad Laboratories), sensitivity was increased from 40% for the antibody test alone to 80%, while specificity increased from 84% to 93% (87). In a retrospective evaluation, Yera et al. (125) compared the results of serial antibody and antigen testing in a group of 45 patients from whom at least one positive blood culture had been obtained. In 73% of cases, the patients had detectable antibodies to mannan and/or mannan antigen by the time the first positive blood culture result was obtained. In some cases, the serologic tests became positive up to 15 days before the blood cultures. The median time intervals between diagnosis by serologic testing and blood culture was seven days for antibody testing and six days for antigen detection. Non-neutropenic surgical patients tended to present first with positive antibody tests, while hematologic patients tended to present with antigenemia (125). These data suggest that regular serologic surveillance might be a useful adjunct to blood cultures in patients at high risk of developing invasive candidiasis. However, prospective studies are needed to determine the benefits of this approach in terms of patient survival and reduction in use of empiric antifungal agents.

Antigen Detection

Antigen detection tests have been extensively evaluated for the rapid diagnosis of invasive forms of candidiasis. The results of these evaluations have been variable, with sensitivities ranging from 0% to 100%, depending on the patient population studied, the detection method used, the number of samples tested, and the target antigen. Test formats that have been investigated include hemagglutination inhibition (126), ELISA (127), RIA (128), LA (129), and dot immunoassay (130). Several antigens have been studied as potential targets, including cell wall mannan and mannoproteins, HSP 90, enolase, proteinase, and other immunodominant cytoplasmic antigens.

   Mannan or mannoprotein is the immunodominant surface antigen of *C. albicans*. It is released from the Candida cell wall during infection, and much effort has been devoted to the development of rapid serologic tests for its detection. However, even in immunocompromised individuals, mannan usually circulates in the form of immune complexes that must first be dissociated for optimal detection of the antigen. This can be accomplished through boiling in the presence of EDTA (131). Mannan is rapidly cleared from the circulation by receptor-mediated endocytosis in the liver and spleen (4). Thus, testing of multiple serum samples is essential to optimize the sensitivity of tests for mannan detection.

   Early tests for mannan detection showed high specificity but poor sensitivity. Using hemagglutination inhibition, Weiner and Yount (126) reported a sensitivity of 31% and a specificity of 100%. Weiner and Coats-Stephen (128) dissociated immune complexes and were able to detect mannan by competitive-binding RIA with a sensitivity of 47% and a specificity of 100%. Initial evaluations of indirect inhibition ELISA were encouraging, but this method was soon superseded by sandwich ELISA, which had the advantage that the results could be converted into concentration, expressed as nanogram of mannan per milliliter of serum. An initial retrospective evaluation of a sandwich ELISA to detect *C. albicans* mannan in cancer patients with invasive candidiasis showed a sensitivity of 65% and a specificity of 100% (132). The highest sensitivity (90%) was reported in a study in which a sandwich ELISA was used to screen cancer patients at weekly intervals (96). Mannan antigenemia was present in nine of 10 patients with invasive candidiasis, but was also detected in two of four patients with oral candidiasis, and one of 36 control subjects. In a subsequent retrospective evaluation, however, a sandwich ELISA had a sensitivity of only 33% (133).

The ICON Candida Assay (Hybritech, Inc., San Diego, California) is a solid-phase sandwich enzyme immunoassay (EIA) that utilizes polyclonal antibodies to detect mannan in serum following pretreatment with heat and protease to dissociate immune complexes. In an initial evaluation, it was reported to have a sensitivity of 86% and a specificity of 92% for the diagnosis of invasive candidiasis in neutropenic and non-neutropenic patients (134). Of note, only a single serum sample was available from each of the two patients with candidiasis who gave false-negative results. The test was rapid and simple to perform, but detectable antigenemia preceded diagnosis by other methods in only 36% of cases. It is no longer commercially available.

Although ELISA is a more sensitive procedure than LA, the latter is easier to perform in a clinical setting. However, experiences with this test format have been very variable with sensitivities ranging from 38% to 81% (135,136). Kahn and Jones (137) used a reverse passive LA test to detect mannan in serial serum samples from neutropenic patients, and observed a sensitivity of 78% and a specificity of 92%. When the test was applied to patients from whom samples were collected only at the time candidiasis was suspected, sensitivity fell to 22%.

Several LA tests for mannan detection have been commercialized. The first of these, the LA-Candida Antigen Detection System (Immuno-Mycologics, Inc., Norman, Oklahoma) utilized polyclonal antimannan antibodies to detect the antigen in serum pretreated with heat and protease. However, several evaluations by different groups indicated that this test was too insensitive to be helpful in the early diagnosis of candidiasis (138,139). A second commercial LA test (Pastorex Candida, Bio-Rad Laboratories), introduced in 1991 (140), has also been found to be highly specific but poorly sensitive. The monoclonal antibody, EB-CA1, used in this test is directed against an epitope derived from *C. albicans* mannan, but it also reacts with several other species including *Candida glabrata*, *Candida parapsilosis*, and *Candida tropicalis* (141). In an initial retrospective evaluation, the test was noted to have a sensitivity of 53% and a specificity of 100% for the diagnosis of invasive candidiasis in immunocompetent patients (142). Although samples were pretreated by boiling in the presence of EDTA to dissociate immune complexes, the test showed low sensitivity in patients who had high titers of antimannan antibodies. Other groups, however, have reported the Pastorex Candida Antigen test to have sensitivities ranging from 0% to only 28% (97,143,144).

More recently, a sandwich ELISA (Platelia Candida Antigen, Bio-Rad Laboratories) has been marketed which employs the same monoclonal antibody, EB-CA1, as the Pastorex Candida Antigen test. Although this test has not been extensively assessed, it appears to be more sensitive than the LA test. A retrospective evaluation showed that the ELISA had a sensitivity of 40%, a specificity of 98%, a PPV of 85%, and a NPV of 84% (97). However, by combining the results of the Platelia Candida Antigen ELISA with those of a commercial ELISA for detection of antimannan antibodies (Platelia Candida Antibody, Bio-Rad Laboratories), sensitivity was increased to 80%, specificity was 93%, PPV was 78%, and NPV was increased to 93% (97). More recently, Prella et al. (145) compared the results of antigen and antibody testing in neutropenic patients at high risk for invasive candidiasis. By combining the results of the Platelia Candida Antigen ELISA with those of the Platelia Candida Antibody ELISA, sensitivity was 89%, specificity was 84%, PPV was 86%, and NPV was 88%. Yera et al. (125) earlier reported that detectable mannan antigen and/or antimannan antibodies could be found in 69% of patients with invasive candidiasis by the time the first positive blood culture was obtained. The median time intervals between diagnosis by serologic testing and blood culture was six days for antigen detection. Non-neutropenic surgical patients tended to present first with positive antibody tests, while hematologic patients tended to present with antigenemia.

Although the Platelia Candida Antigen test appears to be specific, it has to be repeated at frequent intervals for optimal detection of circulating mannan. This is because the α-linked oligomannose residues detected by this test are rapidly cleared from the circulation (141). Sendid et al. (146) have recently improved the sensitivity of mannan detection by combining the Platelia Candida Antigen ELISA with a new ELISA based on the detection of β-linked oligomannose residues. In a retrospective evaluation of 90 serum samples from 26 patients with invasive candidiasis, four had α-mannan antigenemia, four had β-mannanemia, and 14 showed the presence of both. By combining the results of the two ELISAs, sensitivity was increased from 69% to 80%, specificity was 95%, PPV was 79%, and NPV was increased from 94% to 97% (146).

Although mannan is the immunodominant surface antigen of *C. albicans*, cytoplasmic protein antigens have also been detected in serum samples from patients with invasive candidiasis (147,148). Identification of the immunodominant components of Candida cytoplasmic antigen preparations stimulated efforts to develop tests to detect these antigens in serum from patients with invasive candidiasis. Using dot immunobinding, Matthews and Burnie (130) detected the 47 kDa immunodominant antigen of *C. albicans* in 77% of 31 neutropenic and

88% of 56 non-neutropenic patients with invasive *C. albicans* infection. The test was also positive in five of six patients with *C. parapsilosis* infection and four with *C. tropicalis* infection, but negative in four with disseminated *C. glabrata* infection. To increase the sensitivity of the dot immunobinding test, the 47 kDa-specific antibody was later replaced with an antibody to an epitope of *C. albicans* HSP90 that was recognized by all patients who had antibodies to the 47 kDa antigen (149). The epitope-specific antibody was less sensitive, but more specific than the 47 kDa antigen-specific antibody, which recognized multiple epitopes.

A number of Candida enzymes have been investigated as possible targets for antigen detection tests. Initial studies in animal models demonstrated that the 48 kDa enolase antigen of *C. albicans* could be detected in serum by an ELISA using monoclonal antibodies (150). Later, Walsh et al. (151) conducted a prospective clinical trial to assess the usefulness of a commercial double-sandwich liposomal immunoassay (Directigen Disseminated Candidiasis Test, Becton Dickinson, Philadelphia, Pennsylvania) for detecting the enolase antigen in serial serum samples from 170 cancer patients at high risk for invasive candidiasis. Enolase antigenemia was detectable in 85% of patients with deep tissue infection, as well as 64% of patients with bloodstream infection. Overall sensitivity was 75% and specificity was 96%. Unfortunately, the Directigen test is no longer commercially available.

In addition to enolase, detection of several other Candida enzymes has been used for the serologic diagnosis of candidiasis. Ruchel et al. (114,152) developed an ELISA to detect *C. albicans* proteinase. However, the test had a low sensitivity and specificity. The former may be related to the presence of antiproteinase antibodies in patients' serum, since immunodominant protein antigens induce large quantities of antibodies that bind to the antigen and facilitate clearance. More recently, Na and Song (115) developed a monoclonal antibody-based inhibition ELISA to detect a *C. albicans* secreted aspartyl proteinase and reported a sensitivity of 94% and a specificity of 96% for the diagnosis of invasive candidiasis.

The tests described so far have relied on the selection of a specific, well-characterized antigen as the target for detection. In contrast, Gentry et al. (129) adopted a different approach in which an uncharacterized, heat-labile, circulating antigen was detected by reverse passive LA. Serum from rabbits immunized with intact, heat-killed *C. albicans* blastospores was used. The test was later commercialized as the Cand-Tec test (Ramco Laboratories, Inc., Houston, Texas). The antigen does not contain mannan and it has been suggested that the test may detect a neoantigen derived from *C. albicans* after host processing, or it may be a nonspecific host component that is cross-reactive with an antigen of *C. albicans* (153). Although there is an extensive literature, experiences with the Cand-Tec test in the diagnosis of invasive candidiasis have been very variable with sensitivities ranging from 22% to 100% (137,154) and specificities from 29% to 100% (129,155). In general, recent evaluations have concluded that, despite its ease of performance, the test is not acceptable for routine diagnostic use.

In addition to antigen detection, a number of other approaches have been developed for the rapid diagnosis of invasive candidiasis. These include tests to detect the fungal cell wall component, (1-3)-β-D-glucan, and the metabolite, D-arabinitol. In a comparative assessment with two antigen tests for mannan, Fujita and Hashimoto (135) reported sensitivities of 38%, 74%, and 50%, and specificities of 100%, 100%, and 91%, respectively, for LA, ELISA and D-arabinitol detection in the diagnosis of invasive candidiasis. In a second comparison, Mitsutake et al. (144) compared the efficacy of the enolase antigen test (Directigen Disseminated Candidiasis Test), mannan antigen LA test (Pastorex Candida), Cand-Tec LA antigen test and (1-3)-β-D-glucan detection in patients with Candida bloodstream infections. The sensitivity and specificity of the four tests were 72% and 100%, 26% and 100%, 77% and 88%, and 84% and 88%, respectively. More recently, Fujita et al. (156) compared a new EIA for mannan antigen detection (Unimedi Candida monotest, Unitika, Japan) with the Cand-Tec LA antigen test, two commercial ELISA tests (Platelia Candida Antigen and Unimedi Candida), and (1-3)-β-D-glucan detection. The sensitivity and specificity of the five tests were 82% and 96%, 38% and 82%, 53% and 92%, 69% and 89%, and 95% and 84%, respectively.

There have been several head-to-head comparisons of antigen and PCR-based DNA detection methods for the diagnosis of invasive candidiasis. Chryssanthou et al. (157) reported a comparison of the performance of several non-culture-based methods for the diagnosis of invasive candidiasis in HSCT and solid organ transplant recipients. In this study, detection of *C. albicans* DNA by PCR was compared with serum mannan antigen detection, Cand-Tec antigen detection, (1-3)-β-D-glucan detection, and detection of D-arabinitol in urine. Although the tests were positive in some patients, no single test was sufficient to establish the diagnosis in all patients. White et al. (158) performed a retrospective comparison of two commercial mannan detection tests (Pastorex Candida LA test and Platelia Candida Antigen ELISA) with an in-house PCR method in a group of 105 patients at high risk for invasive candidiasis. The sensitivity and specificity of the tests were 25% and 100%, 75% and 97%, and 95% and 97%, respectively.

Isolation of a *Candida* species from a single blood culture is considered to be sufficient evidence for the immediate initiation of antifungal treatment. However, it is well recognized that, despite substantial methodologic improvements, blood cultures can be unreliable in establishing the diagnosis of invasive candidiasis. Although substantial progress has been made in non-culture-based methods, none has achieved widespread use because of the difficulties in obtaining consistent results in patients at high risk for this disease. It is evident that diagnosis based on a test result for a single specimen is unreliable, and it is therefore important to screen serial samples to optimize antigen detection. Nonetheless, it does appear that use of non-culture-based tests, such as antigen detection in combination with blood culture results, can assist in the early diagnosis of invasive candidiasis. However, the benefit of this approach in terms of patient survival, or reduction in use of empiric antifungal agents, remains to be determined.

Cryptococcosis

Antibody Detection

Antibodies to *C. neoformans* have sometimes been detected in persons with cryptococcosis during the early stages of the disease, but they are rapidly neutralized by the large amounts of capsular antigen released during evolution of the infection. Antibodies may subsequently reappear after successful treatment, and it has been suggested that their detection represents a favorable prognostic sign (159). In general, however, agglutination and indirect IF tests for antibody detection are of limited diagnostic usefulness. Using an ELISA to detect IgG and IgA antibodies to *C. neoformans*, Speed et al. (160) found that antibodies are generally not detectable during acute infection in immunocompetent patients. However, antibodies could be detected during antigenemia, and although levels of IgA antibodies diminished after successful treatment, IgG antibodies persisted. More recently, Santangelo et al. (161) observed that IgG antibodies to *C. neoformans* phospholipase B can be detected in many patients with cryptococcosis, and are a sensitive marker for present or past infection.

Antigen Detection

The LA test for detection of *C. neoformans* capsular polysaccharide antigen in serum and CSF (162) is an indispensable tool for the rapid diagnosis of meningeal and disseminated forms of cryptococcosis. The LA test is highly sensitive and specific, giving positive results in around 95% of infected patients (163,164). However, occasional false-positive results can occur, particularly with serum samples (165). Most frequently, these false-positive reactions have been caused by non-specific interference from rheumatoid factor (166,167). This can be eliminated by prior treatment of the sample with the proteolytic enzyme, pronase (168). In some cases, false-positive LA test reactions with serum samples from HIV-infected patients are attributable to other, unidentified interfering factors. These have been eliminated with 2-β-mercaptoethanol, but not with pronase (169). Occasional false positive-reactions have been caused by infection with the related organism, *Trichosporon asahii*, that shares cross-reacting antigens with *C. neoformans* (170), but have also been reported with several bacterial infections (171,172).

It is unusual to obtain false-negative LA test results, but they have been reported in AIDS patients with culture-confirmed cryptococcal meningitis (173–175). False-negative reactions can occur if the organism load is low, or if the organisms are not well encapsulated. False-negative results have also been reported with both serum and CSF specimens owing to a prozone effect, but this can be corrected by dilution of the sample (176).

A number of LA tests for *C. neoformans* antigen detection have been commercialized. These include the CRYPTO-LA system (International Biological Laboratories, Inc., Cranbury, New Jersey), the Cryptococcal Antigen Latex Agglutination system (CALAS, Meridian Bioscience, Inc., Cincinnati, Ohio), and the Latex Crypto Antigen system (Immuno-Mycologics, Inc.). These tests utilize polyclonal antibodies to detect capsular antigen, but a more recent commercial LA test (Pastorex Cryptococcus, Bio-Rad Laboratories) uses a murine monoclonal antibody specific for *C. neoformans* polysaccharide (177). In general, these commercial LA tests have a detection limit of 5 to 20 ng of polysaccharide per ml of sample (164,177). The sensitivity and specificity of these commercial LA tests for CSF samples ranges from 83% to 100%, and 97% to 100%, respectively (164,167,177,178). Of note, LA titer results obtained with kits from different manufacturers can vary considerably with the same sample (164,178). Therefore, if changing antigen titers in sequential samples from an individual case of cryptococcosis are to be interpreted correctly, it is essential for the laboratory to employ one product from a single manufacturer.

Although the LA test for cryptococcal antigen detection remains the most popular test for routine clinical use, other methods have been developed and evaluated. EIA has been shown to detect much lower concentrations of cryptococcal antigen than LA (179), but it has not replaced the older, simpler method in most laboratories. The Premier Cryptococcal Antigen system (Meridian Bioscience, Inc.) is an EIA that utilizes a polyclonal antibody capture system and a monoclonal antibody detection system. This test takes less than 45 minutes to perform without pretreatment of the specimen. It is designed to detect glucuronoxylomannan, the major component of the capsular polysaccharide antigen in either serum or CSF specimens, but not urine. In an initial clinical comparison with the CALAS LA test (Meridian Bioscience, Inc.), the Premier EIA had a sensitivity of 99% and a specificity of 97% (180). Another smaller comparison of the LA and EIA methods reported a lower level of agreement (92%), but concluded that there were fewer false-positive results with the EIA (181). These conclusions were subsequently confirmed in a comparison of four LA procedures with the EIA method (182). The EIA is unaffected by prozone reactions and does not react with rheumatoid factor or require pronase treatment. In general, EIA titers are slightly higher than LA titers for specimens with relatively low antigen concentrations. However, at higher antigen concentrations, EIA titers are frequently 20- to 100-fold higher than LA titers (180).

The cryptococcal antigen test is most commonly employed to screen serum and CSF specimens, but other body fluids can also be tested. In a prospective evaluation, Baughman et al. (183) detected cryptococcal antigen at titers of $\geq 1:8$ in BALFs from all HIV-infected patients with pulmonary cryptococcosis. However, the specificity of the test was poor in that false-positive reactions at titers up to 1:8 were also found in control individuals. Chapin-Robertson et al. (184) compared antigen titers in urine with those in serum and CSF samples from

92 patients with AIDS. In all cases, patients with detectable antigen in CSF and/or serum also had detectable but lower levels of antigen in urine.

Although the cryptococcal antigen test is the most sensitive method for diagnosis of cryptococcosis, serial antigen testing appears to be of limited usefulness in monitoring therapeutic response in AIDS-associated cryptococcal meningitis (185,186). Powderly et al. (185) found serial measurement of serum antigen titers to be unhelpful in detecting failure during initial treatment, or predicting relapse during maintenance treatment. However, when the baseline CSF antigen titer was $\geq 1:8$ and remained unchanged or increased during treatment, it did correlate with clinical and/or microbiological failure to respond to treatment. Furthermore, rising CSF antigen levels during maintenance treatment were predictive of relapse (185). In HIV-negative individuals, high levels of serum and CSF antigen prior to treatment are often predictive of death during treatment, while high antigen levels at the end of treatment are often predictive of later relapse (159).

Like baseline CSF antigen levels, initial quantitative CSF culture results are a useful prognostic factor in patients with AIDS-associated cryptococcal meningitis: high organism loads are usually associated with a poor outcome (187). Brouwer et al. (188) compared baseline values and rates of decline of these two measures of organism load in 68 HIV-seropositive individuals with the disease during the first two weeks of antifungal treatment. There was a significant positive correlation between these markers at baseline, but the rapid decline in CSF counts was not reflected by similar changes in antigen levels. Quantification of CSF cultures appears to be more helpful than serial measurement of antigen titers in monitoring the early response of cryptococcal meningitis to antifungal therapy.

Blastomycosis

Antibody Detection

Although microscopic examination and culture remain the most sensitive means of establishing the diagnosis of blastomycosis, tests for *Blastomyces dermatitidis* antibodies can also provide useful information. The most popular serologic test for blastomycosis is ID, but CF, ELISA, and RIA procedures have also been developed and evaluated. In 1973, Kaufman et al. (189) described an ID test for blastomycosis that utilized an unpurified culture filtrate antigen. The test had a sensitivity of 80% and a specificity of 100%. In contrast, a CF test had a sensitivity of less than 50% and lacked specificity, cross-reacting with serum samples from patients with many other fungal infections, including histoplasmosis and coccidioidomycosis.

Since 1980, substantial effort has been made to improve the specificity and sensitivity of antibody detection tests for blastomycosis by using purified antigens, and by using more sensitive procedures, such as RIA and ELISA. Green et al. (190) isolated and purified an antigen of *B. dermatitidis*, termed the A antigen. ID tests for antibodies to this antigen have been reported to have a sensitivity of 65%, a specificity of 100%, a PPV of 100%, and a NPV of 88% (191). CF tests with this antigen have a sensitivity of only 40%, a specificity of 100%, a PPV of 100% and a NPV of 81% (191).

In an initial evaluation of the A antigen in an ELISA, 93% of sera from patients with blastomycosis were positive (190). The subsequent use of the A antigen in an ELISA test format led to a substantial improvement in sensitivity and specificity of antibody detection tests for blastomycosis resulting in sensitivities of 86% to 100% and specificities of 87% to 92% (192,193). Direct comparison of an ELISA with ID and CF tests during a large point-source outbreak of the disease demonstrated sensitivities of 77%, 28%, and 9%, respectively, with specificities of 92%, 100%, and 100% (194). An ELISA that employed A antigen to detect *B. dermatitidis* antibodies was later marketed (Premier Blastomyces Enzyme Immunoassay, Meridian Bioscience, Inc.), but is no longer available. Two published evaluations indicated that this test had a sensitivity of 85% to 100%, and a specificity of 47% to 86% (195,196).

Klein and Jones (197) described a novel immunodominant surface protein antigen of *B. dermatitidis*, which they named WI-1. It was determined that this was a unique antigen found only in *B. dermatitidis* and not in *Histoplasma capsulatum* or *C. albicans*. Later Klein and Jones (198) purified and characterized WI-1, and compared it with A antigen. WI-1 differed from A antigen in that it was a 120 kDa protein containing no carbohydrate while the latter was a 135 kDa protein containing 37% carbohydrate. Immunological comparison of the two antigens showed that they are very similar, in that monoclonal antibodies made to A antigen also recognized a 25 amino acid tandem repeat molecule that is the major antigenic epitope of the WI-1 antigen. It was also found that an A antigen EIA could be inhibited by preincubation of the A antigen serum with the 25 amino acid tandem repeat antigen (198).

Soufleris et al. (199) developed a RIA that employed WI-1 antigen to detect *B. dermatitidis* antibodies. In an initial evaluation, the method was used to test sera from residents of Wisconsin, where blastomycosis is endemic. A positive result was obtained for at least one sample from 83% of patients with confirmed blastomycosis and from 5% of patients in whom the disease was not confirmed. Less than 1% of samples from random blood donors residing in counties with a high annual incidence of blastomycosis gave a positive result. The RIA method appears to be more sensitive than ID tests, although no direct head-to-head comparisons have been published.

Antigen Detection

Durkin et al. (200) have recently described a sandwich ELISA, which used rabbit polyclonal antibodies, raised against formalinized mycelial-phase *B. dermatitidis*, to detect *B. dermatitidis* antigen in urine. While the clinical usefulness of this test awaits further experience, an initial evaluation showed that it had a sensitivity of 100% for pulmonary blastomycosis, and 89% for disseminated infection. However, cross-reacting antigen was detected in urine samples from 96%, 100%, and 70% of patients with histoplasmosis, paracoccidioidomycosis, and penicilliosis, respectively (200). No cross-reactions were seen for coccidioidomycosis.

Coccidioidomycosis

Antibody Detection

Although the definitive laboratory diagnosis of coccidioidomycosis depends on microscopic examination and culture, tests for *Coccidioides immitis* antibodies are of proven usefulness in diagnosis and management. Despite the fact that sensitive methods, such as RIA and ELISA, have been developed, the CF and ID tests, both of which still utilize unpurified culture filtrate antigens, remain the most reliable methods for the serologic diagnosis of coccidioidomycosis.

In the CF test, a heat-labile protein antigen derived from coccidioidin (a filtrate of autolyzed *C. immitis* mycelial cultures) is used to detect IgG antibodies (201,202). These do not appear until about 4 to 12 weeks after infection, but may persist for long periods in individuals with chronic pulmonary or disseminated disease. In most cases, the CF titer is proportional to the extent of the disease. Smith et al. (201) reported that 98% of patients with disseminated coccidioidomycosis had a positive CF test. Low CF titers of 1:2 to 1:4 are usually indicative of early, residual, or meningeal disease, but are sometimes found in individuals without coccidioidomycosis. Titers of > 1:16 should lead to a careful assessment of the patient for possible spread of the disease beyond the respiratory tract. More than 60% of patients with disseminated coccidioidomycosis have CF titers of > 1:32. However, false-negative results can occur in immunocompromised individuals, such as persons with AIDS (203,204).

The CF titer alone should not be used as the basis for diagnosis of disseminated coccidioidomycosis, but should be considered alongside the results of other clinical and laboratory investigations. In addition to serum, the CF test can be used to test CSF, pleural, and joint fluid samples. The detection of CF antibodies in the CSF is usually diagnostic of coccidioidal meningitis and remains the single most useful test for diagnosis of that infection. Failure of the CF titer to fall during treatment of disseminated coccidioidomycosis is an ominous sign.

Smith et al. (201,202) found that a tube precipitin (TP) test became positive earlier in the infection than did the CF test, usually being positive by the third weeks of illness. The TP test is a qualitative method that detects IgM antibodies reactive against a heat-stable carbohydrate-containing antigen in coccidioidin. With this test, Smith et al. (202) detected precipitins in 91% of patients with primary pulmonary coccidioidomycosis. The antigen reactive in the TP test is heat-stable, differentiating it from the heat-labile antigen reactive in the CF test.

The TP test usually becomes negative within a few months, but this has no prognostic significance.

The TP test has now been replaced by the ID test (205). The simultaneous use of heated and unheated coccidioidin antigens permits this test to be employed to detect either IgM or IgG antibodies to *C. immitis*. The IDTP test utilizes heated coccidioidin as antigen, detects IgM, and gives results comparable to those obtained with the classical TP test. Like that method, it is most useful for diagnosing recent infection (206). The sensitivity of the IDTP test can be improved by 10-fold concentration of serum prior to performing the test. The IDCF test utilizes unheated coccidioidin as antigen, detects IgG antibodies, and gives results comparable to the CF method. It is less sensitive, but more specific than the CF test (206,207). The ID test is useful for initial screening of specimens, and can be followed by other tests if positive (206,207).

Several LA tests, using heated coccidioidin as antigen, have been marketed for the detection of IgM antibodies to *C. immitis* (LA-Cocci Antibody system, Immuno-Mycologics, Inc.; Coccidioides Latex Agglutination system, Meridian Bioscience, Inc.). These qualitative tests are simpler and faster to perform, and more sensitive than the TP or IDTP tests in detecting early infection. Rheumatoid factor is not known to interfere with the LA test. However, it has a false-positive rate of at least 6% (208) and the results should be confirmed using the ID method. It is not recommended for screening CSF specimens because false-positive reactions can occur (209).

A commercial ELISA is available for the qualitative detection of IgM and IgG antibodies to *C. immitis* in serum or CSF specimens (Premier Coccidioides, Meridian Bioscience, Inc.). The antigen used in this test is a mixture of purified TP and CF antigens. Published evaluations suggest this test has a sensitivity of >95%, a specificity of about 95%, and a PPV and NPV of >95% (210–212). However, false-positive reactions have been obtained with some sera from patients with blastomycosis. The results of the ELISA should be confirmed by the IDTP and IDCF tests.

Since 1980, much effort has been devoted to the identification and characterization of the immunodominant components of coccidioidin that react with IgM and IgG antibodies to *C. immitis*. The antigen in coccidioidin reactive with IgM in the TP and IDTP tests is a glycosylated 120 kDa protein containing 3-*O*-methylmannose (213). The antigen reactive in the CF and IDCF tests is a 110 kDa protein that has been identified as a chitinase (214). Yang et al. (215) cloned a cDNA that encoded the CF antigen of *C. immitis*. Although this recombinant chitinase antigen was more sensitive than coccidioidin in detecting IgG antibodies by ELISA in sera from patients with coccidioidomycosis, it also cross-reacted with sera from patients with blastomycosis and histoplasmosis (215). The recombinant clone was later refined to a 290 amino acid peptide (216). Use of this antigen in an EIA enabled antibodies to be detected in 21 of 22 patients with coccidioidomycosis, but no cross-reactions were observed with sera from patients with histoplasmosis or blastomycosis.

Antigen Detection

Tests for antibodies to *C. immitis* are sometimes negative in immunocompromised individuals with coccidioidomycosis (203,204) and this has led to some interest in the development of antigen detection tests for this disease (217–219). An inhibition ELISA that detected antigens derived from spherulin (a filtrate of autolyzed *C. immitis* spherule phase cultures), was positive in 21 of 27 sera obtained from 19 patients within two months of the onset of the illness (218). More recently, Galgiani et al. (219) reported the detection of circulating antigen in sera from 35 patients, 33 of whom had no detectable antibodies to *C. immitis* at that time. Detectable antigen was noted most frequently in sera obtained within the first month of the onset of symptoms. The nature of the antigen that circulates in early primary coccidioidomycosis is not known. At present, coccidioidomycosis antigen testing, while promising, is not available as a routine diagnostic test for immunocompromised individuals or those with early disease.

Histoplasmosis

Antibody Detection

The definitive diagnosis of histoplasmosis can be accomplished by direct microscopic detection of *H. capsulatum* in clinical specimens or its isolation in culture. However, isolation and identification may take two to four weeks. Serologic tests have an important role in the rapid diagnosis of several forms of histoplasmosis, but are most useful for patients with chronic pulmonary or disseminated infection. Because two to six weeks are required for antibodies to appear, they are less helpful for the early diagnosis of acute pulmonary histoplasmosis. However, a rising titer of antibodies to *H. capsulatum* is diagnostic. In disseminated histoplasmosis, serologic tests are positive in only 80% of immunosuppressed patients, compared with 100% of non-immunosuppressed individuals (220). Serologic tests are particularly useful in patients with Histoplasma meningitis. The detection of antibodies to *H. capsulatum* in CSF specimens is sufficient to make a diagnosis in the appropriate clinical setting and often is the only positive diagnostic test (221).

The standard serologic methods for histoplasmosis are the ID and CF tests. The principal antigen used in both these tests is histoplasmin, a soluble filtrate of *H. capsulatum* mycelial cultures (222). Histoplasmin contains two components of particular interest: the H antigen against which antibodies are formed during acute histoplasmosis, and the M antigen, against which antibodies are produced during all phases of the disease. Both H and M antigens are glycoproteins with molecular masses of 116 and 94 kDa, respectively (223). In contrast to the other components of histoplasmin, such as the C antigen, which is a heat-stable galactomannan polysaccharide that is cross-reactive with *B. dermatitidis* and *C. immitis* (224), both the H and M antigens were once thought to be specific proteins for the detection of anti-*H. capsulatum* antibodies. The M antigen, however, was found to be a catalase that was not specific unless used in a deglycosylated form (223,225). The H antigen has been identified as a β-glucosidase (226).

The ID test is a qualitative method that detects antibodies to the H and M antigens of *H. capsulatum* when histoplasmin is used as the antigen. Precipitins first appear between four and eight weeks after exposure. Antibodies to M antigen are the first to appear, and can be detected in up to 75% of patients with acute histoplasmosis. However, they can also be found in nearly all individuals with chronic pulmonary infection, as well as in those who have undergone a recent skin test with histoplasmin. Antibodies to H antigen are specific for active disease, but occur in fewer than 20% of cases (227). They usually disappear within the first six months of infection and are seldom, if ever, found in the absence of M precipitins. The presence of both H and M precipitins is highly suggestive of active histoplasmosis, regardless of other serologic test results. The ID test is more specific, but less sensitive than the CF test and can be used to assess the significance of weakly positive CF results. Only about 1% of patients with histoplasmosis that give negative results in the CF test will have a positive ID result.

The CF test is a quantitative procedure in which two antigens are employed: histoplasmin and an intact *H. capsulatum* yeast cell suspension. The latter is more sensitive but less specific than histoplasmin. Antibodies to the yeast antigen are the first to be observed (about four weeks after exposure) and the last to disappear after resolution of the infection. Antibodies to histoplasmin appear later and reach lower titers than those observed for the yeast antigen. About 95% of patients with histoplasmosis are positive by CF, but 25% of these are positive only at titers of 1:8 or 1:16 (227). Although weakly positive titers are less helpful in differentiating active from past infection, they should not be disregarded, as titers in this range occur in about one-third of cases with active histoplasmosis (202). CF titers of 1:32 or greater and rising titers in serial samples offer stronger evidence of infection.

Antibodies to *H. capsulatum* clear following resolution of the infection but persist in individuals with chronic progressive disease. Antibodies may disappear within a few months following brief exposure but persist for several years following prolonged exposure (227). The significance of persistently elevated or fluctuating CF titers is unclear, as is the effect of antifungal treatment on antibody clearance (228). Because cross-reactions can occur in patients with other fungal infections, care must be taken to exclude these diseases if the clinical signs and symptoms are not typical of histoplasmosis. Cross-reactions occur in up to 40% of patients with blastomycosis and 16% with coccidioidomycosis by CF (229).

A LA test, using histoplasmin as antigen, is commercially available (LA-Histo Antibody system, Immuno-Mycologics, Inc.). This qualitative test is used primarily for the presumptive diagnosis of acute histoplasmosis and is less helpful for the detection of chronic infection. A positive LA test result can be obtained as early as two to three weeks after exposure, and a titer of 1:16 or greater is considered good evidence for active or recent infection. False-positive reactions can occur, and it is recommended that results be confirmed by the ID test.

Since the mid-1970s, attempts have been made to improve the serologic diagnosis of histoplasmosis by replacing the CF test with more sensitive procedures, such as RIA (230–232), ELISA (233,234), or immunoblotting (235). Taken as a whole, the results suggest that RIA and ELISA are more sensitive than CF or ID tests, but their usefulness is limited due to the presence of cross-reactive moieties associated with the H and M antigens of histoplasmin (231). In an initial comparison of a commercial ELISA for the detection of IgG antibodies to *H. capsulatum* (Premier Histoplasma, Meridian Bioscience, Inc.) with the ID test, the two methods had sensitivities of 97% and 100%, and specificities of 84% and 100%, respectively (236). Unfortunately, this test is no longer available.

Most attempts to replace the CF test for histoplasmosis with more sensitive methods, such as ELISA, have been frustrated because of the presence of cross-reactive carbohydrate moieties associated with the H and M antigens, both of which are glycoproteins (223). In a comparison of glycosylated and deglycosylated forms of purified M antigen, cross-reactions with serum from patients with blastomycosis, coccidioidomycosis, paracoccidioidomycosis, and aspergillosis were eliminated after periodate treatment of the antigen (223,237). More recently, Guimaraes et al. (234) compared an ELISA that used glycosylated histoplasmin with one that employed purified deglycosylated histoplasmin as antigen. The two methods had sensitivities and specificities of 57% and 93%, and 93% and 96%, respectively. Pizzini et al. (235) reported a Western blot test using purified, deglycosylated histoplasmin H and M antigens. In an initial evaluation in which the blot method was used to test acute and convalescent sera from an outbreak of histoplasmosis, the test had a sensitivity of 90% to 100% and a specificity of 100%.

The H and M antigens have now been sequenced and nonglycosylated, recombinant antigens have been produced (226,238). A 60 kDa recombinant antigen has also been developed (239). Although the use of specific recombinant antigens in ELISA and other sensitive test formats should lead to improvements in antibody detection tests for histoplasmosis, there will still be problems with false-negative reactions resulting from the development of infection in immunosuppressed individuals, particularly those living with AIDS. Under these circumstances, antigen detection tests may be a more appropriate diagnostic method.

Antigen Detection

Antigen detection has become an essential tool for the rapid diagnosis of several forms of histoplasmosis. Several test formats have been developed, including a solid-phase RIA (240) and a sandwich ELISA (241). Antigen detection complements other diagnostic methods and is particularly useful in immuno-compromised patients with more extensive disease, often providing a rapid diagnosis before positive cultures can be identified. Histoplasma polysaccharide antigen has been detected in serum, urine, CSF, and BALF specimens obtained from individuals with disseminated histoplasmosis.

Wheat et al. (240) used rabbit polyclonal antibodies, raised against formalinized yeast cells of *H. capsulatum*, both as a captor and, in a radiolabeled form, as a detector in a solid-phase RIA. Using this system, it proved possible to detect antigen in 20 of 22 episodes of disseminated histoplasmosis in 16 patients. Antigen was detected in both the urine, where it appeared as a heat-stable, low molecular weight polysaccharide, and in the serum, where it appeared as a higher molecular weight species. In subsequent studies, it was noted that AIDS patients with disseminated histoplasmosis seldom develop antigenemia without antigenuria (242). It was also demonstrated that antigen levels in the urine and serum decline with effective treatment, becoming undetectable in most patients (243,244). Failure of antigen concentrations to fall during treatment suggests therapeutic failure. In patients who have responded to treatment and in whom antigen levels have previously fallen, an increase in antigen in the urine or serum is suggestive of relapse (245). Antigen has been detected in the CSF of patients with Histoplasma meningitis.

Antibodies to *H. capsulatum* require at least four weeks to appear after the initial exposure, limiting their usefulness in the early diagnosis of acute pulmonary histoplasmosis. In immunocompetent patients, urine antigen may often be detectable before antibodies appear, permitting earlier diagnosis and treatment (220). Antigenuria can also be detected in about one-third of patients with subacute pulmonary histoplasmosis, in whom recent exposure cannot be identified (228). Antigen can be found in BALF from immunocompetent patients suffering from acute pulmonary histoplasmosis following heavy inhalation exposure (228).

Initial attempts to replace the RIA for Histoplasma antigen with other test formats, such as ELISA, proved unsuccessful (246). In 1997, however, Durkin et al. (241) developed a sandwich ELISA that used the same polyclonal antibody as captor and detector as did the original RIA. The ELISA had sensitivities with serum and urine from patients with disseminated histoplasmosis of 82% and 92%, respectively, and a specificity of about 98%. More recently, Garringer et al. (247) evaluated an inhibition ELISA, but found that this method showed decreased specificity and inferior reproducibility with control specimens, compared with the standard sandwich ELISA.

Although the initial work suggested that Histoplasma antigen RIA was specific (240), cross-reacting antigens have since been recognized in 65% of patients with blastomycosis, 89% with paracoccidioidomycosis, and 94% with *Penicillium marneffei* infection; however, no cross-reactions were observed with specimens from patients with coccidioidomycosis (5). It has also been reported that sandwich and inhibition ELISA methods for Histoplasma antigen detect cross-reacting antigens in urine samples from patients with blastomycosis (247).

One way in which Histoplasma antigen detection tests might be made more specific is through the application of monoclonal antibodies. Gomez et al. (248) developed an inhibition ELISA that utilizes a murine monoclonal antibody that recognizes an apparently species-specific epitope on a 69 to 70 kDa antigen. The test had sensitivities for acute and chronic forms of histoplasmosis of 89% and 57%, respectively. The specificity was 98% when normal human serum was tested and 85% when serum samples from individuals with chronic fungal or bacterial infections were tested. In contrast to the polyclonal sandwich ELISA, the monoclonal inhibition ELISA detected antigen more frequently in serum than in urine (248). More recently, Gomez et al. (249) used the inhibition ELISA to monitor the response to treatment of patients presenting with different clinical forms of histoplasmosis. Sera from four of five patients with acute pulmonary infection showed a rapid decline in antigenemia, becoming negative after 10 to 16 weeks. In non-AIDS patients with disseminated histoplasmosis, serum antigen levels declined with effective treatment, becoming undetectable in most patients. The effectiveness of the test in AIDS patients with disseminated histoplasmosis is less clear, with high levels of antigen persisting in most patients throughout treatment.

There have been few head-to-head comparisons of antigen and PCR-based molecular detection methods for the diagnosis of histoplasmosis. Tang et al. (250) compared a PCR-EIA for detection of *H. capsulatum* with sandwich ELISA (241) and culture. The PCR-EIA method was positive in only 8% of antigen-positive and 80% of culture-positive urine samples. These results suggest that, while PCR may be useful for the detection of *H. capsulatum* in tissue, it is much less sensitive than antigen detection in urine.

Paracoccidioidomycosis

Antibody Detection

The definitive diagnosis of paracoccidioidomycosis depends on microscopic examination and culture. However, isolation and identification of *Paracocci-dioides brasiliensis* from clinical specimens may take up to four weeks. In this situation, serologic tests are useful for a rapid presumptive diagnosis, particularly in cases of disseminated disease (251). Levels of IgG antibodies to *P. brasiliensis* are usually elevated in immunocompetent patients with untreated infection, and these levels have been shown to be useful for monitoring the response to treatment of patients with acute or chronic forms of the disease (252). Antibody detection is less useful for the diagnosis of paracoccidioidomycosis in persons with AIDS.

As with other dimorphic fungi, the standard serologic tests for paracoccidioidomycosis are ID and CF, but other methods, such as ELISA, have also been employed. The antigens used in these tests have been derived both from whole yeast cells (cell wall and cytoplasmic) and culture filtrates. Cell wall-derived antigens have proved the least useful for serologic diagnosis, largely because they are dominated by cross-reactive galactomannan (251).

However, while cytoplasmic and culture filtrate antigens proved more specific, marked variations were noted in the composition of similar antigen preparations depending on the strains used, culture medium employed, incubation time, and the morphologic form of the fungus (251). With the introduction of more rigorous standardization of antigen production methods during the 1980s, it proved possible to prepare more consistent cytoplasmic and culture filtrate antigens (253,254).

ID is more specific than CF for the diagnosis of paracoccidioidomycosis, and the use of better-characterized antigens should further improve its performance. The ID test is positive in 65% to 100% of patients with acute or chronic pulmonary infection, or with disseminated paracoccidioidomycosis (255). CIE gives similar results (228). The CF test with yeast-form culture-filtrate antigen is positive in 70% to 100% of patients, higher titers being obtained in those with more severe disease (255,256). Titers of at least 1:8 are considered presumptive evidence of paracoccidioidomycosis. However, 85% to 95% of patients with active disease have CF titers of 1:32 or greater. The CF test is not altogether specific, and cross-reactions can occur with serum from patients with histoplasmosis (256). Several reports have suggested that falling CF titers are predictive of successful treatment, and high or fluctuating CF titers are suggestive of a poor prognosis (255,256). Other reports, however, have indicated that ID and CF results do not correlate well with the clinical status of the patient (257,258).

Since the mid-1980s, much effort has been devoted to the purification and characterization of defined antigenic components within both cytoplasmic and culture filtrate antigens of *P. brasiliensis*. These include a 43 kDa glycoprotein (259), a 22 to 25 kDa protein (260), a 58 kDa glycoprotein (261), a 70 kDa HSP (262), and an 87 kDa protein that has been purified and characterized as an HSP70 (263). The 43 kDa glycoprotein was the first *P. brasiliensis* antigen to be cloned (264); however, the clone was lost, and only prepared anew by Cisalpino et al. (265). Shortly thereafter, McEwen et al. (266) cloned and sequenced a specific 27 kDa protein from *P. brasiliensis* that appeared to be free of significant cross-reactions (267). More recently, a recombinant HSP60 antigen was cloned and characterized (268).

Efforts to develop more sensitive and specific tests to detect antibodies to *P. brasiliensis* have also intensified since the 1980s. Although ELISA has proved a sensitive procedure (269–271), cross-reactions with sera from patients with histoplasmosis have been a problem, even when the purified 43 kDa glycoprotein antigen of *P. brasiliensis* was employed (272). Camargo et al. (273) developed a monoclonal antibody capture EIA that measures IgG antibodies against the 43 kDa glycoprotein antigen of *P. brasiliensis*. In an initial retrospective evaluation, the capture EIA had a sensitivity of 100% and a specificity of 97%. Ortiz et al. (274) used the 27 kDa recombinant protein antigen in an indirect ELISA, and reported a sensitivity of 73%, and a PPV of 90%, for all forms of paracoccidioidomycosis. The ELISA had a specificity of 59% when tested with serum from patients with other mycotic infections, largely as a result of cross-reactions with sera from patients with histoplasmosis and aspergillosis (73% and 40%, respectively). More recently, Diez et al. (275) used a combination of the 27 kDa recombinant protein antigen and purified 87 kDa HSP antigen in an ELISA. The results demonstrated a significant increase in sensitivity (92%) and specificity (90%) compared to results using the antigens separately.

In 1994, Taborda and Camargo (276) described a rapid dot immunobinding assay for the detection of antibodies to *P. brasiliensis* 43 kDa antigen (in its periodate-treated form). The test had a sensitivity and specificity of 100%. Despite its potential as a simple and rapid screening method, no reports of its further development have appeared.

Antigen Detection

Antigen detection may be useful for the diagnosis of paracoccidioidomycosis, particularly in immunocompromised individuals. In addition, antigen detection may be helpful in situations where antibody detection has proved inconclusive, and it may also be useful in monitoring the response of patients to antifungal treatment. Mendez-Giannini et al. (277) were the first to demonstrate that the 43 kDa glycoprotein antigen of *P. brasiliensis* could be detected in the serum of patients with both the acute and chronic forms of paracoccidioidomycosis. Later, Gomez et al. (278) described an inhibition ELISA, which utilized a monoclonal antibody directed against the 87 kDa HSP antigen of *P. brasiliensis*. In a retrospective evaluation, the ELISA detected circulating antigen in 100% of patients with the acute form of paracoccidioidomycosis, and in 83% and 60% of patients with chronic multifocal and unifocal forms of the disease. The test had a specificity of 80%, but cross-reactions were common with sera from patients with aspergillosis (100%) and histoplasmosis (40%).

Although antigen testing has most commonly been employed to screen serum specimens, other body fluids can also be tested. Salina et al. (279) detected the presence of 43 kDa and 70 kDa antigens of *P. brasiliensis* in urine samples of patients with untreated paracoccidioidomycosis. Both antigens can also be detected in BALF and CSF (280–282). Marques da Silva et al. (280) used a monoclonal antibody-based inhibition ELISA to detect the 43 kDa glycoprotein antigen in CSF and BALF samples. The ELISA showed 100% sensitivity and specificity for samples from patients with meningitis or unifocal pulmonary paracoccidioidomycosis. More recently, the same group used this inhibition ELISA to detect the 43 kDa and 70 kDa glycoprotein antigens in all CSF samples from patients with neurologic paracoccidioidomycosis (281). Using a conventional ELISA, antibodies to both antigens were also found in all CSF samples.

Several reports have described the usefulness of serial antigen testing in the assessment of therapeutic response of patients with paracoccidioidomycosis. Gomez et al. (258) noted that levels of the 87 kDa HSP antigen of *P. brasiliensis* in serum diminished or even disappeared during successful treatment. Marques da Silva (257,282) monitored levels of the 43 kDa and 70 kDa antigens for up to 12 months in serum samples from 23 patients who responded to treatment with itraconazole. In all cases, clinical improvement was followed by a decrease in levels of circulating antigens. Salina et al. (279) reported that the 43 kDa antigen remained present in the urine during treatment, although levels decreased in those who responded and increased in those who relapsed.

Penicilliosis

Antibody Detection

The laboratory diagnosis of disseminated *P. marneffei* infection is usually accomplished by isolation in culture of the organism or its microscopic detection in tissue specimens or body fluids. However, the tissue form of this fungus can be confused with those of *H. capsulatum* and *C. neoformans*, and cultures often require at least three days of incubation before definitive identification is possible. Serologic methods have also been developed. In one of the earliest reports, Yuen et al. (283) evaluated an indirect IF method using serum samples from 103 patients with persistent fever and 78 normal individuals. Eight patients with documented infection had titers of IgG antibodies to *P. marneffei* of $\geq 1{:}160$, while the other patients and control subjects had titers of $\leq 1{:}40$. In contrast, Kaufman et al. (284) detected antibodies by ID in only two of 17 (12%) HIV-seropositive patients.

A number of *P. marneffei* antigens have been characterized and evaluated as potential serodiagnostic reagents. These include antigens with molecular masses of 38 kDa (285), and 50 and 54 kDa (286). Antibodies to the 38 kDa antigen were detected in 45% of serum samples from HIV-positive individuals with penicilliosis (285), while IgG antibodies to the 50 and 54 kDa antigens were detected in 58% and 61% of patients, respectively (286). Jeavons et al. (287) described the identification and purification of two antigens with molecular masses of 54 and 61 kDa, and the partial purification of a 50 kDa antigen. Using immunoblotting, the purified antigens were recognized by 71% and 86% of sera from patients with *P. marneffei* infection, respectively. The 61 kDa antigen appears to be a catalase, but the identity of the 54 kDa antigen and its relationship to the antigen described by Vanittanakom et al. (286) has not been determined.

A *P. marneffei* gene that encodes a cell wall mannoprotein, Mp1p, has been cloned and studied as a potential diagnostic antigen (288). Immunoblot analysis demonstrated that this antigen contains two predominant components with molecular masses of 58 and 90 kDa. In a subsequent report, the purified recombinant antigen was used to develop an ELISA for detection of antibodies to *P. marneffei* (289). In an initial retrospective evaluation, the ELISA had a sensitivity of 82% and a specificity of 100%. The results of larger prospective evaluations of this test are awaited with interest.

Antigen Detection

A recent approach to the diagnosis of *P. marneffei* infection in HIV-positive patients has been the development of methods for detection of circulating antigens. Thus, Kaufman et al. (284) used rabbit polyclonal antibodies raised against concentrated culture filtrate antigens to develop ID and LA tests. These tests had sensitivities of 59% and 76.5% respectively. Perhaps surprisingly, both tests appeared to be specific, since no false-positive reactions were obtained in tests with sera from patients with cryptococcosis or histoplasmosis. Cao et al. (290) described the development and evaluation of an ELISA that detects the Mp1p cell wall mannoprotein antigen of *P. marneffei*. The test had a sensitivity of 65% and a specificity of 100%. However, when these investigators combined the results of the antigen ELISA with those of an ELISA for anti-Mp1p antibodies, the sensitivity increased to 88%, with a specificity of 100%, a PPV of 100%, and a NPV of 96%.

Desakorn et al. (291) described the development and prospective evaluation of a polyclonal antibody-based ELISA for detection of *P. marneffei* antigen in urine. This test had a sensitivity of 97%, a specificity of 98%, a PPV of 84%, and a NPV of 100%. In a subsequent report, Desakorn et al. (292) described a simplified dot blot ELISA and a LA test for detecting *P. marneffei* antigenuria that both utilized the polyclonal anti-*P. marneffei* antibody used in their previous work. In a comparison with the ELISA, urine specimens from 37 patients with penicilliosis and 300 control subjects were tested. The sensitivity and specificity of the dot blot ELISA, ELISA, and LA tests were 95% and 97%, 97% and 98%, and 100% and 99%, respectively (292). The antigen detected by these tests has not been characterized, but the LA procedure appears to be simple, rapid, robust, and convenient, and could prove to be an important addition to existing diagnostic tests for penicilliosis in developing countries. Its role in monitoring the response of patients to treatment needs to be evaluated.

Trewatcharegon et al. (293) described the production and characterization of four clones of murine monoclonal antibodies to *P. marneffei*. One of these clones, 8C3, was later used to develop a sandwich ELISA capable of detecting antigen in serum or urine (294). With serum, the ELISA had a sensitivity of 72%, a specificity of 100%, a PPV of 100%, and a NPV of 97%. When five sets of paired serum and urine specimens from patients with penicilliosis were tested, all the serum samples were positive, as were four of the five urines. This group of investigators has also described the development and prospective evaluation of an antigen-capture ELISA in which two of their murine monoclonals, 8C3 and 8B11, were used (295). The test was evaluated using serum samples from 53 HIV-positive patients with penicilliosis, as well as 38 samples from HIV-positive patients with candidiasis, cryptococcosis, or histoplasmosis, and 202 samples from control subjects. The ELISA had a sensitivity of 92%, a specificity of 97.5%, a PPV of 89%, and a NPV of 98%.

At present, antigen detection appears to be a highly promising approach to the rapid diagnosis of penicilliosis in patients at high risk of developing the disease. However, it remains to be established whether prospective screening of serum or urine samples will be of benefit in monitoring the response to antifungal treatment, or detecting later relapse.

Other Fungal Infections

Blumer et al. (296) compared five serologic tests for sporotrichosis using serum samples from 55 cases of localized cutaneous and subcutaneous infection, and 25 cases of localized deep or disseminated infection. A LA test had a sensitivity and specificity of 94% and 100%, respectively, and was recommended for routine clinical use because of its ease of performance. A LA test for sporotrichosis is commercially available (LA-Sporo Antibody system, Immuno-Mycologics, Inc.), but there have been few formal evaluations of its performance. Using this test, Scott et al. (297) detected antibodies to *Sporothrix schenckii* in CSF and serum samples from seven patients with chronic meningeal sporotrichosis. Thirty patients with other forms of fungal meningitis, and 100 with bacterial or viral meningitis all gave negative results, as did 170 patients with other neurological disorders. Scott et al. (297) compared the commercial LA test with an in-house ELISA, and showed that titers of antibodies were higher with the latter method. Both LA and ELISA showed a decline in titers after amphotericin B treatment was begun.

Using immunoblotting and ELISA, Scott and Muchmore (298) investigated the serologic response of patients with various forms of sporotrichosis. Sera from 40 patients with the infection had IgG antibody titers of 1:128 to 1:65,200 by ELISA, while none of 300 control sera or 100 sera from patients with systemic fungal infections had titers of >1:64. Antibodies to 40 and 70 kDa antigenic components were detected by immunoblotting in sera from all patients with sporotrichosis, while antibodies to 22 and 36 kDa components were detected in 13 of 15 patients with extracutaneous disease but not in patients with cutaneous sporotrichosis. More recently, Mendoza et al. (299) noted marked variations in the composition of mycelial culture filtrate antigen preparations depending on the composition of the medium employed. In a defined medium, a 90 kDa component was expressed that reacted with sera from three patients with sporotrichosis, but did not cross-react with sera from patients with paracoccidioidomycosis, coccidioidomycosis, or histoplasmosis. Purification of this 90 kDa component could provide the basis of more specific and sensitive serologic tests for sporotrichosis.

Several serologic methods have been described for zygomycosis (300,301), but these tests have not been extensively evaluated. Laboratory diagnosis of this disease continues to depend on the isolation of the etiologic agents in culture and/ or their histopathologic demonstration in tissue or other clinical specimens. Of the different serologic methods that have been studied for invasive forms of zygomycosis, ELISA appears to be a more sensitive procedure than ID (301). Nevertheless, with the unpurified antigens that were used in this work, false-positive reactions were obtained with sera from patients with other fungal infections, including aspergillosis and candidiasis.

The definitive diagnosis of subcutaneous and gastrointestinal forms of basidiobolomycosis and conidiobolomycosis (also termed entomophthoramycosis or subcutaneous zygomycosis) depends on microscopic examination and culture. However, ID has proved useful as an adjunctive method for the detection of these uncommon infections (302,303). The ID test appears to be specific for *Basidiobolus ranarum*, but its sensitivity has not been determined. It also appears to be useful for monitoring the response to treatment (304).

CONCLUSIONS

This chapter reviewed the wide range of serologic tests that are now available for the diagnosis of invasive fungal infections. Tests for the detection of fungal antibodies have long had an important role in the diagnosis of endemic fungal infections, such as histoplasmosis, coccidioidomycosis, and paracoccidio-idomycosis, as well as the different forms of aspergillosis that occur in non-immunocompromised individuals. However, despite strenuous efforts to develop more sensitive methods, these tests remain less useful for the opportunistic infections, such as aspergillosis and candidiasis, which occur in immunocom-promised individuals. In the future, antibody detection methods should benefit from the use of purified and well-characterized antigens, some of which are now derived from the application of recombinant molecular biological procedures.

Antigen detection has long been an established method for the diagnosis of cryptococcosis, and the last few years have seen the advent of similar approaches for the detection of histoplasmosis, paracoccidioidomycosis, and penicilliosis. Although the use of monoclonal antibodies has enabled antigen detection tests to be marketed for the diagnosis of aspergillosis and candidiasis, finding circulating antigens that are not transient in nature remains an elusive goal. The antigen detection tests that are now being introduced for these diseases appear promising, but continued evaluation will be essential if their full potential is to be realized and if the results obtained are to be of most benefit to patients.

The inability of most antigen detection tests to detect fungi other than the target species or genus is an important limitation. Molecular diagnosis, using panfungal PCR primers and species-specific probes, offers a potential solution to this problem. Numerous "in-house" protocols have been developed and evaluated for the detection of fungal DNA in clinical specimens, but there has been no standardization of test procedures, and the risk of contamination of specimens or reagents should not be underestimated. Although this approach appears promising, the temporal relationship between DNA detection and other diagnostic signs has not been clearly established. Until such time as these molecular procedures are standardized and commercialized, serologic tests will remain essential for the rapid diagnosis of invasive fungal infections.

REFERENCES

1. Chen SC, Halliday CL, Meyer W. A review of nucleic acid-based diagnostic tests for systemic mycoses with an emphasis on polymerase chain reaction-based assays. Med Mycol 2002; 40:333–57.
2. Yeo SF, Wong B. Current status of nonculture methods for diagnosis of invasive fungal infections. Clin Microbiol Rev 2002; 15:465–84.
3. Bennett JE, Friedmann MM, Dupont B. Receptor mediated clearance of Aspergillus galactomannan. J Infect Dis 1987; 155:1005–10.
4. Kappe R, Muller J. Rapid clearance of *Candida albicans* mannan antigen by liver and spleen in contrast to prolonged circulation of *Cryptococcus neoformans* antigens. J Clin Microbiol 1991; 29:1665–9.
5. Wheat J, Wheat H, Connolly P, et al. Cross-reactivity in *Histoplasma capsulatum* variety *capsulatum* antigen assays of urine samples from patients with endemic mycoses. Clin Infect Dis 1997; 24:1169–71.
6. Ascioglu S, de Pauw BE, Donnelly JP, Collette L. Reliability of clinical research on invasive fungal infections: a systematic review of the literature. Med Mycol 2001; 39:35–40.
7. Dupont B, Improvisi L, Prevost F. Detection de galactomannane dans les aspergilloses invasives humaines et animales avec un test au latex. Bull Soc Fr Mycol Med 1990; 19:35–41.
8. Sulahian A, Tabouret M, Ribaud P, et al. Comparison of an enzyme immunoassay and latex agglutination test for detection of galactomannan in the diagnosis of invasive aspergillosis. Eur J Clin Microbiol Infect Dis 1996; 15:139–45.
9. Ascioglu S, Rex JH, de Pauw B, et al. Defining opportunistic invasive fungal infections in immunocompromised patients with cancer and hematopoietic stem cell transplants: an international consensus. Clin Infect Dis 2002; 34:7–14.
10. Bennett JE, Kauffman C, Walsh T, et al. Forum report: issues in the evaluation of diagnostic tests, use of historical controls, and merits of the current multicenter collaborative groups. Clin Infect Dis 2003; 36(Suppl. 1):S123–7.
11. Herbrecht R, Letscher-Bru V, Oprea C, et al. Aspergillus galactomannan detection in the diagnosis of invasive aspergillosis in cancer patients. J Clin Oncol 2002; 20:1898–906.
12. Kurup VP, Kumar A. Immunodiagnosis of aspergillosis. Clin Microbiol Rev 1991; 4:439–56.
13. Hearn VM. Antigenicity of *Aspergillus* species. J Med Vet Mycol 1992; 30:11–25.
14. Wilson EV, Hearn VM. Comparison of partially purified mycelial and culture filtrate antigens of *Aspergillus fumigatus* by enzyme-linked immunosorbent assay. Sabouraudia 1983; 21:195–203.
15. Schonheyder H, Anderson P. IgG antibodies to purified *Aspergillus fumigatus* antigens determined by enzyme-linked immunosorbent assay. Int Arch Allergy Appl Immunol 1984; 74:262–9.
16. Kurup VP, Greenberger PA, Fink JN. Antibody response to low-molecular-weight antigens of *Aspergillus fumigatus* in allergic bronchopulmonary aspergillosis. J Clin Microbiol 1989; 27:1312–6.
17. Latge JP. *Aspergillus fumigatus* and aspergillosis. Clin Microbiol Rev 1999; 12:310–50.

18. Latge JP, Moutaouakil M, Debeaupuis JP, Bouchara JP, Haynes K, Prevost MC. The 18-kilodalton antigen secreted by *Aspergillus fumigatus*. Infect Immun 1991; 59:2586–94.

19. Lopez-Medrano R, Ovejero MC, Calera JA, Puente P, Leal F. An immunodominant 90-kilodalton *Aspergillus fumigatus* antigen is the subunit of a catalase. Infect Immun 1995; 63:4774–80.

20. Beauvais A, Monod M, Debeaupuis JP, Diaquin M, Kobayashi H, Latge JP. Biochemical and antigenic characterization of a new dipeptidyl-peptidase isolated from *Aspergillus fumigatus*. J Biol Chem 1997; 272:6238–44.

21. Bennett JE, Bhattacharjee AK, Glaudemans CP. Galactofuranosyl groups are immunodominant in *Aspergillus fumigatus* galactomannan. Mol Immunol 1985; 22:251–4.

22. Latge JP, Kobayashi H, Debeaupuis JP, et al. Chemical and immunological characterization of the extracellular galactomannan secreted by *Aspergillus fumigatus*. Infect Immun 1994; 62:5424–33.

23. Crameri R, Hemmann S, Ismail C, Menz G, Blaser K. Disease-specific recombinant allergens for the diagnosis of allergic bronchopulmonary aspergillosis. Int Immunol 1998; 10:1211–6.

24. Hemmann S, Nikolaizik WH, Schoni MH, Blaser K, Crameri R. Differential IgE recognition of recombinant *Aspergillus fumigatus* allergens by cystic fibrosis patients with allergic bronchopulmonary aspergillosis or Aspergillus allergy. Eur J Immunol 1998; 28:1155–60.

25. Kurup VP, Banerjee B, Hemmann S, Greenberger PA, Blaser K, Crameri R. Selected recombinant *Aspergillus fumigatus* allergens bind specifically to IgE in ABPA. Clin Exp Allergy 2000; 30:988–93.

26. Sarfati J, Monod M, Recco P, et al. Recombinant antigens as diagnostic markers for aspergillosis. Diagn Microbiol Infect Dis 2006; 55:279–91.

27. Crameri R. Recombinant *Aspergillus fumigatus* allergens: from the nucleotide sequences to clinical applications. Int Arch Allergy 1998; 115:99–114.

28. Knutsen AP, Hutcheson PS, Slavin RG, Kurup VP. IgE antibody to *Aspergillus fumigatus* recombinant allergens in cystic fibrosis patients with allergic bronchopulmonary aspergillosis. Allergy 2004; 59:198–203.

29. Holmberg K, Berdischewsky M, Young LS. Serologic immunodiagnosis of invasive aspergillosis. J Infect Dis 1980; 141:656–64.

30. Young RC, Bennett JE. Invasive aspergillosis: absence of detectable antibody response. Am Rev Respir Dis 1971; 104:710–6.

31. Trull AK, Parker J, Warren RE. IgG enzyme linked immunosorbent assay for diagnosis of invasive aspergillosis: retrospective study over 15 years of transplant recipients. J Clin Pathol 1985; 38:1045–51.

32. Tommee JF, Mannes GP, van der Bij W, et al. Serodiagnosis and monitoring of Aspergillus infection after lung transplantation. Ann Intern Med 1996; 125:197–201.

33. Yuen KY, Chan CM, Chan KM, et al. Characterization of *AFMP1*: a novel target for serodiagnosis of aspergillosis. J Clin Microbiol 2001; 39:3830–7.

34. Chan CM, Woo PC, Leung AS, et al. Detection of antibodies specific to an antigenic cell wall galactomannoprotein for serodiagnosis of *Aspergillus fumigatus* aspergillosis. J Clin Microbiol 2002; 40:2041–5.

35. Weiner MH, Talbot GH, Gerson SL, Filice G, Cassileth PA. Antigen detection in the diagnosis of invasive aspergillosis: utility in controlled, blinded trials. Ann Intern Med 1983; 99:777–82.

36. Talbot GH, Weiner MH, Gerson SL, Provencher M, Hurwitz S. Serodiagnosis of invasive aspergillosis in patients with hematologic malignancy: validation of *Aspergillus fumigatus* antigen radioimmunoassay. J Infect Dis 1987; 155:12–27.

37. Sabetta JR, Miniter P, Andriole VT. The diagnosis of invasive aspergillosis by an enzyme-linked immunosorbent assay for circulating antigen. J Infect Dis 1985; 152:946–53.

38. Rogers TR, Haynes KA, Barnes RA. Value of antigen detection in predicting invasive pulmonary aspergillosis. Lancet 1990; 336:1210–3.

39. Stynen D, Goris A, Sarfati J, Latge JP. A new sensitive sandwich enzyme-linked immunosorbent assay to detect galactofuran in patients with invasive aspergillosis. J Clin Microbiol 1995; 33:497–500.

40. Patterson TF, Miniter P, Ryan JL, Andriole VT. Effect of immunosuppression and amphotericin B on Aspergillus antigenemia in an experimental model. J Infect Dis 1988; 158:415–22.

41. Hurst SF, Reyes GH, McLaughlin DW, Reiss E, Morrison CJ. Comparison of commercial latex agglutination and sandwich enzyme immunoassays with a competitive binding inhibition enzyme immunoassay for detection of antigenemia and antigenuria in a rabbit model of invasive aspergillosis. Clin Diagn Lab Immunol 2000; 7:477–85.

42. Marr KA, Balajee A, McLaughlin L, Tabouret M, Bentsen C, Walsh TJ. Detection of galactomannan antigenemia by enzyme immunoassay for the diagnosis of invasive aspergillosis: variables that affect performance. J Infect Dis 2004; 190(3):641–9.

43. Ansorg R, Heintschel von Heinegg E, Rath PM. Aspergillus antigenuria compared to antigenemia in bone marrow transplant recipients. Eur J Clin Microbiol Infect Dis 1994; 13:582–9.

44. Haynes K, Rogers TR. Retrospective evaluation of a latex agglutination test for diagnosis of invasive aspergillosis in immunocompromised patients. Eur J Clin Microbiol Infect Dis 1994; 13:670–4.

45. Manso E, Montillo M, De Sio G, D'Amico S, Discepoli G, Leoni P. Value of antigen and antibody detection in the serological diagnosis of invasive aspergillosis in patients with hematological malignancies. Eur J Clin Microbiol Infect Dis 1994; 13:756–60.

46. Hopwood V, Johnson EM, Cornish JM, Foot ABM, Evans EGV, Warnock DW. Use of the Pastorex Aspergillus antigen latex agglutination test for the diagnosis of invasive aspergillosis. J Clin Pathol 1995; 48:210–3.

47. Verweij PE, Rijs AJ, De Pauw BE, Horrevorts AM, Hoogkamp-Korstanje JA, Meis JF. Clinical evaluation and reproducibility of the Pastorex Aspergillus antigen latex agglutination test for diagnosing invasive aspergillosis. J Clin Pathol 1995; 48:474–6.

48. Caillot D, Casasnovas O, Bernard A, et al. Improved management of invasive aspergillosis in neutropenic patients using early thoracic computed tomographic scan and surgery. J Clin Oncol 1997; 15:139–47.

49. Verweij PE, Stynen D, Rijs AJ, De Pauw BE, Hoogkamp-Korstanje JAA, Meis JF. Sandwich enzyme-linked immunosorbent assay compared with Pastorex latex agglutination test for diagnosing invasive aspergillosis in immunocompromised patients. J Clin Microbiol 1995; 33:1912–4.

50. Marr KA, Laverdiere M, Gugel A, Leisenring W. Antifungal therapy decreases sensitivity of the Aspergillus galactomannan enzyme immunoassay. Clin Infect Dis 2005; 40:1762–9.

51. Verweij PE, Erjavec Z, Sluiters W, et al. Detection of antigen in sera of patients with invasive aspergillosis: intra- and interlaboratory reproducibility. J Clin Microbiol 1998; 36:1612–6.

52. Maertens J, Verhaegen J, Demuynck H. Autopsy-controlled prospective evaluation of serial screening for circulating galactomannan by a sandwich enzyme-linked immunosorbent assay for hematological patients at risk for invasive aspergillosis. J Clin Microbiol 1999; 37:3223–8.

53. Sulahian A, Boutboul F, Ribaud P, Leblanc T, Lacroix C, Derouin F. Value of antigen detection using an enzyme immunoassay in the diagnosis and prediction of invasive aspergillosis in two adult and pediatric hematology units during a 4-year prospective study. Cancer 2001; 91:311–8.

54. Maertens J, Theunissen K, Verbeken E, et al. Prospective clinical evaluation of lower cut-offs for galactomannan detection in adult neutropenic cancer patients and haematological stem cell transplant recipients. Br J Haematol 2004; 126:852–60.

55. Maertens J, Verhaegen J, Lagrou K, Van Eldere J, Boogaerts M. Screening for circulating galactomannan as a noninvasive diagnostic tool for invasive aspergillosis in prolonged neutropenic patients and stem cell transplantation recipients: a prospective validation. Blood 2001; 97:1604–10.

56. Pfeiffer CD, Fine JP, Safdar N. Diagnosis of invasive aspergillosis using a galactomannan assay: a meta-analysis. Clin Infect Dis 2006; 42:1417–27.

57. Weisser M, Rausch C, Droll A, et al. Galactomannan does not precede major signs on a pulmonary computerized tomographic scan suggestive of invasive aspergillosis in patients with hematological malignancies. Clin Infect Dis 2005; 41:1143–9.

58. George D, Miniter P, Andriole VT. Efficacy of U.K.-109496, a new azole antifungal agent, in an experimental model of invasive aspergillosis. Antimicrob Agents Chemother 1996; 40:86–91.

59. Petraitiene R, Petraitis V, Groll AH, et al. Antifungal activity and pharmacokinetics of posaconazole (SCH 56592) in treatment and prevention of experimental invasive pulmonary aspergillosis: correlation with galactomannan antigenemia. Antimicrob Agents Chemother 2001; 45:857–69.

60. Boutboul F, Alberti C, Leblanc T, et al. Invasive aspergillosis in allogeneic stem cell transplant recipients: increasing antigenemia is associated with progressive disease. Clin Infect Dis 2002; 34:939–43.

61. Petraitiene R, Petraitis V, Groll AH, et al. Antifungal efficacy of caspofungin (MK-0991) in experimental pulmonary aspergillosis in persistently neutropenic rabbits: pharmacokinetics, drug disposition, and relationship to galactomannan antigenemia. Antimicrob Agents Chemother 2002; 46:12–23.

62. Klont RR, Mennink-Kersten MA, Ruegebrink D, et al. Paradoxical increase in circulating Aspergillus antigen during treatment with caspofungin in a patient with pulmonary aspergillosis. Clin Infect Dis 2006; 43:e23–5.

63. Maertens J, Glasmacher A, Selleslag D, et al. Evaluation of serum sandwich enzyme-linked immunosorbent assay for circulating galactomannan during caspofungin therapy: results from the caspofungin invasive aspergillosis study. Clin Infect Dis 2005; 41:e9–14.

64. Husain S, Kwak EJ, Obman A, et al. Prospective assessment of Platelia Aspergillus galactomannan for the diagnosis of invasive aspergillosis in lung transplant recipients. Am J Transplant 2004; 4:1–7.

65. Kwak EJ, Husain S, Obman A, et al. Efficacy of galactomannan antigen in the Platelia Aspergillus enzyme immunoassay for diagnosis of invasive aspergillosis in liver transplant recipients. J Clin Microbiol 2004; 42:435–8.

66. Stynen D, Sarfati J, Goris A, et al. Rat monoclonal antibodies against Aspergillus galactomannan. Infect Immun 1992; 60:2237–45.

67. Kappe R, Schulze-Berge A. New cause for false-positive results with the Pastorex Aspergillus antigen latex agglutination test. J Clin Microbiol 1993; 31:2489–90.

68. Swanink CM, Meis JF, Rijs AJ, Donnelly JP, Verweij PE. Specificity of a sandwich enzyme-linked immunosorbent assay for detecting Aspergillus galactomannan. J Clin Microbiol 1997; 35:257–60.

69. Gangneux JP, Lavarde D, Bretagne S, Guiguen C, Gandemer V. Transient Aspergillus antigenaemia: think of milk. Lancet 2002; 359:1251.

70. Mennink-Kersten MA, Ruegebrink D, Klont RR, et al. Bifidobacterial lipoglycan as a new cause for false-positive Platelia Aspergillus enzyme-linked immunosorbent assay reactivity. J Clin Microbiol 2005; 43:3925–31.

71. Murashige N, Kami M, Kishi Y, Fujisaki G, Tanosaki R. False-positive results of Aspergillus enzyme-linked immunosorbent assays for a patient with gastrointestinal graft-versus-host disease taking a nutrient containing soybean protein. Clin Infect Dis 2005; 40:333–4.

72. Ansorg R, van den Boom R, Rath PM. Detection of Aspergillus galactomannan antigen in foods and antibiotics. Mycoses 1997; 40:353–7.

73. Sulahian A, Touratier S, Ribaud P. False-positive test for Aspergillus antigenemia related to concomitant administration of piperacillin and tazobactam. N Engl J Med 2003; 349:2366–7.

74. Adam O, Auperin A, Wilquin F, Bourhis JH, Gachot B, Chachaty E. Treatment with piperacillin–tazobactam and false-positive Aspergillus galactomannan antigen test results for patients with hematological malignancies. Clin Infect Dis 2004; 38:917–20.

75. Viscoli C, Machetti M, Cappellano P, et al. False-positive galactomannan Platelia Aspergillus test results for patients receiving piperacillin–tazobactam. Clin Infect Dis 2004; 38:913–6.

76. Maertens J, Theunissen K, Verhoef G, Van Eldere J. False-positive Aspergillus galactomannan antigen test results. Clin Infect Dis 2004; 39:289–90.

77. Mattei D, Rapezzi D, Mordini N, et al. False-positive Aspergillus galactomannan enzyme-linked immunosorbent assay results in vivo during amoxicillin–clavulanic acid treatment. J Clin Microbiol 2004; 42:5362–3.

78. Bart-Delabesse E, Basile M, Al Jijakli A, et al. Detection of Aspergillus galactomannan antigenemia to determine biological and clinical implications of beta-lactam treatments. J Clin Microbiol 2005; 43:5214–20.

79. Walsh TJ, Shoham S, Petraitiene R, et al. Detection of galactomannan antigenemia in patients receiving piperacillin–tazobactam and correlations between in vitro, in vivo, and clinical properties of the drug-antigen interaction. J Clin Microbiol 2004; 42:4744–8.

80. Aubry A, Porcher R, Bottero J, et al. Occurrence and kinetics of false-positive Aspergillus galactomannan test results following treatment with beta-lactam antibiotics in patients with hematological disorders. J Clin Microbiol 2006; 44:389–94.

81. Verweij PE, Latge JP, Rijs AJ, et al. Comparison of antigen detection and PCR assay using bronchoalveolar lavage fluid for diagnosing invasive pulmonary aspergillosis in patients receiving treatment for hematological malignancies. J Clin Microbiol 1995; 33:3150–3.

82. Becker MJ, Lugtenburg EJ, Cornelissen JJ, Van Der Schee C, Hoogsteden HC, De Marie S. Galactomannan detection in computerized tomography-based bronchoalveolar lavage fluid and serum in haematological patients at risk for invasive pulmonary aspergillosis. Br J Haematol 2003; 121:448–57.

83. Sanguinetti M, Posteraro B, Pagano L, et al. Comparison of real-time PCR, conventional PCR, and galactomannan antigen detection by enzyme-linked immunosorbent assay using bronchoalveolar lavage fluid samples from hematology patients for diagnosis of invasive pulmonary aspergillosis. J Clin Microbiol 2003; 41:3922–5.

84. Musher B, Fredricks D, Leisenring W, Balajee SA, Smith C, Marr KA. Aspergillus galactomannan enzyme immunoassay and quantitative PCR for diagnosis of invasive aspergillosis with bronchoalveolar lavage fluid. J Clin Microbiol 2004; 42:5517–22.

85. Verweij PE, Brinkman K, Kremer HP, Kullberg BJ, Meis JF. Aspergillus meningitis: diagnosis by non-culture-based microbiological methods and management. J Clin Microbiol 1999; 37:1186–9.

86. Kami M, Ogawa S, Kanda Y, et al. Early diagnosis of central nervous system aspergillosis using polymerase chain reaction, latex agglutination test, and enzyme-linked immunosorbent assay. Br J Haematol 1999; 106:536–7.

87. Klont RR, Mennink-Kersten MA, Verweij PE. Utility of Aspergillus antigen detection in specimens other than serum specimens. Clin Infect Dis 2004; 39:1467–74.

88. Kawazu M, Kanda Y, Nannya Y, et al. Prospective comparison of the diagnostic potential of real-time PCR, double-sandwich enzyme-linked immunosorbent assay for galactomannan, and a (1-3)-β-D-glucan test in weekly screening for invasive aspergillosis in patients with hematological disorders. J Clin Microbiol 2004; 42:2733–41.

89. Pazos C, Ponton J, Del Palacio A. Contribution of (1-3)-β-D-glucan chromogenic assay to diagnosis and therapeutic monitoring of invasive aspergillosis in neutropenic adult patients: a comparison with serial screening for circulating galactomannan. J Clin Microbiol 2005; 43:299–305.

90. Bretagne S, Costa JM, Bart-Delabesse E, Dhedin N, Rieux C, Cordonnier C. Comparison of serum galactomannan antigen detection and competitive polymerase chain reaction for diagnosing invasive aspergillosis. Clin Infect Dis 1998; 26:1407–12.

91. Costa C, Costa JM, Desterke C, Botterel F, Cordonnier C, Bretagne S. Real-time PCR coupled with automated DNA extraction and detection of galactomannan antigen in serum by enzyme-linked immunosorbent assay for diagnosis of invasive aspergillosis. J Clin Microbiol 2002; 40:2224–7.

92. Maertens J, Theunissen K, Verhoef G, et al. Galactomannan and computed tomography-based preemptive antifungal therapy in neutropenic patients at high risk for invasive fungal infection: a prospective feasibility study. Clin Infect Dis 2005; 41:1242–50.

93. Evans EGV, Forster RA. Antibodies to Candida after operations on the heart. J Med Microbiol 1976; 9:303–8.
94. Warnock DW, Speller DCE, Finan PJ, Vellacott KD, Phillips MN. Antibodies to *Candida* species after operations on the large intestine: observations on the association with oral and faecal yeast colonization. Sabouraudia 1979; 17:405–14.
95. Greenfield RA, Bussey MJ, Stephens JL, Jones JM. Serial enzyme-linked immunosorbent assays for antibody to Candida antigens during induction chemotherapy for acute leukemia. J Infect Dis 1983; 148:275–83.
96. Fujita S, Matsubara F, Matsuda T. Enzyme-linked immunosorbent assay measurement of fluctuations in antibody titer and antigenemia in cancer patients with and without candidiasis. J Clin Microbiol 1986; 23:568–75.
97. Sendid B, Tabouret M, Poirot JL, Mathieu D, Fruit J, Poulain D. New enzyme immunoassays for sensitive detection of circulating *Candida albicans* mannan and antimannan antibodies: useful combined test for diagnosis of systemic candidiasis. J Clin Microbiol 1999; 37:1510–7.
98. Greenfield RA, Jones JM. Purification and characterization of a major cytoplasmic antigen of *Candida albicans*. Infect Immun 1981; 34:469–77.
99. Strockbine NA, Largen MT, Zweibel SM, Buckely HR. Identification and molecular weight characterization of antigens from *Candida albicans* that are recognized by human sera. Infect Immun 1984; 43:715–21.
100. Matthews RC, Burnie JP, Tabaqchali S. Immunoblot analysis of the serological response in systemic candidiasis. Lancet 1984; 2:1415–8.
101. Au Young JK, Troy FA, Goldstein E. Serologic analysis of antigen-specific reactivity in patients with systemic candidiasis. Diagn Microbiol Infect Dis 1985; 3:419–32.
102. Gatermann S, Heessemann S, Laufs R. Identification of *Candida albicans* antigens recognized by sera of patients with candidiasis. Mykosen 1986; 29:343–54.
103. Matthews RC, Burnie JP. Cloning of a cDNA sequence encoding a major fragment of the 47 kilodalton stress protein homologue of *Candida albicans*. FEMS Microbiol Lett 1989; 60:25–30.
104. Mason AB, Brandt ME, Buckley HR. Enolase activity associated with a *Candida albicans* cytoplasmic antigen. Yeast 1989; 5:S231–40.
105. Franklyn KM, Warmington JR, Ott AK, Ashman RB. An immunodominant antigen of *Candida albicans* shows homology to the enzyme enolase. Immunol Cell Biol 1990; 68:173–8.
106. Matthews RC, Burnie JP, Tabaqchali S. Isolation of immunodominant antigens from the sera of patients with systemic candidosis and characterization of the serological response to *Candida albicans*. J Clin Microbiol 1987; 25:230–7.
107. Weis C, Kappe R, Sonntag HG. Western blot analysis of the immune response to *Candida albicans* antigens in 391 long-term intensive care patients. Mycoses 1997; 40:153–7.
108. Van Deventer AJ, van Vliet HJ, Hop WC, Goessens WH. Diagnostic value of anti-Candida enolase antibodies. J Clin Microbiol 1994; 32:17–23.
109. Mitsutake K, Kohno S, Miyazaki T, Miyazaki H, Maesaki S, Koga H. Detection of Candida enolase antibody in patients with candidiasis. J Clin Lab Anal 1994; 8:207–10.

110. Staib F, Focking M, Frohlich B, Blisse A. *Candida albicans*-serumprazipitine bei blutspendern: auffallige serologische und kulturelle *Candida albicans*-befunde bei alkoholikern. Mykosen 1977; 20:423–30.

111. Staib F, Mishra SK, Abel TL. Serodiagnostic value of extracellular antigens of an actively proteolysing culture of *Candida albicans* (immunodiffusion test). Zbl Bakt Hyg I Abt Orig A 1977; 238:284–7.

112. Macdonald F, Odds FC. Inducible proteinase of *Candida albicans* in diagnostic serology and in the pathogenesis of systemic candidosis. J Med Microbiol 1980; 13:423–35.

113. Macdonald F, Odds FC. Purified *Candida albicans* proteinase in the serological diagnosis of systemic candidosis. JAMA 1980; 243:2409–11.

114. Ruchel R, Bonning-Stutzer B, Mari A. A synoptical approach to the diagnosis of candidosis relying on serological antigen and antibody tests, on culture, and on evaluation of clinical data. Mycoses 1988; 31:87–106.

115. Na BK, Song CY. Use of monoclonal antibody in diagnosis of candidiasis caused by *Candida albicans*: detection of circulating aspartyl proteinase antigen. Clin Diagn Lab Immunol 1999; 6:924–9.

116. El Moudni B, Rodier MH, Daniault G, Jacquemin JL. Improved immunodiagnosis of human candidiasis by an enzyme-linked immunosorbent assay using a *Candida albicans* 52-kilodalton metallopeptidase. Clin Diagn Lab Immunol 1998; 5:823–5.

117. Evans EGV, Richardson MD, Odds FC, Holland KT. Relevance of antigenicity of *Candida albicans* growth phases to diagnosis of systemic candidiasis. Br Med J 1973; 4:86–7.

118. Smail EH, Jones JM. Demonstration and solubilization of antigens expressed primarily on the surfaces of *Candida albicans* germ tubes. Infect Immun 1984; 45:74–81.

119. Sundstrom PG, Kenny GE. Characterization of antigens specific to the surface of germ tubes of *Candida albicans* by immunofluorescence. Infect Immun 1984; 43:850–5.

120. Casanova M, Gil ML, Cardeneso L, Martinez JP, Sentandreu R. Identification of wall-specific antigens synthesized during germ-tube formation by *Candida albicans*. Infect Immun 1989; 57:262–71.

121. Ponton J, Jones JM. Identification of two germ tube specific cell wall antigens of *Candida albicans*. Infect Immun 1986; 54:864–8.

122. Quindos G, Ponton J, Cisterna R. Detection of antibodies to *Candida albicans* germ tube in the diagnosis of systemic candidiasis. Eur J Clin Microbiol 1987; 6:142–6.

123. Quindos G, Ponton J, Cisterna J, Mackenzie DWR. Value of detection of antibodies to *Candida albicans* germ tube in the diagnosis of systemic candidosis. Eur J Clin Microbiol Infect Dis 1990; 9:178–83.

124. Ponton J, Quindos G, Arilla MC, Mackenzie DWR. Simplified adsorption method for detection of antibodies to *Candida albicans* germ tubes. J Clin Microbiol 1994; 32:217–9.

125. Yera H, Sendid B, Francois N, Camus D, Poulain D. Contribution of serological tests and blood culture to the early diagnosis of systemic candidiasis. Eur J Clin Microbiol Infect Dis 2001; 20:864–70.

126. Prella M, Bille J, Pugnale M, et al. Early diagnosis of invasive candidiasis with mannan antigenemia and antimannan antibodies. Diagn Microbiol Infect Dis 2005; 51:95–101.

127. Weiner MH, Yount WJ. Mannan antigenemia in the diagnosis of invasive Candida infections. J Clin Invest 1976; 58:1045–53.
128. Segal E, Berg RA, Pizzo PA, Bennett JE. Detection of Candida antigen in sera of patients with candidiasis by an enzyme-linked immunosorbent assay-inhibition technique. J Clin Microbiol 1979; 10:116–8.
129. Weiner MH, Coats-Stephen M. Immunodiagnosis of systemic candidiasis: mannan antigenemia detected by radioimmunoassay in experimental and human infection. J Infect Dis 1979; 140:989–93.
130. Gentry LO, Wilkinson ID, Lea AS, Price MF. Latex agglutination test for detection of Candida antigenemia in patients with disseminated disease. Eur J Clin Microbiol 1983; 2:122–8.
131. Matthews RC, Burnie JP. Diagnosis of systemic candidosis by an enzyme-linked dot immunobinding assay for a circulating immunodominant 47-kilodalton antigen. J Clin Microbiol 1988; 26:459–63.
132. Reiss E, Stockman L, Kuykendall RS, Smith SJ. Dissociation of mannan-serum complexes and detection of *Candida albicans* mannan by enzyme immunoassay variations. Clin Chem 1982; 28:306–10.
133. de Repentigny L, Marr LD, Keller JW, et al. Comparison of enzyme immunoassay and gas–liquid chromatography for the rapid diagnosis of invasive candidiasis in cancer patients. J Clin Microbiol 1985; 21:972–9.
134. Lemieux C, St. Germain G, Vincelette J, Kaufman L, de Repentigny L. Collaborative evaluation of antigen detection by a commercial latex agglutination test and enzyme immunoassay in the diagnosis of invasive candidiasis. J Clin Microbiol 1990; 28:249–53.
135. Pfaller MA, Cabezudo I, Buschelman B, et al. Value of the Hybritech ICON Candida assay in the diagnosis of invasive candidiasis in high-risk patients. Diagn Microbiol Infect Dis 1993; 16:53–60.
136. Fujita SI, Hashimoto T. Detection of serum Candida antigens by enzyme-linked immunosorbent assay and a latex agglutination test with anti-*Candida albicans* and anti-*Candida krusei* antibodies. J Clin Microbiol 1992; 30:3132–7.
137. Bailey JW, Sada E, Brass C, Bennett JE. Diagnosis of systemic candidiasis by latex agglutination for serum antigen. J Clin Microbiol 1985; 21:749–52.
138. Kahn FW, Jones JM. Latex agglutination tests for detection of Candida antigens in sera of patients with invasive candidiasis. J Infect Dis 1986; 153:579–85.
139. Bisbe J, Miro JM, Torres JM, et al. Diagnostic value of serum antibody and antigen detection in heroin addicts with systemic candidiasis. Rev Infect Dis 1989; 11:310–5.
140. Phillips P, Dowd A, Jewesson P, et al. Nonvalue of antigen detection immunoassays for diagnosis of candidemia. J Clin Microbiol 1990; 28:2320–6.
141. Georges E, Garrigues ML, Stynen D, Poirot JL. Specificite in vitro d'un anticorps monoclonal (Acm) anti-mannane et du latex sensibilise par cet anticorps au cours de la candidose disseminee experimentale. J Mycol Med 1991; 1:21–4.
142. Jacquinot PM, Plancke Y, Sendid B, Strecker G, Poulain D. Nature of *Candida albicans*-derived carbohydrate antigen recognized by a monoclonal antibody in patient sera and distribution over *Candida* species. FEMS Microbiol Lett 1998; 169:131–8.
143. Herent P, Stynen D, Hernando F, Fruit J, Poulain D. Retrospective evaluation of two latex agglutination tests for detection of circulating antigen during invasive candidosis. J Clin Microbiol 1992; 30:2158–64.

144. Gutierrez J, Maroto C, Piedrola G, Martin E, Perez JA. Circulating Candida antigens and antibodies: useful markers of candidemia. J Clin Microbiol 1993; 31:2550–2.

145. Mitsutake K, Miyazaki T, Tashiro T, et al. Enolase antigen, mannan antigen, Cand-Tec antigen, and β-glucan in patients with candidemia. J Clin Microbiol 1996; 34:1918–21.

146. Sendid B, Jouault T, Coudriau R, et al. Increased sensitivity of mannanemia detection tests by joint detection of α- and β-linked oligomannosides during experimental and human systemic candidiasis. J Clin Microbiol 2004; 42:164–71.

147. Stevens P, Huang S, Young LS, Berdischewsky M. Detection of Candida antigenemia by a new solid phase radioimmunoassay. Infection 1980; 8(Suppl. 3):S334–8.

148. Araj GF, Hopfer RL, Chesnut S, Fainstein V, Bodey GP. Diagnostic value of the enzyme-linked immunosorbent assay for detection of *Candida albicans* cytoplasmic antigen in sera of cancer patients. J Clin Microbiol 1982; 16:46–52.

149. Matthews RC, Burnie JP, Lee W. The application of epitope mapping to the development of a new serological test for systemic candidosis. J Immunol Methods 1991; 143:73–9.

150. Strockbine NA, Largen MT, Buckley HR. Production and characterization of three monoclonal antibodies to *Candida albicans* proteins. Infect Immun 1984; 43:1012–8.

151. Walsh TJ, Hathorn JW, Sobel JD, et al. Detection of circulating Candida enolase by immunoassay in patients with cancer and invasive candidiasis. N Engl J Med 1991; 324:1026–31.

152. Ruchel R, Boning B. Detection of Candida proteinase by enzyme immunoassay and interaction of the enzyme with alpha-2-macroglobulin. J Immunol Methods 1983; 61:107–16.

153. de Repentigny L. Serodiagnosis of candidiasis, aspergillosis, and cryptococcosis. Clin Infect Dis 1992; 14(Suppl. 1):S11–22.

154. Fung JC, Donta ST, Tilton RC. Candida detection system (CAND-TEC) to differentiate between *Candida albicans* colonization and disease. J Clin Microbiol 1986; 24:542–7.

155. Ness MJ, Vaughan WP, Woods GL. Candida antigen latex test for detection of invasive candidiasis in immunocompromised patients. J Infect Dis 1989; 159:495–502.

156. Fujita S, Takamura T, Nagahara M, Hashimoto T. Evaluation of a newly developed down-flow immunoassay for detection of serum mannan antigens in patients with candidaemia. J Med Microbiol 2006; 55:537–43.

157. Chryssanthou E, Klingspor L, Tollemar J, et al. PCR and other non-culture methods for diagnosis of invasive Candida infections in allogeneic bone marrow and solid organ transplant recipients. Mycoses 1999; 42:239–47.

158. White PL, Archer AE, Barnes RA. Comparison of non-culture-based methods for detection of systemic fungal infections, with an emphasis on invasive Candida infections. J Clin Microbiol 2005; 43:2181–7.

159. Diamond RD, Bennett JE. Prognostic factors in cryptococcal meningitis. A study of 111 cases. Ann Intern Med 1974; 80:176–81.

160. Speed BR, Kaldor J, Cairns B, Pegorer M. Serum antibody response to active infection with *Cryptococcus neoformans* and its varieties in immunocompetent subjects. J Med Vet Mycol 1997; 34:187–93.

161. Santangelo RT, Chen SC, Sorrell TC, Wright LC. Detection of antibodies to phospholipase B in patients infected with *Cryptococcus neoformans* by enzyme-linked immunosorbent assay (ELISA). Med Mycol 2005; 43:335–41.

162. Bloomfield N, Gordon MA, Elmendorf DF. Detection of *Cryptococcus neoformans* antigen in body fluids by latex particle agglutination. Proc Soc Exp Biol Med 1963; 114:64–7.

163. Snow RM, Dismukes WE. Cryptococcal meningitis: diagnostic value of cryptococcal antigen in cerebrospinal fluid. Arch Intern Med 1975; 135:1155–7.

164. Wu T, Koo SY. Comparison of three commercial cryptococcal latex kits for detection of cryptococcal antigen. J Clin Microbiol 1983; 18:1127–30.

165. Bennett JE, Bailey JW. Control for rheumatoid factor in the latex test for cryptococcosis. Am J Clin Pathol 1970; 56:360–5.

166. Gordon MA, Lapa EW. Elimination of rheumatoid factor in the latex test for cryptococcosis. Am J Clin Pathol 1974; 60:488–94.

167. Gray LD, Roberts GD. Experience with the use of pronase to eliminate interference factors in the latex agglutination test for cryptococcal antigen. J Clin Microbiol 1988; 26:2450–1.

168. Stockman L, Roberts GD. Corrected version. Specificity of the latex test for cryptococcal antigen: a rapid, simple method for eliminating interference factors. J Clin Microbiol 1983; 17:945–7.

169. Whittier S, Hopfer RL, Gilligan P. Elimination of false-positive serum reactivity in latex agglutination test for cryptococcal antigen in human immunodeficiency virus-infected population. J Clin Microbiol 1994; 32:2158–61.

170. McManus EJ, Jones JM. Detection of a *Trichosporon beigelii* antigen cross-reactive with *Cryptococcus neoformans* capsular polysaccharide in serum from a patient with disseminated trichosporon infection. J Clin Microbiol 1985; 21:681–5.

171. Westerink MA, Amsterdam D, Petell RJ, Stram MN, Apicella MA. Septicemia due to DF-2. Cause of a false-positive cryptococcal latex agglutination result. Am J Med 1987; 83:155–8.

172. Chanock SJ, Toltzis P, Wilson C. Cross-reactivity between *Stomatococcus mucilaginosus* and latex agglutination for cryptococcal antigen. Lancet 1993; 342:1119–20.

173. Chuck SL, Sande MA. Infections with *Cryptococcus neoformans* in the acquired immunodeficiency syndrome. N Engl J Med 1989; 321:794–9.

174. Currie BP, Freundlich LF, Soto MA, Casadevall A. False-negative cerebrospinal fluid cryptococcal latex agglutination tests for patients with culture-positive cryptococcal meningitis. J Clin Microbiol 1993; 31:2519–22.

175. Taelman H, Bogaerts J, Batungwanayo J, Van de Perre P, Lucas S, Allen S. Failure of the cryptococcal serum antigen test to detect primary pulmonary cryptococcosis in patients infected with human immunodeficiency virus. Clin Infect Dis 1994; 18:119–20.

176. Stamm AM, Polt SS. False-negative cryptococcal antigen test. JAMA 1980; 244:1359.

177. Temstet A, Roux P, Poirot JL, Ronin O, Dromer F. Evaluation of a monoclonal antibody-based latex agglutination test for diagnosis of cryptococcosis: comparison with two tests using polyclonal antibodies. J Clin Microbiol 1992; 30:2544–50.

178. Hamilton JR, Noble A, Denning DW, Stevens DA. Performance of *Cryptococcus* antigen latex agglutination kits on serum and cerebrospinal fluid specimens of AIDS patients before and after pronase treatment. J Clin Microbiol 1991; 29:333–9.

179. Scott EN, Muchmore HG, Felton FG. Comparison of enzyme immunoassay and latex agglutination methods for detection of *Cryptococcus neoformans* antigen. Am J Clin Pathol 1980; 73:790–4.

180. Gade W, Hinnefeld SW, Babcock LS, et al. Comparison of the PREMIER cryptococcal antigen enzyme immunoassay and the latex agglutination assay for detection of cryptococcal antigens. J Clin Microbiol 1991; 29:1616–9.

181. Knight FR. New enzyme immunoassay for detecting cryptococcal antigen. J Clin Pathol 1992; 45:836–7.

182. Tanner DC, Weinstein MP, Fedorciw B, Joho KL, Thorpe JJ, Reller LB. Comparison of commercial kits for detection of cryptococcal antigen. J Clin Microbiol 1994; 32:1680–4.

183. Baughmann RP, Rhodes JC, Dohn MN, Henderson H, Frame PT. Detection of cryptococcal antigen in bronchoalveolar lavage fluid: a prospective study of diagnostic utility. Am Rev Respir Dis 1992; 145:1226–9.

184. Chapin-Robertson K, Bechtel C, Waycott S, Kdontnick C, Edberg SC. Crypto-coccal antigen detection from urine of AIDS patients. Diagn Microbiol Infect Dis 1993; 17:197–201.

185. Powderly WG, Cloud GA, Dismukes WE, Saag MS. Measurement of cryptococcal antigen in serum and cerebrospinal fluid: value in the management of AIDS-associated cryptococcal meningitis. Clin Infect Dis 1994; 18:789–92.

186. Antinori S, Radice A, Galimberti L, Magni C, Fasan M, Parravicini C. The role of cryptococcal antigen assay in diagnosis and monitoring of cryptococcal meningitis. J Clin Microbiol 2005; 43:5828–9.

187. Brouwer AE, Rajanuwong A, Chierakul W, et al. Combination antifungal therapies for HIV-associated cryptococcal meningitis: a randomized trial. Lancet 2004; 363:1764–7.

188. Brouwer AE, Teparrukkul P, Pinpraphaporn S, et al. Baseline correlation and comparative kinetics of cerebrospinal fluid colony-forming unit counts and antigen titers in cryptococcal meningitis. J Infect Dis 2005; 192:681–4.

189. Kaufman L, McLaughlin DW, Clark MJ, Blumer S. Specific immunodiffusion test for blastomycosis. Appl Microbiol 1973; 26:244–7.

190. Green JH, Harrell WK, Johnson J, Benson R. Isolation of an antigen from *Blasto-myces dermatitidis* that is specific for the diagnosis of blastomycosis. Curr Microbiol 1980; 4:293–6.

191. Kaufman L. Laboratory methods for the diagnosis and confirmation of systemic mycoses. Clin Infect Dis 1992; 14(Suppl. 1):S23–9.

192. Klein BS, Kuritsky JN, Chappell WA, et al. Comparison of the enzyme immunoassay, immunodiffusion, and complement fixation tests in detecting antibody in human serum to the A antigen of *Blastomyces dermatitidis*. Am Rev Respir Dis 1986; 133:144–8.

193. Turner S, Kaufman L, Jalbert M. Diagnostic assessment of an enzyme-linked immunosorbent assay for human and canine blastomycosis. J Clin Microbiol 1986; 23:294–7.

194. Klein BS, Vergeront JM, Kaufman L, et al. Serological tests for blastomycosis: assessments during a large point-source outbreak in Wisconsin. J Infect Dis 1987; 155:262–8.

195. Sekhon AS, Kaufman L, Kobayashi GS, Moledina NH, Jalbert M. The value of the Premier enzyme immunoassay for diagnosing *Blastomyces dermatitidis* infections. J Med Vet Mycol 1995; 33:123–5.

196. Bradsher RW, Pappas PG. Detection of specific antibodies in human blastomycosis by enzyme immunoassay. South Med J 1995; 88:1256–9.

197. Klein BS, Jones JM. Isolation, purification, and radiolabeling of a novel 120-kD surface protein on *Blastomyces dermatitidis* yeasts to detect antibody in infected patients. J Clin Invest 1990; 85:152–61.

198. Klein BS, Jones JM. Purification and characterization of the major antigen WI-1 from *Blastomyces dermatitidis* yeasts and immunological comparison with A antigen. Infect Immun 1994; 62:3890–900.

199. Soufleris AJ, Klein BS, Courtney BT, Proctor ME, Jones JM. Utility of anti-WI-1 serological testing in the diagnosis of blastomycosis in Wisconsin residents. Clin Infect Dis 1994; 19:87–92.

200. Durkin M, Witt J, LeMonte A, Wheat B, Connolly P. Antigen assay with the potential to aid in diagnosis of blastomycosis. J Clin Microbiol 2004; 42:4873–5.

201. Smith CE, Saito MT, Beard RR, Kepp R, Clark RW, Eddie BU. Serological tests in the diagnosis and prognosis of coccidioidomycosis. Am J Hyg 1950; 52:1–21.

202. Smith CE, Saito MT, Simons SA. Pattern of 39,500 serologic tests in coccidioidomycosis. JAMA 1956; 160:546–52.

203. Bronniman DA, Adam RD, Galgiani JN, et al. Coccidioidomycosis in the acquired immunodeficiency syndrome. Ann Intern Med 1987; 106:372–9.

204. Antoniskis D, Larsen RA, Akil B, Rarik MU, Leedom JM. Seronegative disseminated coccidioidomycosis in patients with HIV infection. AIDS 1990; 4:691–3.

205. Huppert M, Bailey JW. The use of immunodiffusion tests in coccidioidomycosis. II. An immunodiffusion test as a substitute for the tube precipitin test. Am J Clin Pathol 1965; 44:369–73.

206. Pappagiannis D, Zimmer BL. Serology of coccidioidomycosis. Clin Microbiol Rev 1990; 3:247–68.

207. Kaufman L, Clark MJ. Value of the concomitant use of complement fixation and immunodiffusion tests in the diagnosis of coccidioidomycosis. Appl Microbiol 1974; 28:641–3.

208. Huppert M, Peterson ET, Sun SH, Chitjian PA, Derrevere WJ. Evaluation of a latex particle agglutination test for coccidioidomycosis. Am J Clin Pathol 1968; 49:96–102.

209. Pappagianis D, Krasnow I, Beall S. False-positive reactions of cerebrospinal fluid and diluted sera with the coccidioidal latex agglutination test. Am J Clin Pathol 1976; 66:916–21.

210. Kaufman L, Sekhon AS, Moledina N, Jalbert M, Pappagianis D. Comparative evaluation of commercial Premier EIA and microimmunodiffusion and complement fixation tests for *Coccidioides immitis* antibodies. J Clin Microbiol 1995; 33:618–9.

211. Martins TB, Jaskowski TD, Mouritsen CL, Hill HR. Comparison of commercially available enzyme immunoassay with traditional serological tests for detection of antibodies to *Coccidioides immitis*. J Clin Microbiol 1995; 33:940–3.

212. Zartarian M, Peterson EM, de la Maza LM. Detection of antibodies to *Coccidioides immitis* by enzyme immunoassay. Am J Clin Pathol 1997; 107:148–53.
213. Cole GT, Kruse D, Seshan KR. Antigen complex of *Coccidioides immitis* which elicits a precipitin antibody response in patients. Infect Immun 1991; 59:2434–46.
214. Johnson SM, Pappagianis D. The coccidioidal complement fixation and immunodiffusion-complement fixation antigen is a chitinase. Infect Immun 1992; 60:2588–92.
215. Yang MC, Magee DM, Kaufman L, Zhu Y, Cox RA. Recombinant *Coccidioides immitis* complement-fixation antigen: detection of an epitope shared by *C. immitis*, *Histoplasma capsulatum*, and *Blastomyces dermatitidis*. Clin Diagn Lab Immunol 1997; 4:19–22.
216. Yang MC, Magee DM, Cox RA. Mapping of a *Coccidioides immitis*-specific epitope that reacts with complement-fixing antibody. Infect Immun 1997; 65:4068–74.
217. Weiner MH. Antigenemia detected in human coccidioidomycosis. J Clin Microbiol 1983; 18:136–42.
218. Galgiani JN, Dugger KO, Ito JI, Wieden MA. Antigenemia in primary coccidioidomycosis. Am J Trop Med Hyg 1984; 33:645–9.
219. Galgiani JN, Grace GM, Lundergan LL. New serologic tests for early detection of coccidioidomycosis. J Infect Dis 1991; 163:671–4.
220. Williams B, Fojtasek M, Connolly-Stringfield P, Wheat J. Diagnosis of histoplasmosis by antigen detection during an outbreak in Indianapolis, Ind. Arch Pathol Lab Med 1994; 118:1205–8.
221. Wheat J, French M, Batteiger B, Kohler R. Cerebrospinal fluid Histoplasma antibodies in central nervous system histoplasmosis. Arch Intern Med 1985; 145:1237–40.
222. Pine L. Histoplasma antigens: their production, purification and uses. Contrib Microbiol Immunol 1977; 3:138–68.
223. Zancope-Oliveira RM, Bragg SL, Reiss E, Peralta JM. Immunochemical analysis of the H and M glycoproteins from *Histoplasma capsulatum*. Clin Diagn Lab Immunol 1994; 1:563–8.
224. Reiss E, Knowles JB, Bragg SL, Kaufman L. Monoclonal antibodies against the M-protein and carbohydrate antigens of histoplasmin characterized by the enzyme-linked immunoelectrotransfer blot method. Infect Immun 1986; 53:540–6.
225. Hamilton AJ, Bartholomew MA, Figueroa J, Fenelon LE, Hay RJ. Evidence that the M antigen of *Histoplasma capsulatum* var. *capsulatum* is a catalase which exhibits cross-reactivity with other dimorphic fungi. J Med Vet Mycol 1990; 28:479–85.
226. Deepe GS, Durose GG. Immunological activity of recombinant H antigen from *Histoplasma capsulatum*. Infect Immun 1995; 63:3151–7.
227. Wheat J, French ML, Kohler RB, et al. The diagnostic laboratory tests for histoplasmosis: analysis of experience in a large urban outbreak. Ann Intern Med 1982; 97:680–5.
228. Wheat LJ. Current diagnosis of histoplasmosis. Trends Microbiol 2003; 11:488–94.
229. Wheat J, French ML, Kamel S, Tewari RP. Evaluation of cross-reactions in *Histoplasma capsulatum* serologic tests. J Clin Microbiol 1986; 23:493–9.
230. Reiss E, Hutchinson H, Pine L, Ziegler DW, Kaufman L. Solid-phase competitive-binding radioimmunoassay for detecting antibody to the M antigen of histoplasmin. J Clin Microbiol 1977; 6:598–604.

231. George DB, Lambert RS, Bruce MJ, Pickering TW, Wolcott RM. Radioimmunoassay: a sensitive screening test for histoplasmosis and blastomycosis. Am Rev Respir Dis 1981; 124:407–10.
232. Wheat LJ, Kohler RB, French ML, et al. Immunoglobulin M and G histoplasmal antibody response in histoplasmosis. Am Rev Respir Dis 1983; 128:65–70.
233. Lambert RS, George RB. Evaluation of enzyme immunoassay as a rapid screening test for histoplasmosis and blastomycosis. Am Rev Respir Dis 1987; 136:316–9.
234. Guimaraes AJ, Pizzini CV, De Matos Guedes HL, et al. ELISA for early diagnosis of histoplasmosis. J Med Microbiol 2004; 53:509–14.
235. Pizzini CV, Zancope-Oliveira RM, Reiss E, Hajjeh R, Kaufman L, Peralta JM. Evaluation of a Western blot test in an outbreak of acute pulmonary histoplasmosis. Clin Diagn Lab Immunol 1999; 6:20–3.
236. Sekhon AS, Kaufman L, Kobayashi GS, Moledina N, Jalbert M, Notenboom RH. Comparative evaluation of the Premier enzyme immunoassay, micro-immunodiffusion and complement fixation tests for the detection of *Histoplasma capsulatum* var. *capsulatum* antibodies. Mycoses 1994; 37:313–6.
237. Zancope-Oliveira RM, Bragg SL, Reiss E, Wanke B, Peralta JM. Effects of histoplasmin M antigen chemical and enzymatic deglycosylation on cross-reactivity in the enzyme-linked immunoelectrotransfer blot method. Clin Diagn Lab Immunol 1994; 1:390–3.
238. Zancope-Oliveira RM, Reiss E, Lott TJ, Mayer LW, Deepe GS. Molecular cloning, characterization, and expression of the M antigen of *Histoplasma capsulatum*. Infect Immun 1999; 67:1947–53.
239. Chandrashekar R, Curtis KC, Rawot BW, Kobayashi GS, Weil GJ. Molecular cloning and characterization of a recombinant *Histoplasma capsulatum* antigen for antibody-based diagnosis of human histoplasmosis. J Clin Microbiol 1997; 35:1071–6.
240. Wheat LJ, Kohler RB, Tewari RP. Diagnosis of disseminated histoplasmosis by detection of *Histoplasma capsulatum* antigen in serum and urine specimens. N Engl J Med 1986; 314:83–8.
241. Durkin MM, Connolly PA, Wheat LJ. Comparison of radioimmunoassay and enzyme-linked immunoassay methods for detection of *Histoplasma capsulatum* var. *capsulatum* antigen. J Clin Microbiol 1997; 35:2252–5.
242. Wheat LJ, Connolly-Stringfield P, Kohler RB, Frame PT, Gupta MR. *Histoplasma capsulatum* polysaccharide antigen detection in diagnosis and management of disseminated histoplasmosis in patients with acquired immunodeficiency syndrome. Am J Med 1989; 87:396–400.
243. Wheat LJ, Connolly-Stringfield P, Blair R, et al. Effect of successful treatment with amphotericin B on *Histoplasma capsulatum* variety *capsulatum* polysaccharide antigen levels in patients with AIDS and histoplasmosis. Am J Med 1992; 92:153–60.
244. Wheat LJ, Connolly P, Haddad N, Le Monte A, Brizendine E, Hafner R. Antigen clearance during treatment of disseminated histoplasmosis with itraconazole versus fluconazole in patients with AIDS. Antimicrob Agents Chemother 2002; 46:248–50.
245. Wheat LJ, Connolly-Stringfield P, Blair R, Connolly K, Garringer T, Katz BP. Histoplasmosis relapse in patients with AIDS: detection using *Histoplasma capsulatum* variety *capsulatum* antigen levels. Ann Intern Med 1991; 115:936–41.

246. Zimmerman SE, Stringfield PC, Wheat LJ, French ML, Kohler RB. Comparison of sandwich solid-phase radioimmunoassay and two enzyme-linked immunosorbent assays for detection of *Histoplasma capsulatum* polysaccharide antigen. J Infect Dis 1989; 160:678–85.

247. Garringer TO, Wheat LJ, Brizendine EJ. Comparison of an established antibody sandwich method with an inhibition method of *Histoplasma capsulatum* antigen detection. J Clin Microbiol 2000; 38:2909–13.

248. Gomez BL, Figueroa JI, Hamilton AJ, et al. Development of a novel antigen detection test for histoplasmosis. J Clin Microbiol 1997; 35:2618–22.

249. Gomez BL, Figueroa JI, Hamilton AJ, et al. Detection of the 70-kilodalton *Histoplasma capsulatum* antigen in serum of histoplasmosis patients: correlation between antigenemia and therapy during follow-up. J Clin Microbiol 1999; 37:675–80.

250. Tang YW, Li H, Durkin MM, et al. Urine polymerase chain reaction is not as sensitive as urine antigen for the diagnosis of disseminated histoplasmosis. Diagn Microbiol Infect Dis 2006; 54:283–7.

251. Brummer E, Castenada E, Restrepo A. Paracoccidioidomycosis: an update. Clin Microbiol Rev 1993; 6:89–117.

252. Bueno JP, Mendes-Giannini MJ, del Negro GM, Assis CM, Takiguti CK, Shikanai-Yasuda MA. IgG, IgM and IgA antibody response for the diagnosis and follow-up of paracoccidioidomycosis: comparison of counterimmuno-electrophoresis and complement fixation. J Med Vet Mycol 1997; 35:213–7.

253. Blumer SO, Jalbert M, Kaufman L. Rapid and reliable method for production of a specific *Paracoccidioides brasiliensis* immunodiffusion test antigen. J Clin Microbiol 1984; 19:404–7.

254. McGowan KL, Buckley HR. Preparation and use of cytoplasmic antigens for the serodiagnosis of paracoccidioidomycosis. J Clin Microbiol 1985; 22:39–43.

255. Cano LE, Restrepo A. Predictive value of serologic tests in the diagnosis and follow-up of patients with paracoccidioidomycosis. Rev Inst Med Trop Sao Paulo 1987; 29:276–83.

256. Del Negro GM, Garcia NM, Rodrigues EG, et al. The sensitivity, specificity and efficiency values of some serological tests used in the diagnosis of paracoccidioidomycosis. Rev Inst Med Trop Sao Paulo 1991; 33:277–80.

257. Marques da Silva SH, Queiroz-Telles F, Colombo AL, Blotta MH, Lopes JD, Camargo ZP. Monitoring of gp43 antigenemia in paracoccidioidomycosis patients during therapy. J Clin Microbiol 2004; 42:2419–24.

258. Gomez BL, Figueroa JI, Hamilton AJ, et al. Antigenemia in patients with paracoccidioidomycosis: detection of the 87-kilodalton determinant during and after antifungal therapy. J Clin Microbiol 1998; 36:3309–16.

259. Puccia R, Schenkman S, Gorin PA, Travassos LR. Exocellular components of *Paracoccidioides brasiliensis*: identification of a specific antigen. Infect Immun 1986; 53:199–206.

260. Figueroa JI, Hamilton A, Allen M, Hay R. Immunohistochemical detection of a novel 22- to 25- kilodalton glycoprotein of *Paracoccidioides brasiliensis* in biopsy material and partial characterization by using species-specific monoclonal antibodies. J Clin Microbiol 1994; 32:1566–74.

261. Figueroa JI, Hamilton AJ, Allen MH, Hay RJ. Isolation and partial characterization of a *Paracoccidioides brasiliensis* 58 kDa extracellular glycoprotein which is recognized by human immune sera. Trans R Soc Trop Med Hyg 1995; 89:566–72.

262. Bisio LC, Silva SP, Pereira IS, et al. A new *Paracoccidioides brasiliensis* 70-kDa heat shock protein reacts with sera from paracoccidioidomycosis patients. Med Mycol 2005; 43:495–503.

263. Diez S, Gomez BL, Restrepo A, Hay RJ, Hamilton AJ. *Paracoccidioides brasiliensis* 87-kilodalton antigen, a heat shock protein useful in diagnosis: characterization, purification, and detection in biopsy material via immunohistochemistry. J Clin Microbiol 2002; 40:359–65.

264. Taba MR, da Silveira JF, Travassos LR, Schenkman S. Expression in *Escherichia coli* of a gene encoding for epitopes of a diagnostic antigen of *Paracoccidioides brasiliensis*. Exp Mycol 1989; 13:223–30.

265. Cisalpino PS, Puccia R, Yamauchi LM, Cano MI, da Silveira JF, Travassos LR. Cloning, characterization, and epitope expression of the major diagnostic antigen of *Paracoccidioides brasiliensis*. J Biol Chem 1996; 271:4553–60.

266. McEwen JG, Ortiz BL, Garcia AM, Florez AM, Botero S, Restrepo A. Molecular cloning, nucleotide sequencing, and characterization of a 27 kDa antigenic protein from *Paracoccidioides brasiliensis*. Fungal Genet Biol 1996; 20:125–31.

267. Ortiz BL, Garcia AM, Restrepo A, McEwen JG. Immunological characterization of a recombinant 27-kilodalton antigenic protein from *Paracoccidioides brasiliensis*. Clin Diagn Lab Immunol 1996; 3:239–41.

268. Izacc SM, Gomez FJ, Jesuino RS, et al. Molecular cloning, characterization and expression of the heat shock protein 60 gene from the human pathogenic fungus *Paracoccidioides brasiliensis*. Med Mycol 2001; 39:445–55.

269. Mendes-Giannini MJ, Camargo ME, Lacaz CS, Ferreira AW. Immunoenzymatic absorption test for serodiagnosis of paracoccidioidomycosis. J Clin Microbiol 1984; 20:103–8.

270. Camargo ZP, Unterkircher C, Drouhet E. Comparison between magnetic enzyme-linked immunosorbent assay (MELISA) and complement fixation test (CF) in the diagnosis of paracoccidioidomycosis. J Med Vet Mycol 1986; 24:77–9.

271. Cano LE, Brummer E, Stevens DA, Restrepo A. An evaluation of the enzyme-linked immunosorbent assay (ELISA) for quantitation of antibodies to *Paracoccidioides brasiliensis*. J Med Vet Mycol 1986; 24:467–75.

272. Puccia R, Travassos LR. 43-kilodalton glycoprotein from *Paracoccidioides brasiliensis*: immunochemical reactions with sera from patients with paracoccidioidomycosis, histoplasmosis, or Jorge Lobo's disease. J Clin Microbiol 1991; 29:1610–5.

273. Camargo ZP, Gesztesi JL, Saraiva EC, Taborda CP, Vicentini AP, Lopes JD. Monoclonal antibody capture enzyme immunoassay for detection of *Paracoccidioides brasiliensis* antibodies in paracoccidioidomycosis. J Clin Microbiol 1994; 32:2377–81.

274. Ortiz BL, Diez S, Uran ME, et al. Use of the 27-kilodalton recombinant protein from *Paracoccidioides brasiliensis* in serodiagnosis of paracoccidioidomycosis. Clin Lab Diagn Immunol 1998; 5:826–30.

275. Diez S, Gomez BL, McEwen JG, Restrepo A, Hay RJ, Hamilton AJ. Combined use of *Paracoccidioides brasiliensis* recombinant 27-kilodalton and purified 87-kilodalton antigens in an enzyme-linked immunosorbent assay for serodiagnosis of paracoccidioidomycosis. J Clin Microbiol 2003; 41:1536–42.

276. Taborda CP, Camargo ZP. Diagnosis of paracoccidioidomycosis by dot immunobinding assay for antibody detection using the purified and specific antigen gp43. J Clin Microbiol 1994; 32:554–6.

277. Mendez-Giannini MJ, Bueno JP, Shikanai-Yasuda MA, Ferreira AW, Masuda A. Detection of the 43,000-molecular-weight glycoprotein in sera of patients with paracoccidioidomycosis. J Clin Microbiol 1989; 27:2842–5.

278. Gomez BL, Figueroa JI, Hamilton AJ, et al. Use of monoclonal antibodies in diagnosis of paracoccidioidomycosis: new strategies for detection of circulating antigens. J Clin Microbiol 1997; 35(12):3278–83.

279. Salina MA, Shikanai-Yasuda MA, Mendes RP, Barraviera B, Mendes-Giannini MJ. Detection of circulating *Paracoccidioides brasiliensis* antigen in urine of paracoccidioidomycosis patients before and during treatment. J Clin Microbiol 1998; 36:1723–8.

280. Marques da Silva SH, Colombo AL, Blotta MH, Lopes JD, Queiroz-Telles F, de Camargo ZP. Detection of circulating gp43 antigen in serum, cerebrospinal fluid, and bronchoalveolar lavage fluid of patients with paracoccidioidomycosis. J Clin Microbiol 2003; 41:3675–80.

281. Marques da Silva SH, Colombo AL, Blotta MH, Queiroz-Telles F, Lopes JD, de Camargo ZP. Diagnosis of neuroparacoccidioidomycosis by detection of circulating antigen and antibody in cerebrospinal fluid. J Clin Microbiol 2005; 43:4680–3.

282. Marques da Silva SH, de Mattos Grosso D, Lopes JD, et al. Detection of *Paracoccidioides brasiliensis* gp70 circulating antigen and follow-up of patients undergoing antimycotic therapy. J Clin Microbiol 2004; 42:4480–6.

283. Yuen KY, Wong SS, Tsang DN, Chau PY. Serodiagnosis of *Penicillium marneffei* infection. Lancet 1994; 344:444–5.

284. Kaufman L, Standard PG, Jalbert M, Kantipong P, Limpakarnjanarat K, Mastro TD. Diagnostic antigenemia tests for penicilliosis marneffei. J Clin Microbiol 1996; 34:2503–5.

285. Chongtrakool P, Chaityaroj SC, Vithayasai V, et al. Immunoreactivity of a 38-kilodalton *Penicillium marneffei* antigen with human immunodeficiency virus-positive sera. J Clin Microbiol 1997; 35:2220–3.

286. Vanittanakom N, Mekaprateep M, Sittisombut N, et al. Western immunoblot analysis of protein antigens of *Penicillium marneffei*. J Med Vet Mycol 1997; 35:123–31.

287. Jeavons L, Hamilton AJ, Vanittanakom N, et al. Identification and purification of specific *Penicillium marneffei* antigens and their recognition by human immune sera. J Clin Microbiol 1998; 36:949–54.

288. Cao L, Chan CM, Lee C, Wong SS, Yuen KY. *MP1* encodes an abundant and highly antigenic cell wall mannoprotein in the pathogenic fungus *Penicillium marneffei*. Infect Immun 1998; 66:966–73.

289. Cao L, Chen DL, Lee C, et al. Detection of specific antibodies to an antigenic mannoprotein for diagnosis of *Penicillium marneffei penicilliosis*. J Clin Microbiol 1998; 36:3028–31.

290. Cao L, Chan KM, Chen D, et al. Detection of cell wall mannoprotein Mp1p in culture supernatants of *Penicillium marneffei* and in sera of penicilliosis patients. J Clin Microbiol 1999; 37:981–6.

291. Desakorn V, Smith MD, Walsh AL, et al. Diagnosis of *Penicillium marneffei* infection by quantitation of urinary antigen by using an enzyme immunoassay. J Clin Microbiol 1999; 37:117–21.

292. Desakorn V, Simpson AJ, Wuthiekanun V, et al. Development and evaluation of rapid urinary antigen detection tests for diagnosis of penicilliosis marneffei. J Clin Microbiol 2002; 40:3179–83.

293. Trewatcharegon S, Chaiyaroj SC, Chongtrakool P, Sirisinha S. Production and characterization of monoclonal antibodies reactive with the mycelial and yeast phases of *Penicillium marneffei*. Med Mycol 2000; 38:91–6.

294. Pnaichakul T, Chawengkirttikul R, Chaiyaroj SC, Sirisinha S. Development of a monoclonal antibody-based enzyme-linked immunosorbent assay for the diagnosis of *Penicillium marneffei* infection. Am J Trop Med Hyg 2002; 67:443–7.

295. Chaiyaroj SC, Chawengkirttikul R, Sirisinha S, Watkins P, Srinoulprasert Y. Antigen detection assay for identification of *Penicillium marneffei* infection. J Clin Microbiol 2003; 41:432–4.

296. Blumer SO, Kaufman L, Kaplan W, McLaughlin DW, Kraft DE. Comparative evaluation of five serological methods for the diagnosis of Sporotrichosis. Appl Microbiol 1973; 26:4–8.

297. Scott EN, Kaufman L, Brown AC, Muchmore HG. Serologic studies in the diagnosis and management of meningitis due to *Sporothrix schenckii*. N Engl J Med 1987; 317:935–40.

298. Scott EN, Muchmore HG. Immunoblot analysis of antibody responses to *Sporothrix schenckii*. J Clin Microbiol 1989; 27:300–4.

299. Mendoza M, Diaz AM, Hung MB, Zambrano EA, Diaz E, de Albornoz MC. Production of culture filtrates of *Sporothrix schenckii* in diverse culture media. Med Mycol 2002; 40:447–54.

300. Jones KW, Kaufman L. Development and evaluation of an immunodiffusion test for diagnosis of systemic zygomycosis (mucormycosis): preliminary report. J Clin Microbiol 1978; 7:97–103.

301. Kaufman L, Turner LF, McLaughlin DW. Indirect enzyme-linked immunosorbent assay for zygomycosis. J Clin Microbiol 1989; 27:1979–82.

302. Kaufman L, Mendoza L, Standard PG. Immunodiffusion test for serodiagnosing subcutaneous zygomycosis. J Clin Microbiol 1990; 28:1887–90.

303. Lyon GM, Smilack JD, Komatsu KK, et al. Gastrointestinal basidiobolomycosis in Arizona: clinical and epidemiological characteristics and review of the literature. Clin Infect Dis 2001; 32:1448–55.

304. Pasha TM, Leighton JA, Smilack JD, Heppell J, Colby TV, Kaufman L. Basidiobolomycosis: an unusual fungal infection mimicking inflammatory bowel disease. Gastroenterology 1997; 112:250–4.

5

Detection of Fungal Metabolites

Tania C. Sorrell

Centre for Infectious Diseases and Microbiology and Westmead Millennium Institute, University of Sydney, and Department of Infectious Diseases, Westmead Hospital, Westmead, New South Wales, Australia

INTRODUCTION

Detection of fungal metabolites in infected tissues and body fluids is a potentially attractive approach to rapid diagnosis and monitoring of deep mycoses. Secondary metabolites and other macromolecular compounds, such as proteins, lipids, or carbohydrates isolated from respective groups of microorganisms, are utilized in chemotaxonomic approaches to the classification and identification of fungi and lichenized fungi (1). In human mycoses, most investigators have focused on two acyclic polyols, D-arabinitol and D-mannitol (2). To date, only the 5-carbon compound, D-arabinitol, has been validated as a practical diagnostic marker of an invasive mycosis, namely, candidiasis. This test is specific for species within the genus *Candida* (2). It can yield a positive result within a few hours (3), in contrast to the slower, more cumbersome and labor-intensive battery of conventional culture, morphology, and assimilation tests. Rapid, polyphasic methods for simultaneous identification of chemicals in complex solutions, biofluids, or tissues, for example, nuclear magnetic resonance (NMR) spectroscopy and gas chromatography-mass spectrometry (GC-MS), have recently been developed. With this advance and the development of sophisticated computer-based methods for analysis of complex data, new, rapid, simple-to-perform, phenotypic approaches to fungal diagnosis have become feasible. In this chapter, current and experimental methods for detection of fungal metabolites in biofluids and tissues are discussed.

Polyols

Polyols are polyhydric alcohols derived from sugars and are present in almost all living organisms (4). Pathogenic yeasts and filamentous fungi produce acyclic polyols including D-mannitol, D-arabinitol, erythritol, and glycerol in culture. The relative abundance of each polyol depends on the fungal genus and growth conditions. For example, D-arabinitol is the predominant polyol produced by *Candida albicans* (5) and large amounts of D-mannitol are produced by *Cryptococcus neoformans* (6,7) and *Aspergillus* spp. (4,8). *C. albicans* is a net producer of D-arabinitol during the logarithmic phase of growth, with most being released into the medium, whereas synthesis and secretion of D-mannitol by *C. neoformans* is maximal in the stationary phase. In *Aspergillus* spp. most of the D-mannitol produced remains cell-associated. The serum and urine of human subjects also contains low concentrations of polyols that are produced by metabolism of endogenous or dietary substrates or ingested in food. L-arabinitol is the most abundant, followed by erythritol, D-mannitol, and threitol (9). Serum levels of the polyols arabinitol, mannitol, sorbitol, myoinositol, and anhydroglucitol vary significantly between healthy individuals and the variation is greatest for mannitol. Polyol levels are also influenced by diet, renal dysfunction, and metabolic disorders such as diabetes mellitus, meningitis, sepsis, and cerebral atrophy (9,10). The L-enantiomer of arabinitol is the form produced by mammalian cells, whereas fungi produce the D-enantiomer; thus, quantitation of D-arabinitol will identify arabinitol of fungal origin (4,5,11).

Arabinitol: A Marker of Invasive Candidiasis

The possibility that fungal sugars might be diagnostic markers of candidemia and invasive candidiasis (IC) was first raised in 1974 (12). Miller et al. detected four water-soluble compounds, two with chromatographic characteristics of isomers of mannose and two that were not identified, in sera from patients with candidemia when analyzed by gas liquid chromatography (GLC). Diagnostic levels of arabinitol, the major polyol produced by *C. albicans*, were subsequently identified by GLC in sera of patients with IC but also in patients with renal failure (13). It was then shown that arabinitol is excreted in urine quantitatively at a rate equal to creatinine clearance (14) and that serum levels could be corrected for renal dysfunction by expressing them as the ratio of arabinitol to creatinine clearance (15,16). In experimental animals with candidemia and other forms of IC (15,17,18), arabinitol levels correlated with fungal load and declined after institution of effective therapy, suggesting a potential use in both diagnosis and monitoring therapeutic response. Furthermore, levels were not increased in animals that were heavily colonized but not infected (19). The potential value of arabinitol as a diagnostic marker of candidiasis was improved following recognition that the D-enantiomer is the form produced by fungi, whereas the L-enantiomer is the form produced by vertebrates. Diagnoses of candidiasis based on analytic methods that distinguish D-arabinitol from the L-arabinitol produced by the host are more accurate than those which measure total arabinitol (2,20).

Technical and sampling issues have limited introduction of arabinitol assays into clinical practice. Specifically, initial investigations used sophisticated instrumentation not commonly present in routine diagnostic laboratories and/or cumbersome and time-consuming methods. Furthermore, obtaining repeated blood samples from low birth weight neonates, a group at significant risk of IC, is problematic. Simple, rapid, enzyme-based colorimetric or fluorometric assays that are amenable to automation were subsequently developed, based on metabolism of arabinitol by the nicotinamide adenine dinucleotide (NAD)-dependent enzyme, D-arabinitol dehydrogenase (ArDH), obtained from *Enterobacter aerogenes* (21). The specificity of this assay (mannitol, which is produced by other fungi and is present in human serum is an alternative substrate for this enzyme—see below) was improved by using ArDR prepared from *Candida tropicalis* (22), then recombinant ArDR from *C. albicans* (23). These two latter assays are not affected by L-arabinitol, D-mannitol, or other polyols in human serum (except for 3% cross-reactivity with xylitol, which is present in sera from healthy humans at a fivefold lower concentration than D-arabinitol). Nor were they affected by 17 therapeutic drugs likely to be present in serum of patients at high risk of IC (22). Of advantage to routine laboratories is the fact that both assays can be automated and read in a standard clinical chemistry analyzer but neither is available commercially. The problem of blood sampling in neonates was resolved by using urine samples that had been collected on to filter paper, extracting the polyols, derivatizing them, and measuring the ratio of D-/L-arabinitol (which is not affected by renal function) by GC-MS (24). Though promising results were obtained, such equipment is not available in routine laboratories, little is known about L-arabinitol distribution and excretion in humans, and only a small proportion of samples from infected patients was positive (see below).

Clinical Studies

Salient findings of nine published clinical trials are summarized in Table 1. It should be noted that the method of patient selection and type of controls varied and that five of these studies were conducted in patients with cancer. Only one, the most recent, involved an unselected cohort of patients from a population-based study of candidemia (25). The early studies did not distinguish between D- and L-arabinitol or correct for renal function. In addition, serum or urine was used as the test sample in different studies and different cut-offs were used to identify a positive result. Only three studies included more than 17 patients with proven IC. Because of the small sample sizes, 95% confidence intervals for sensitivity and specificity were calculated from data given in the published studies and are included in Table 1.

Despite methodological differences, it is evident that the sensitivity of the tests is higher for patients with candidemia (76–100% in five studies and 83% for persisting fungemia and 50% for transient fungemia in one) than in those with

Table 1 Clinical Studies of Arabinitol in Patients with IC

Method	Parameter	Cut-off	Host	IC[a] (+)/total cases	Sensitivity	Colonized (+)/total	Control (+)/total	Specificity	Refs. (year)
Serum									
GLC	Arabinitol	1 µg/mL	Cancer	4/8	50% (16–84)	0/20	0/65	100% (96–100)	13 (1979)
				11/12 RF[b]	92% (62–100)	3/8 RF[b]	0/0 RF	63% (25–92)	
GC-MS	Arabinitol	1.2 µg/mL	Not stated	9/11	81% (48–98)	0/6		100% (54–100)	17 (1980)
GLC	Arabinitol/creatinine	1.51	Cancer	16/25 (11/11 BC+)	64% (43–82) (BC+) (100%)	Included in controls	3/88 (cancer patients)	97% (90–99)	16 (1983)
Enzyme assay	D-arabinitol/creatinine	≥4.0 µmol/L	Cancer-inpatient	11/26 IC tissue BC+	42% (23–63)	19/66 (high-risk)	9/140 (low-risk)	71% (59–82) (by high-risk patient)	3 (1995)
				6/12 transient	50% (21–79)		1/404 (blood donors)	94% (88–97) (by low-risk patient)	
				25/30 persistent	83% (65–94)			99.7% (99–100) (by blood donors)	
Enzyme assay	D-arabinitol/creatinine	Not stated	Immuno-competent	1.64–2.23 µmol/mg/dL (n=11, all BC+)			1.1–1.58 (n=10)		23 (2000)
Enzyme assay	D-arabinitol/creatinine	≥3.9 µM/ng/dL	Unselected	40/83 (initial sample)	48%	Not known	11/100 (hospital patients)	89%	25 (2006)
				63/83 (all samples)	76%		0/30 (healthy controls)	100%	

Urine

Method	Metabolite		Group						Ref.
GC-MS	D-/L-arabinitol ratio	4.0	Hematol. malignancies	15/17 (creatinine raised in 2)	88% (64–99) (by patient)	2/22	1/22 (neutropenic)	91% (79–98) (by patient)	26 (1996)
				32/53 (samples)	60% (46–74) (by sample)		0/50 (healthy adults)	95% (89–98) (by sample) 100% (93–100) (healthy controls)	
GC	D-/L-arabinitol ratio	4.6	Cancer+ neutropenia	10/10 (IC)	100% (69–100)	Included with controls	4/63	94% (85–98)	27 (1997)
				12/23 (empiric therapy group)	52% (31–73)		16/86 (with empiric therapy)	81% (72–89)	
				22/33 (both)	67% (48–82)		4/63		
GC-MS	D-/L-arabinitol ratio	4.8	NICU pre- term neonates	6/6 (IC)	100% (54–100)	2/22 (MCC)	0/81	100% (96–100)	24 (2000)
				5/8 (empiric therapy)	79% (49–95)		2/103 (includes MCC)	98% (93–100)	
				11/14 (both)					

In an additional study (27) in neutropenic patients receiving empirical amphotericin B, urine D-/L-arabinitol was positive in one patient with persistent candidemia and in 0/4 with transient candidemia.

[a] IC, biopsy or autopsy-proven, with or without BC+.
[b] Renal failure.

Abbreviations: BC+, positive blood culture; GC-MS, gas chromatography mass spectrometry; GLC, gas liquid chromatography; IC, invasive candidiasis; MCC, mucocutaneous candidiasis; NICU, Neonatal Intensive Care Unit; RF, renal failure.

blood culture (BC) negative IC [40–44% (3) and 36% (16)]. The sensitivity of the assay is influenced by the number of samples, for example D-/L-arabinitol ratios were elevated in 71% of initial urine samples from patients with IC, rising to 88% with an average of 3.5 samples (26). The timing of the urine collections was not stated in this study and it is possible that the assay sensitivity would have been improved by testing concentrated early morning samples. In unselected patients with candidemia, the overall sensitivity of the assay increased from 48% in an initial serum sample to 76% based on multiple samples (25). The sensitivity of serum arabinitol as an indicator of occult IC is unknown as there is no gold standard for diagnosis. Furthermore, the result may be influenced by empirical antifungal therapy as shown in a study of neutropenic patients receiving empirical amphotericin B for presumed invasive fungal infection (28). The largest study of the effect of antifungal therapy on D-arabinitol, performed in patients with proven IC, showed that serum arabinitol levels declined or became negative during therapy [85–89% correlation with response (3)]. Smaller studies showed similar trends (22,24).

After correction for renal function, the specificity is high in most studies when calculated using healthy controls (97–100%), slightly lower using cancer patient populations or hospitalized patients suspected of having an infection as controls, and possibly as low as 71% (95% CI = 59–82%) in high-risk cancer patients. Exclusion of patients receiving empiric therapy (3,24,27) from specificity calculations on the grounds that they have occult IC increased the specificity from 71% to 94–100%. Notably, the specificity of the test for high-risk hematology patients also increased (to 93%) in one study when based on total serum samples rather than individual patients (3). In this study, false positives occurred in 17% of patients with bacteremia, three of eight with aspergillosis, but none of four with cryptococcosis and none of 60 with herpes virus infection. False positives were also noted in the presence of rapidly deteriorating renal function and pre-terminal multi-organ failure. Others have observed positive D-arabinitol/creatinine ratios in infants receiving long-term antibiotic therapy (29) and adults with bacteremia or other infections (who were presumably also receiving antibiotic therapy) (25). Some of the adult patients had multi-organ failure and deteriorating renal function. Though causality has not been established, observations in rats are consistent with an additional hypothesis, namely, that increased serum levels of D-arabinitol result from antibiotic-induced suppression of gastrointestinal bacteria, which usually metabolize D-arabinitol from the diet or that derived from colonizing *Candida* strains (19).

D-Arabinitol in IC due to Non-albicans Species of *Candida*

C. albicans remains the commonest cause of IC in many series. Of the major pathogenic yeast species, *C. albicans* produces the most D-arabinitol in vitro, followed by *Candida parapsilosis*, *Candida pseudotropicalis*, and *C. tropicalis*, whereas none is either assimilated or produced by *Candida glabrata* or *Candida krusei* (5,30). Data from only two clinical studies have been analyzed by species.

Walsh et al. reported that the sensitivity of the serum assay was similar for *C. albicans, C. tropicalis, C. glabrata,* and *C. parapsilosis* but negative in single cases of fungemia due to *C. krusei, Candida lusitaneae,* and *Candida guilliermondii.* (3). The urinary D-/L-arabinitol ratio was unexpectedly positive in two patients with candidiasis due to *C. glabrata* and *C. krusei,* respectively (26,28), since these species produce only trace amounts or no D-arabinitol in vitro (5). However, a larger study confirmed that the serum D-arabinitol/creatinine ratio was positive in a substantially smaller proportion of patients with fungemia due to *C. glabrata* than other species (*C. krusei* was not included in this analysis) (25).

Serum D-Arabinitol in Clinical Practice

There are no recent or prospective studies comparing the sensitivity and specificity of D-arabinitol detection with antigen/antibody assays or DNA-based tests, nor are there studies in critically ill patients, which comprise one of the groups at highest risk [e.g., (31)]. As with DNA based tests, the methods and interpretation of D-arabinitol measurements have not been standardized, although promising results have been obtained in different laboratories. Arabinitol detection is fast, methods suitable for automated measurement in routine clinical laboratories have been developed, and the range of sensitivity and specificity of the test appears comparable with antigen-antibody detection and polymerase chain reaction (PCR) for patients with candidemia. Exclusive of the instrumentation required, the test is cheap and applicable to readily obtained body fluids (serum and urine). As with other methods of detection of candidemia, false-positives occur in some patients deemed on clinical grounds to be colonized, but not infected (Table 1).

As a specific diagnostic test, measurement of serum D-arabinitol is limited by the inability to distinguish between *Candida* spp. and hence guide antifungal drug selection based on species association. It is not reliable for detection of *C. glabrata* or *C. krusei* infections, as these species either do not produce D-arabinitol or the amount secreted is below the limit of detection.

False positives have been noted in a minority of febrile neutropenic patients with bacteremia or invasive aspergillosis (3) and in hospitalized patients with bacterial infection of the blood or other body sites (25). However, except in units with a high incidence of *C. krusei* or *C. glabrata* infections, D-arabinitol shows promise as a screening test since it is less labor intensive and less costly than PCR and cheaper than antigen-antibody based assays and could therefore be done more frequently. In a study involving twice-weekly screening of high-risk febrile neutropenic patients, 53% of candidemias were identified before the results of BC became available (3). In comparison, the Platelia antigen-antibody assay was positive in 60% of samples prior to growth of yeast in a hematology/intensive care population (32). Screening by detection of fungal beta-D-glucan (commercial Glucatell and Fungitec-G assays) may be more sensitive (discussed in detail in chap. 9). A recent report showed that these tests were positive before the clinical diagnosis of proven or probable invasive fungal infection (*Candida* and non-*Candida* spp.) in 100% of patients with acute myeloid leukemia or myelodysplastic syndrome and 70% of those with proven, probable, or possible infection (33). Notably, all patients were receiving antifungal prophylaxis at the time of study. D-arabinitol/creatinine clearance ratios are of potential value in monitoring the efficacy of antifungal therapy, since they parallel the therapeutic response; conversely, mortality is increased in patients whose levels fail to decrease after three days of antifungal therapy (25).

Mannitol

Aspergillosis

As BC are typically negative in disseminated aspergillosis, rapid detection of specific antigens or secreted metabolites in serum is a potentially attractive diagnostic strategy. The *Aspergillus* spp. that are responsible for most cases of human aspergillosis produce large amounts of mannitol in vitro, though most remains cell-associated (4,8). Serum and tissue levels were elevated in rats with experimental aspergillosis; however, preliminary data from cases of human aspergillosis have not been promising (2).

Cryptococcal Meningitis

Detection of cryptococcal polysaccharide antigen in cerebrospinal fluid (CSF) (and serum) is a rapid, sensitive, specific, and readily available diagnostic test. However, it is a poor indicator of microbiological response to therapy because the antigen is cleared slowly from the CSF in vivo. Large quantities of D-mannitol and glycerol, small amounts of glucitol and erythritol, and no arabinitol, are secreted by actively metabolizing strains of *C. neoformans* during the stationary phase of growth in vitro (6,7). Small quantities of five polyols (arabinitol, anhydroglucitol, mannitol, sorbitol, and myoinositol) arising from neural tissue are present in human CSF (10). In a steroid-treated rabbit model of acute cryptococcal meningitis, CSF mannitol levels correlated with fungal load and cryptococcal Ag titers. CSF kinetic studies in the rabbit indicated that continued production of significant amounts of mannitol is needed to maintain high levels and that quantification may therefore be of value in monitoring the microbiological response to therapy. In a single study of HIV-infected patients with cryptococcal meningitis, elevated mannitol concentrations of 1.5 to 26.2 mg/L were recorded in 20/22 CSF samples but did not correlate with cryptococcal antigen titers (0–1:2048). This might be explained in part by the differences in CSF kinetics between rabbits and humans. In rabbits, approximately 90% of CSF produced per day is absorbed into the lymph (34) whereas in humans most is reabsorbed through arachnoid villi and cerebral granulations. Alternatively, because most CSF samples were obtained during maintenance antifungal therapy for meningitis, the lack of correlation may reflect the different kinetics of clearance of mannitol and capsular polysaccharide from the CSF. In this study, mannitol levels were determined by gas chromatography (35). The practicality and value of quantifying

CSF mannitol as an objective measure of response to therapy in cryptococcal meningitis requires prospective study and development of a simple method that is suitable for use in a routine diagnostic laboratory.

THE FUTURE: POLYPHASIC METHODS OF METABOLITE PROFILING—PROTON NMR SPECTROSCOPY

NMR spectroscopy identifies a broad range of metabolites in solution rapidly and simultaneously and can be applied to living microbial cells, body tissues, and fluids, and to non-invasive diagnosis of pathological lesions in the clinic, as in neurospectroscopy (30,36–41). Practical use of such methods requires the initial development of a reference data set. Sensitivity and specificity are maximized by analysis of the full NMR spectrum using computerized pattern recognition techniques that may involve data reduction by automated selection of the most discriminatory regions of the spectra, followed by linear discriminant analytical methods (42,43). Pathogenic *Candida* and *Cryptococcus* spp. have been distinguished by such methods. In this case the major differences relied on the yeast species-specific profiles of polyols and carbohydrates (30). The unique cryptococcal metabolite profile was identified in biopsy material from animal models of cryptococcoma using ^{1}H NMR spectroscopy (37,38,41) and is under investigation in cryptococcal meningitis (Himmelreich and Sorrell, submitted for publication). The ease of sample preparation, which requires no processing, and the rapid turnaround time (less than five minutes per sample), is attractive for clinical applications.

A potentially exciting application of NMR spectroscopy lies in the linkage of magnetic resonance imaging (MRI) and magnetic resonance (MR) spectroscopy, which can be achieved in a single examination in the clinic. Neurospectroscopy is already in use for the non-invasive diagnosis of cerebral tumors, stroke, and pyogenic brain abscesses, and characteristic polyol resonances have been identified in a case of cerebral cryptococcoma (41).

CONCLUSION

Characteristics of an assay for fungal metabolite(s) suitable for introduction into in the routine clinical microbiology laboratory include the following: (*i*) metabolite(s) of interest is/are present in serum in amounts proportional to the viable fungal load; (*ii*) it is selective for fungi and preferably for a fungal genus or species; (*iii*) the assay is simple, rapid, sensitive, and specific; and (*iv*) it is of diagnostic value as well useful for monitoring therapeutic response. To date measurement of D-arabinitol for the diagnosis of IC has demonstrated that this approach is feasible. Metabolite profiling ("metabolomics") using methods such as NMR spectroscopy or other polyphasic approaches (infrared spectroscopy, GC-MS) amenable to automated statistical analysis by pattern recognition methods offer promise for the future.

REFERENCES

1. Frisvad JC, Bridge PD, Arora DK. Chemical Fungal Taxonomy. New York: Marcel Dekker, 1998.
2. Yeo SF, Wong B. Non-culture methods for diagnosis of fungal infections. Clin Microbiol Rev 2002; 15:465–84.
3. Walsh TJ, Merz WG, Lee JW, et al. Diagnosis and therapeutic monitoring of invasive candidiasis by rapid enzymic detection of serum D-arabinitol. Am J Med 1995; 99:164–72.
4. Touster O, Shaw DRD. Biochemistry of the acyclic polyols. Physiol Rev 1962; 42:181–225.
5. Bernard EM, Christiansen KJ, Tsang SF, Kiehn TE, Armstrong D. Rate of arabinitol production by pathogenic yeast species. J Clin Micro 1981; 14:189–94.
6. Wong B, Perfect JR, Beggs S, Wright KA. Production of the hexitol D-mannitol by *Cryptococcus neoformans* in vitro and in rabbits with experimental meningitis. Infect Immun 1990; 58:1664–70.
7. Bubb WA, Wright LC, Cagney M, Santangelo RT, Sorrell TC, Kuchel PW. Heteronuclear NMR studies of metabolites produced by *Cryptococcus neoformans* in culture media: identification of possible virulence factors. Magn Reson Med 1999; 42:442–53.
8. Dijkema C, Kester HCM, Visser J. ^{13}C NMR studies of carbon metabolism in the hyphal fungus *Aspergillus nidulans*. Proc Natl Acad Sci USA 1985; 82:14–18.
9. Roboz J, Kappatos C, Greaves J, Holland J. Determination of polyols in serum by selected ion monitoring. Clin Chem 1984; 30:1611–5.
10. Servo C, Palo J, Pitkanen E. Gas chromatographic separation and mass spectrometric identification of polyols in human cerebrospinal fluid and plasma. Acta Neurol Scand 1997; 56:111–6.
11. Bernard EM, Wong B, Armstrong D. Stereoisomeric configuration of arabinitol in serum, urine and tissues in invasive candidiasis. J Infect Dis 1985; 151:711–5.
12. Miller GG, Witwer MW, Braude AI, Davis CE. Rapid identification of *Candida albicans* septicemia in man by gas–liquid chromatography. J Clin Invest 1974; 54:1235–40.
13. Kiehn TE, Bernard EM, Gold JWM, Armstrong D. Candidiasis: detection by gas–liquid chromatography of D-arabinitol, a fungal metabolite, in human serum. Science 1979; 206:577–80.
14. Wong B, Bernard EM, Gold JW, Fong D, Armstrong D. The arabinitol appearance rate in laboratory animals and humans; estimation from the arabinitol/creatinine ratio and relevance to the diagnosis of candidiasis. J Infect Dis 1982; 146:353–9.
15. Wong B, Bernard EM, Gold JW, Fong D, Silber A, Armstrong D. Increased arabinitol levels in experimental candidiasis in rats: arabinitol appearance rates, arabinitol/creatinine ratios and severity of infection. J Infect Dis 1982; 146:346–52.
16. Gold JW, Wong B, Bernard EM, Kiehn TE, Armstrong D. Serum arabinitol concentrations and arabinitol/creatinine ratios in invasive candidiasis. J Infect Dis 1983; 147:504–13.
17. Roboz J, Suzuki R, Holland JF. Quantification of arabinitol in serum by selected ion monitoring as a diagnostic technique in invasive candidiasis. J Clin Microbiol 1980; 12:594–602.

18. Walsh TJ, Lee JW, Sien T, et al. Serum D-arabinitol measured by automated quantitative enzymatic assay for detection and therapeutic monitoring of experimental disseminated candidiasis: correlation with tissue concentrations of *Candida albicans*. J Med Vet Mycol 1994; 32:205–15.

19. Wong B, Brauer KL, Clemens JR, Beggs S. Effects of gastrointestinal candidiasis, antibiotics, dietary arabinitol and cortisone acetate on levels of the *Candida* metabolite D-arabinitol in rat serum and urine. Infect Immun 1990; 58:283–8.

20. Wong B, Brauer KL. Enantioselective measurement of fungal D-arabinitol in the sera of normal adults and patients with candidiasis. J Clin Microbiol 1988; 26:1670–4.

21. Soyama K, Ono E. Improved procedure for determining serum D-arabinitol by reazurin-coupled method. Clin Chim Acta 1987; 168:259–60.

22. Switchenko AC, Miyada CG, Goodman TC, et al. An automated enzymatic method of measurement of D-arabinitol, a metabolite of pathogenic *Candida* species. J Clin Microbiol 1994; 32:92–7.

23. Yeo SF, Zhang Y, Schafer D, Campbell S, Wong B. A rapid, automated enzymatic fluorometric assay for determination of D-arabinitol in serum. J Clin Microbiol 2000; 38:1439–43.

24. Sigmundsdottir G, Christensson B, Bjorklund LJ, Hakansson K, Pehrson C, Larsson L. Urine D-arabinitol/L-arabinitol ratio in diagnosis of invasive candidiasis in newborn infants. J Clin Microbiol 2000; 38:3039–42.

25. Yeo SF, Huie S, Sofair AN, Campbell S, Durante A, Wong B. Sensitivity, specificity, timeliness, and correlation with outcome of serum D-arabinitol/creatinine ratios in an unselected, population-based sample of patients with *Candida* fungemia. J Clin Microbiol 2006 (epub ahead of print 6th September); 44:3894–9.

26. Lehtonen L, Anttila VJ, Ruutu T, et al. Diagnosis of disseminated candidiasis by measurement of urine D-arabinitol/L-arabinitol ratio. J Clin Microbiol 1996; 34:2175–9.

27. Christensson B, Wiebe T, Pehrson C, Larsson L. Diagnosis of invasive candidiasis in neutropenic children with cancer by determination of D-arabinitol/L-arabinitol ratios in urine. J Clin Microbiol 1997; 35:636–40.

28. Salonen JH, Rimpilainin M, Lehtonen L, Lehtonen OP, Nikoskelainen J. Measurement of D-arabinitol/L-arabinitol ratio in urine of neutropenic patients treated empirically with amphotericin B. Eur J Clin Microbiol Infect Dis 2001; 20:179–84.

29. Stradomska TJ, Bobula-Milewska B, Bauer A, et al. Urinary D-arabinitol/L-arabinitol levels in infants undergoing long-term antibiotic therapy. J Clin Microbiol 2005; 43:5351–4.

30. Himmelreich U, Somorjai RL, Dolenko B, et al. Rapid identification and chemical characterization of *Candida* species using nuclear magnetic resonance spectroscopy and a statistical classification strategy. Appl Environ Microbiol 2003; 69:4566–74.

31. Chen S, Slavin M, Nguyen Q, et al. Active surveillance for candidemia, Australia. Emerg Infect Dis 2006; 12:1508–16.

32. Sendid B, Poirot JL, Tabiouret M, et al. Combined detection of mannanaemia and antimannan antibodies as a strategy for the diagnosis of systemic infection caused by pathogenic *Candida* species. J Med Microbiol 2002; 51:433–42.

33. Odabasi Z, Mattiuzzi G, Estey E, et al. 1,3 beta-D-Glucan as a diagnostic adjunct for invasive fungal infections: validation, cutoff development, and performance in patients with acute myelogenous leukemia and myelodysplastic syndrome. Clin Infect Dis 2004; 39:199–205.
34. Erlich SS, McComb JG, Hyman S, Weiss MH. Ultrastructural morphology of the olfactory pathway for cerebrospinal fluid drainage in the rabbit. J Neurosurg 1989; 70:926–31.
35. Megson GM, Stevens DA, Hamilton JR, Denning DW. D-Mannitol in cerebrospinal fluid of patients with AIDS and cryptococcal meningitis. J Clin Microbiol 1996; 34:218–21.
36. Bourne R, Himmelreich U, Sharma A, Mountford C, Sorrell T. Identification of *Enterococcus, Streptococcus*, and *Staphylococcus* by multivariate analysis of proton magnetic resonance spectroscopic data from plate cultures. J Clin Microbiol 2001; 39:2916–23.
37. Himmelreich U, Dzendrowskyj T, Allen C, et al. Cryptococcomas distinguished from gliomas with MR spectroscopy: an experimental rat and cell culture study. Radiology 2001; 220:122–8.
38. Himmelreich U, Allen C, Dowd S, et al. Identification of metabolites of importance in the pathogenesis of pulmonary cryptococcoma using nuclear magnetic resonance spectroscopy. Microb Infect 2003; 5:285–90.
39. Himmelreich U, Accurso R, Malik R, et al. Identification of *Staphylococcus aureus* brain abscesses: rat and human studies using ^{1}H magnetic resonance spectroscopy. Radiology 2005; 236:261–70.
40. Howe FA, Opstad KS. ^{1}H MR spectroscopy of brain tumours and masses. NMR Biomed 2003; 16:123–31.
41. Himmelreich U, Sorrell TC, Dzendrowskyj T, Malik R, Mountford CE. Identification of *Cryptococcus neoformans* by magnetic resonance spectroscopy. Microbiol Aust 2002; 23:31–3.
42. Lean CL, Somorjai RL, Smith ICP, Russell P, Mountford CE. Accurate diagnosis and prognosis of human cancers by proton MRS and a three-stage classification strategy. Annu Rep NMR Spectrosc 2002; 48:71–111.
43. Baumgartner R, Somorjai R, Bowen C, Sorrell TC, Mountford CE, Himmelreich U. Unsupervised feature dimension reduction for classification of MR spectra. Magn Reson Imaging 2004; 22:251–6.

6

Molecular Diagnostics: Present and Future

Holger Hebart, Juergen Loeffler, and Hermann Einsele

*Department of Hematology and Oncology, Medizinische Klinik,
Tübingen, Germany*

INTRODUCTION

Invasive fungal infections have become the major cause of infectious morbidity and mortality in immunosuppressed patients. Despite many efforts to develop sensitive detection methods, the diagnosis of invasive fungal infections still remains difficult in many cases. Several reasons are responsible for these limitations, such as unspecific and variable clinical signs that occur late in the course of disease, broad differences between patient cohorts with respect to individual risk periods ranging for a short period of time or for years, and, especially, a lack of diagnostic methods with sufficient sensitivity and specificity. In consequence, invasive fungal infections are often diagnosed late, leading to a delayed initiation of antifungal therapy, which is often fatal.

This review discusses and compares the tools that are available today for molecular diagnosis of invasive fungal infections. Because *Candida* and *Aspergillus* account for more than 80% of all fungal episodes in stem cell and solid organ transplantation, this chapter will focus on developments of molecular methods for invasive candidiasis and invasive aspergillosis (IA).

GENERAL ASPECTS OF NUCLEIC ACID BASED DIAGNOSTIC

Although a large number of manuscripts dealing with the detection of fungal DNA in clinical samples has been published since the first presentation of the polymerase chain reaction (PCR) by Saiki et al. (1) in the year 1988, up to now, no commercially nucleic acid-based detection system is available.

The critical and important issues for the detection of fungal DNA by PCR from clinical material are the type of clinical material and its sampling, the DNA extraction protocol, the PCR design, the detection and specification of the amplicon, the need for appropriate controls (especially to exclude contamination), and whether quantitation of the fungal DNA load by real-time PCR assays is beneficial.

Clinical Material and Collection of Specimens

The choice of the clinical specimen to be analyzed to make a diagnosis of invasive infection is a key question in medical microbiology. For diagnosis of an invasive fungal infection, the ideal material should be easily assessable and be free of fungal DNA in a healthy individual. Moreover, the clinical material should be taken from a body site affected by the infection.

Blood and blood fractions are potentially free of fungal DNA and can be easily collected. In patients affected by an invasive fungal infection this material may contain phagocytes with phagocyted conidia and hyphae, free fungal cell elements, and/or free circulating fungal DNA. Various groups, including ours, have addressed the question whether cell-free blood components such as serum or plasma or whole blood should be preferentially used for analysis. In a previous study, we examined the detection limit on plasma and whole blood samples and found that the assay was more sensitive when performed on whole blood rather than on plasma (2). In line with these results, PCR on serum samples was found to be not more or even less sensitive compared to the galactomannan detection method (3–6). However, the lower amount of fungal DNA in cell-free blood components did not affect the diagnostic sensitivity if highly sensitive nested PCR protocols were applied (7,8).

Bronchoalveolar lavage (BAL) is a method that allows for the detection of fungal DNA directly from sites of pulmonary infection. However, interpretation of PCR results from BAL might be hampered by distinguishing invasive infection from colonization (9). The negative predictive value of PCR from BAL samples was found to be consistently high in different reports using a variety of PCR protocols (10–12). In one study, the sensitivity correlated with the certainty of diagnosis based on histopathology (10).

Sputum samples show a very low specificity. Cerebrospinal fluid (CSF) can be used in selected cases with suspected invasive fungal infections (13). Hendolin et al. developed a panfungal PCR for the detection of *Aspergillus* DNA in tissue specimens from the paranasal sinuses (14). Jaeger et al. described an assay based on a nested PCR for fungal endophthalmitis (15). Moreover, biopsies of any potentially affected organ can be taken and analyzed by PCR (16,17).

In addition, clinical materials have to be collected according to defined rules. Blood samples should be collected using the anticoagulants ethylenediamintetraacetate (EDTA) or sodium citrate. The use of heparin is problematic, as heparin might inhibit the action of the Taq polymerase during PCR. Blood as well as plasma and serum should be transported to the laboratory and processed as fast as possible (18). Tissue samples that are paraffinized must be processed with a xylol–ethanol treatment prior to DNA extraction, and tissue treated with formalin should be extensively washed with sterile saline because formalin is an inhibitor of Taq polymerase. If possible, specimens should be transported to the laboratory frozen on ice or dry ice.

DNA Extraction

DNA extraction is the first and one of the most critical steps in designing fungal PCR protocols. Fungal DNA extraction should aim to reduce the amount of human and enrich for target fungal DNA, to eliminate potential Taq-inhibitors, and to avoid contamination with airborne spores. To achieve this goal, all published protocols for the extraction of fungal DNA involve red and white blood cell lysis, the disruption of the fungal cell wall, the release of fungal DNA, and the purification of the DNA (Fig. 1).

The lysis of red and white blood cells in whole blood specimens has to be performed prior to the fungal DNA extraction and can be efficiently achieved by the use of hypotonic buffers and proteinase K digestion. These steps are not needed for the analysis of serum and plasma specimens.

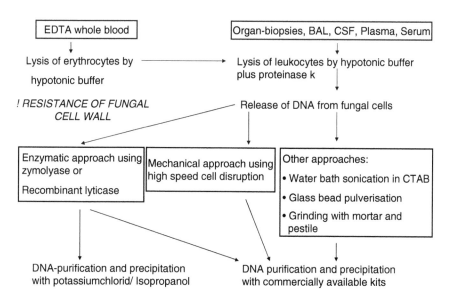

Figure 1 Extraction of DNA from *Aspergillus* spp. in clinical samples. *Abbreviations*: BAL, bronchoalveolar larage; CSF, cerebrospinal fluid; CTAB, cetyl trimethyl amonium aromide; EDTA, ethylenediamintetraacetate.

The release of fungal DNA can be achieved by enzymatic or mechanical approaches. Many investigators have used zymolyase and lyticase, β-1,3-glucanases to generate fungal spheroplasts (19). However, an efficient release of DNA from many molds, such as *Aspergillus niger*, *Aspergillus terreus*, *Mucorales*, and *Fusarium* spp. requires additional preparation steps such as boiling of the samples with NaOH (20), high-speed cell disruption, grinding with mortar and pestle, or repeated freeze-thawing using liquid nitrogen (21). Zymolyase, an enzyme extracted from brewery sewage, may contain traces of yeast DNA. Therefore, recombinant enzymes, such as recombinant lyticase should be preferably used for diagnostic assays.

For fungal DNA release and purification, phenol–chloroform extraction procedures were successfully applied (22). However, these protocols were time-consuming and rely on toxic chemicals. Furthermore, the cationic detergent cetyl trimethyl amonium aromide (CTAB) was successfully used to release *Aspergillus*-DNA (23) from blood and sputum specimens. The use of commercially available kits shortened the duration of DNA extraction (24). Investigators should keep in mind that the sensitivity of these kits varies widely. In our experience, only the Qiamp Tissue Kit® (Qiagen, Hilden, Germany) showed a comparable sensitivity of 10 cells/mL blood to the in-house method, whereas the lowest sensitivity was seen with the DNAzol kit (1000 cells/mL blood). The commercial kits are more expensive than any of the in-house methods. In another study, different DNA extraction methods were compared for the extraction of fungal DNA from sera artificially spiked with genomic DNA from *Candida* species (25). DNA purity and the detection limit were superior for the QIAamp DNA blood kit (Qiagen) and boiling of sera in an alkaline guanidine–phenol–Tris reagent compared to proteinase K digestion followed by organic extraction, the HighPure PCR template kit (Roche, Mannheim, Germany) and DNAzol (Sigma, Deissenhofen, Germany).

To make molecular diagnostics more reliable to routine clinical use, to reduce the risk of cross-contamination and to improve standardization of these diagnostic assays, automation of the complex extraction process is highly warranted (4). In a recently published study, fully automated DNA extraction from fungal cultures and from blood specimens was compared using the MagNA Pure LC technique to manual extraction (26). Fully automated extraction from cultures was achieved within one hour compared to four hours by manual extraction and within three hours from blood samples compared to seven hours by manual extraction. Thus, combining automated DNA extraction and real-time PCR permits results to be obtained within one working day.

Amplicon Detection

After amplification of fungal DNA by PCR, the underlying fungal pathogen needs to be identified to a species or genus level. The traditional methods include gel electrophoresis followed by hybridization protocols (Southern blot), Slot

Blots, or PCR-ELISA using species- or genus-specific probes. PCR protocols providing the amplification of a broad range of DNA from fungal pathogens using panfungal primer sets rely on these methods. Alternatively, a second amplification step using species-specific primers can be applied (nested PCR). Southern Blot assays were successfully applied to the detection of different *Aspergillus* species (10,27). The commercially available PCR-ELISA format from Roche was able to specifically detect *Aspergillus* DNA extracted from 10 CFU (20). In another study, the sensitivity of a plate hybridization assay and Southern Blotting showed an identical sensitivity of 1.5 pg; however, by plate assay, results were obtained within three hours (28). Sequence analysis for species identification of PCR amplicons from maxillary sinus aspirates was reported recently to be the most sensitive technique (success rate of 90.3%) compared with hybridization with a range of specific probes (77.4%) and culture of these aspirates (51.6%) (29). The differentiation of fungi by sequencing analysis has also been successfully explored by Turenne et al., who perform an automated fluorescent capillary electrophoresis system (30). Meletiadis et al. combined a PCR amplification of the ITS1 region with a reverse-hybridization line probe assay (LiPA). The authors were able to simultaneously detect and identify different *Aspergillus* species present in pure or mixed populations within six hours in a single assay (31).

Real-Time PCR

These recently developed PCR assays combine rapid in vitro amplification of DNA with real-time speciation and quantification of DNA load. The number of protocols for the detection of *Aspergillus*-DNA by real-time PCR tests is still limited. We have established a quantitative PCR protocol for the detection of *Aspergillus fumigatus* (32). The sensitivity of the assay was comparable to previously described PCR protocols (5 CFU/mL). The LightCycler® (Roche) allowed a quantification of fungal load in a limited number of clinical specimens from patients with hematological malignancies and histologically proven invasive fungal infection. Five out of nine positive samples showed a fungal load between 5 CFU/mL and 10 CFU/mL, 2/9 samples between 10 CFU/mL and 100 CFU/mL, and 2/9 samples were positive with more than 100 CFU/mL blood. The same assay was used to quantify the fungal burden in PCR-positive blood samples from animal models (33). None of 68 blood cultures from mice and rabbits were positive for *A. fumigatus*, whereas PCR detected *Aspergillus* DNA in 17 of 68 blood samples. Quantitative RT-PCR analysis of blood samples showed a fungus load of 10^1 to 10^2 CFU/mL of blood. The low fungal burden in the blood of patients with proven/probable IA and in experimental models of IA further highlights the need for a high sensitivity of a clinically valuable assay. Spiess and colleagues (34) reported a LightCycler assay for the detection of *A. fumigatus* DNA that demonstrated a lower clinical sensitivity compared to a nested PCR developed by the same investigators (35).

Bowman et al. developed a PCR to monitor disease progression and to measure the efficacy of caspofungin acetate in a murine model of disseminated aspergillosis. Because of its much larger dynamic range and its higher sensitivity, the quantitative PCR assay was concluded to be superior to traditional CFU determination for monitoring the progression of disseminated aspergillosis and evaluating the activity of antifungal compounds (36). Costa et al. developed two TaqMan® PCR tests (Applera, Norwalk, Connecticut, U.S.A.), targeting the mt gene and the FKS gene of *A. fumigatus* including a quantification of the fungal DNA load in spiked blood samples (37). Pham et al. report the design and evaluation of a real-time PCR assay for the detection of mould DNA in serum. The test permitted a cut-off of 110 fg (3 genomes). Quantitative analysis of the positive serum samples showed a mean fungal load of 1.6×10^5 genomes and a maximum fungal load of 4.2×10^7 genomes (38).

In a recent publication, real-time PCR targeting the 28S rRNA gene of *A. fumigatus* was reported to be as sensitive as the galactomannan sandwich ELISA; however, real-time PCR seemed to be more specific (6). In another study, real-time PCR on plasma samples was compared to the galactomannan sandwich ELISA and an assay for the detection of β-D-glucan (5). In this report, the galactomannan sandwich ELISA provided a higher sensitivity compared with RT-PCR, indicating that whole blood instead of plasma might be the preferred clinical sample. This assumption is further supported by the work of Kami et al. (39), which reports a superior diagnostic sensitivity of a RT-PCR assay on whole blood compared to ELISA methods for galactomannan and β-D-glucan.

Real-time quantitative PCR assays have been also developed for the rapid identification of *Candida* species. Targeting the ITS2 gene region, Guiver et al. reported a real-time TaqMan assay that allowed for the identification of six different *Candida* species (40). Loeffler and colleagues reported the rapid detection of point mutations by fluorescence resonance energy transfer and probe melting curves in *Candida* species (41). Maaroufi and colleagues described a rapid and reproducible PCR assay for quantitation of the *Candida albicans* ribosomal DNA (ITS region) in clinical blood samples based on the TaqMan principle (25). The TaqMan-based PCR assay for *C. albicans* exhibited a low limit of detection (5 CFU/mL of blood) and an excellent reproducibility (96–99%). In 11 culture and PCR positive samples, *C. albicans* loads extending from 5 to 100,475 CFU/mL of blood were reported. The sensitivity and specificity of the assay were 100% and 97%, respectively, compared with the results of blood culture. The same gene region was targeted for the rapid identification of commonly encountered *Candida* species from blood culture bottles using the LightCycler (42). Another potential application for real-time quantitative PCR is the expression analysis of genes mediating antifungal drug resistance (43).

In summary, various real-time PCR protocols have been developed that provide a rapid quantification of the fungal load in clinical specimens. As the clinical experience with these assays is still limited, prospective studies in large patient cohorts are warranted. Potential questions to be answered will be whether quantification of the fungal DNA load in BAL samples might be beneficial in helping to differentiate colonization from tissue-invasive infection and whether fungal load measurements in blood samples are of clinical value. In addition, these assays need to be evaluated for their clinical sensitivity and specificity in multi-center trials.

Contamination

Fungal spores such as conidia from *Aspergillus* spp. and other molds might be present in the air. Thus, airborne spore inoculation during the DNA extraction process could potentially lead to false-positive results, especially when panfungal primers are used. However, our experiences show that the frequency of contamination does not seem to be higher in fungal PCR than in diagnostic PCR-based techniques targeting non-fungal pathogens (44). Nevertheless, precautions to prevent airborne contamination as well as the use of sufficient negative controls have to be performed carefully. To monitor for contamination, aliquots of saline or DNA from healthy control persons should be prepared concurrently. For each 10 clinical samples analyzed, one extraction control and one PCR negative control should be included.

In a typical PCR amplification reaction, 10^{12} identical amplicons can be generated. As these amplicons may serve as targets for further reactions, carry-over contamination has to be excluded. Post-PCR treatment of the amplicons with UV light and 8-methoxypsoralen or pre-PCR uracil-DNA-glycosylase digestion have been proven to efficiently inactivate amplicons from previous PCR reactions. To minimize the risk of carry-over contamination, DNA extraction, amplification, and detection should be performed in separate rooms with equipment (pipettes, aerosol resistant tips, glassware) used exclusively for these purposes. Workers performing PCR assays should wear single use gowns, sterile gloves, and face masks and should not be allowed to move from the detection into the extraction area on the same day (45).

MOLECULAR DIAGNOSIS OF INVASIVE CANDIDIASIS

Candida species are among the most common pathogens isolated in immunosuppressed and intensive care unit (ICU) patients. *Candida* is the foremost common isolate in blood cultures, and candidemia is observed in the majority of patients with organ-invasive candidiasis. However, the fungal burden in the blood might be very low, such as in patients suffering from chronic disseminated candidiasis. In contrast to IA, bloodstream infections are the rule. Conventional blood cultures have a low sensitivity and many patients are diagnosed at autopsy only. The development of sensitive, specific, and rapid detection methods is thus of major importance to improve diagnosis of candida infections.

In 1990, Buchman et al. described the successful amplification of the gene encoding the *Candida*-specific enzyme lanosterol-14α-demethylase (46). The lower detection limit reported was 100 fungal cells/mL blood. The technique allowed detection of fungal genomes in a variety of clinical materials (urine, blood, sputum, wound drainage). Major disadvantages of this approach were its limitation to a restricted number of *Candida* species and its low sensitivity due to the fact that lanosterol-14α-demethylase is a single copy gene. Thus, the authors developed a nested PCR method with a higher sensitivity of 2 fungal cells/mL blood (47). Despite the improved sensitivity of the assay, only 76% of culture-positive blood samples were also PCR-positive. Moreover, the assay is restricted to *C. albicans*, *Candida glabrata*, *Candida krusei*, *Candida parapsilosis*, and *Candida tropicalis*, and therefore samples of a patient with septicemia due to *Candida kefyr* were persistently PCR-negative (47). Other groups developed PCR-based detection systems targeting gene sequences of the *C. albicans* heat shock protein 90 (48); Candida actin (49); EO3, a mitochondrial gene (50); and ribosomal DNA (51–53). For various reasons, all these assays lacked sensitivity and/or specificity when applied to clinical materials. Major factors responsible for the low sensitivity and specificity may be technical problems with the PCR assay as well as problems to extract enriched and very pure fungal DNA of clinical samples.

To determine whether a panfungal PCR assay allows one to identify patients at risk for invasive fungal infections, we performed a prospective monitoring once per week during 92 neutropenic episodes in patients receiving chemotherapy for acute leukemia or high-dose therapy followed by allogeneic or autologous stem cell transplantation, with the investigators blinded to clinical and microbiological data (54). PCR positivity was documented in 34 out of 92 risk episodes. In 17 out of these 34 PCR positive episodes *Candida* species were identified: *C. albicans* in 8, *C. albicans + Aspergillus* spp. in 4, and *C. glabrata* in 5 episodes. Systemic antifungal therapy was given in 12 out of 17 PCR positive episodes: in 4 patients for a previous history of invasive fungal infection, in 2 for proven invasive fungal infection (culture positive candidemia preceded by PCR by 14 days), and in 6 patients for possible fungal infection. These data indicate that patients with a previous history of candidemia as well as patients who later developed proven candidiasis were correctly identified by the panfungal PCR screening program. We concluded from this experience that prospective panfungal PCR screening for *Candida* DNA in the peripheral blood allows for the identification of patients at high risk for invasive candidiasis. In a prospective randomized trial comparing PCR-based versus empirical antifungal therapy, PCR-based intervention during the neutropenic episode was associated with a very low rate of fatal *Candida* infections (unpublished observation of the authors).

In another study by Lin and colleagues, the use of nested PCR to make therapeutic decisions was studied (55). Sequential blood samples obtained from 42 pediatric patients with neutropenia and cancer were tested by nested PCR targeting the 18S rRNA gene and culture. The sensitivity of the PCR assay was 1 fg for *C. albicans* and 10 fg for *A. fumigatus*. Instead of the empirical antifungal therapy strategy, amphotericin B treatment was initiated for patients who had two consecutive positive results by nested PCR. The second positive PCR result was available earlier than the final blood culture results (range, 1–8 days). The nested PCR approach was able to correctly identify patients with evidence for chronic disseminated candidiasis. Four of 22 patients with an episode of candidemia died. Thus, this study and results from our group indicate a potential utility for the use of sensitive PCR assays for early detection of fungal infection in febrile patients with neutropenia as a guideline for antifungal therapy. Prospective randomized studies comparing a targeted PCR-based approach to more traditional approaches such as empirical antifungal therapy in patients at high risk for invasive candidiasis are warranted.

MOLECULAR DIAGNOSIS OF INVASIVE ASPERGILLOSIS

The selection of a target gene followed by the design of the primers and probes are the most important issues when creating a PCR assay. In contrast to *Candida* spp. where a variety of PCR protocols based on single copy genes (lanosterol-14-alpha-demethylase, actin, chitin synthase) exist, the detection of mold DNA has been largely achieved by targeting multi-copy genes. More recently, Kanbe et al. described a nested PCR assay using specific primers binding to the DNA topoisomerase II gene (56). Primers targeting multi-copy genes bind to the 18S or 28S subunits of the ribosomal DNA (12,57,58) or to the highly variable intergenic transcribed spacer regions (ITS1-4) that are flanking the ribosomal gene regions (30,59,60). Furthermore, mitochondrial genes have been used for the design of primers for diagnostic assays (61). Luo et al. described a multiplex PCR with five sets of species-specific primers binding to the ITS1 and ITS2 regions. They found that this multiplex PCR method provided 100% sensitivity and specificity in testing a total of 242 fungal isolates (60).

Different PCR protocols have been evaluated on blood and BAL samples in patients with clinical evidence of IA (Table 1). Raad et al. performed a study on whole blood specimens from 54 patients with cancer. A PCR assay targeting the *A. fumigatus* mitochondrial DNA and the alkaline protease gene was performed on the day the patients underwent diagnostic bronchoscopy for newly developed pulmonary infiltrates. The sensitivity, specificity, and positive and negative predictive value were 100% for proven IA and 57%, 100%, 100% and 92%, respectively, for each of the probable and possible IA cases, indicating the high sensitivity of their PCR assay (62).

Ferns et al. described a PCR assay based on the amplification of a 135 bp fragment in the mitochondrial region of *A. fumigatus* or *Aspergillus flavus*. A high sensitivity of the nested PCR assay was described, and 6 of 7 patients supposed to have clinical evidence of IA were found to be PCR positive (66). Buchheidt et al. developed a nested PCR assay enabling the authors to detect

Table 1 PCR-Based Diagnosis of Invasive Aspergillosis

Authors	Method of PCR amplification and detection	Study population	Type and number of clinical specimen analyzed	Sensitivity	Specificity
Raad et al. (62)	*Aspergillus* mitochondrial, agarose gel electrophoresis	Cancer	Whole blood 54 patients	100% (with proven IA)	100% (with proven IA)
Hebart et al. (63)	Panfungal PCR, 18S rRNA Slot Blot	Stem cell transplantation	Whole blood (*n*=1193)	100%	65%
Lass-Florl et al. (64)	Panfungal PCR ITS1, ITS4 PCR-ELISA	Hematological malignancies, stem cell transplantation	Whole blood (*n*=619)	75%	84% (2 specimens) 96%
Buchheidt et al. (58)	*Aspergillus*-specific nested PCR 18S rRNA	Hematological malignancies	Whole blood (*n*=907) BAL (*n*=105)	91.7% 100%	81.3% 90.2%
Raad et al. (10)	*Aspergillus* mitochondrial polyacrylamide gel, Southern Blot	Cancer	BAL (*n*=249)	80%	93%
Buchheidt et al. (11)	*Aspergillus*-specific nested PCR 18S rRNA	Hematological malignancies	BAL (*n*=197)	93.9%	94.4%
Jones et al. (61)	*Aspergillus* mitochondrial PCR-ELISA	Hematological malignancies	BAL (*n*=75)	100%	100%
Einsele et al. (67)	Panfungal primers, 18s rRNA, Slot Blot	Allogeneic stem cell transplantation	BAL (*n*=261)	63%	98%

Abbreviations: BAL, bronchoalveolar lavage; ELISA, enzyme-linked immunosorbent assay; PCR, polymerase chain reaction.

10 fg of *Aspergillus*-DNA, corresponding to 1 to 5 CFU/mL of spiked samples in vitro (11).

Einsele and coworkers developed a PCR assay targeting the 18S rDNA region (57). The sensitivity of the assay in 21 patients with clinical evidence of an invasive fungal infection was 100% if two samples were analyzed. The sensitivity of the assay was improved from 88% to 100% if two instead of only one blood sample were analyzed, indicating that repetitive sampling is necessary to correctly identify patients with IA. In a prospective study, the same assay was used to prospectively screen 84 recipients of an allogeneic stem cell transplant 2 to 4 times/wk. *Aspergillus* spp.-specificity was achieved by oligonucleotide hybridization (63). The aim of this study was to assess the potential of prospective PCR screening for early diagnosis of IA. Of 1193 blood samples analyzed, 169 (14.2%) were positive by PCR. In patients with newly diagnosed IA ($n = 7$), PCR positivity preceded the first clinical signs by a median of two days (range, 1–23 days) and preceded clinical diagnosis of IA by a median of nine days (range, 2–34 days). Pre-transplantation IA, acute graft-versus-host disease, and corticosteroid treatment were associated with PCR positivity, factors known to be associated with a high risk for IA. The PCR assay had a sensitivity of 100% and a specificity of 65%. The specificity increased to 84% if calculations were based on 2 positive PCR results without a decrease in sensitivity. None of the PCR-negative patients developed IA during the study period. We concluded from this study that prospective PCR screening allows for the identification of patients at high risk for IA. These results were confirmed by independent investigators using the same PCR assay, in a study in which sensitivity and specificity estimates were 75% and 96%, respectively, (64).

An excellent sensitivity for a nested PCR assay in patients with clinical evidence of IA was reported by Skladny (35). They reported a 100% correlation between positive histology, culture, and high-resolution computed tomography findings and PCR results.

Recently, de Aguirre et al. described a PCR-enzyme immunoassay that utilized a single probe directed to the internal transcribed spacer 2 region of seven of the most medically important *Aspergillus* species (*A. fumigatus*, *A. flavus*, *A. nidulans*, *A. niger*, *A. terreus*, *Aspergillus ustus*, *Aspergillus versicolor*) (67). The assay gave no false-positive reactions with 33 other medically important molds and yeast species, including *Fusarium*, *Mucor*, and *Penicillium* species. The lower detection limit of this assay was 0.5 pg of fungal DNA.

Several clinical studies have clearly shown that PCR performed on BAL samples could be useful in the diagnosis of invasive pulmonary aspergillosis (9–12). Despite the fact that different PCR assays were evaluated, all these studies consistently demonstrated a high negative predictive value and good sensitivity and specificity. However, the positive predictive values of the assays varied considerably, reflecting differences in patient characteristics, certainty of diagnosis of invasive pulmonary aspergillosis, transient colonization of the respiratory tract, and other factors. In a large number of allogeneic stem cell transplant recipients, PCR positivity in BAL samples at the time of transplantation were found to be associated with the subsequent development of invasive pulmonary aspergillosis during episodes of intensive immunosuppression (65).

In addition, PCR has been successfully applied on CSF fluid (13), tissue specimens from the paranasal sinuses (14), ocular samples (15), and biopsies of any potentially affected organ (16,17).

Taken together, these results indicate a potential value of PCR assays to allow for a non-invasive diagnosis of IA. Further standardization of these assays and prospective evaluations in clinical trials are needed.

MOLECULAR DIAGNOSIS OF OTHER FUNGAL INFECTIONS

The number of opportunistic species reported to be involved in fungal infections in immunocompromised patients is increasing rapidly. Zygomycetes cause very severe and often fatal infections and therefore these infections pose difficult diagnostic and therapeutic challenges. In addition, these strains usually fail to sporulate under normal laboratory conditions, thereby making morphological identification difficult.

Voigt et al. described a PCR identification system based on a molecular database for most of the clinically important zygomycetes (68). The database was constructed from nucleotide sequences from the small (18S) and large (28S) subunits of the ribosomal DNA. The primers described were able to rapidly and accurately identify zygomycetes DNA.

Wedde et al. described a specific PCR assay enabling the detection and discrimination of *Scedosporium* spp., fungi that can cause severe infections in immunocompromised and accidentally injured persons (69). In view of the difficult treatment, especially of *Scedosporium proliferans*, it was essential for the authors to establish hybridization probes for genus or species-specific identification.

Recently, quantitative PCR assays were developed for the detection of different *Aspergillus*, *Penicillium* and *Paecilomyces* species (70). The PCR assay described is based on the TaqMan chemistry and directed against the internal transcribed spacer regions. Additionally, a generic assay for all target species was developed. Conidia detection limits ranged from less than one to several hundred per sample for the different assays.

For the detection of DNA from *Scedosporium* spp., a specific PCR was developed by Williamson et al. based on the amplification of a part of the ITS gene region (71). Since infections with *Scedosporium* spp. occurring post-transplantation are usually untreatable, respiratory tract colonization with *Scedosporium* spp. in patients with chronic lung disease is a significant concern for lung transplantation candidates.

For the detection of Fusarium DNA, different PCR protocols were described. However, as *Fusarium* spp. are often detected in vitreous specimens, these reports were focused on ocular samples. Fungal corneal infections occur most frequently in agricultural workers as well as in patients with diabetes mellitus and AIDS. Gaudio et al. investigated corneal scrapings from 30 patients with presumed fungal keratitis by PCR and culture assays (72). They found that PCR and fungal culture matched in 74% of the samples, 23% were PCR positive but negative by fungal culture, and only 3% showed a PCR negative but culture-positive result.

Also, different PCR assays for the detection of *Histoplasma capsulatum* were described. This slow-growing, dimorphic fungus causes disease ranging from focal and self-limited to disseminated and rapidly fatal. Immunocompromised patients, especially those with advanced AIDS, are at risk for disseminated histoplasmosis. Martagon-Villamil et al. designed and tested a real-time PCR assay by LightCycler, which was able to correctly identify 34 *H. capsulatum* isolates and additionally in clinical specimens from 3 patients (73). De Matos Guedes et al. also described a *Histoplasma*-specific PCR assay (74). Their PCR test correctly identified the 31 *H. capsulatum* var. *capsulatum* strains isolated from human, animal, and soil specimens and 1 *H. capsulatum* var. *duboisii* isolate. The specificity of the PCR using M-antigen-derived primers was confirmed by the absence of amplification products when genomic DNA from *Paracoccidioides brasiliensis*, *Candida* spp., *Sporothrix schenckii*, *Cryptococcus neoformans*, *Blastomyces dermatitidis*, *Coccidioides immitis*, *A. niger*, and *A. fumigatus* was analyzed.

Besides *H. capsulatum*, *B. dermatitidis* is a relevant, thermally dimorphic fungus. It produces mycelia and forms aleurioconidia at 25°C, whereas at 37°C it takes the form of a broad-based budding yeast. Human disease is acquired by inhaling conidia, which causes local pulmonary infection, often accompanied by extrapulmonary dissemination. Lindsley et al. developed specific oligonucleotide probes which are able to identify *B. dermatitidis* as well as *Coccidioides immitis*, *Paracoccidioides brasiliensis*, *Penicillium marneffei*, *Sporothrix schenckii*, *Cryptococcus neoformans*, five *Candida* species, and *Pneumocystis jiroveci* using universal fungal primers ITS1 and ITS4 (75). In addition, a probe to detect all dimorphic, systemic pathogens was developed.

NON–PCR-BASED MOLECULAR DETECTION METHODS

Nucleic Acid Sequence Based Amplification

Nucleic acid sequence based amplification (NASBA) is an isothermal amplification technology that specifically amplifies RNA sequences in a DNA background by using T7 RNA polymerase. The NASBA assay offers practical advantages compared to PCR or RT-PCR. PCR requires rapid temperature changes for which thermal cyclers are required, whereas NASBA is an isothermal amplification process. Unlike RT-PCR, it allows detection of unspliced mRNA, and as thermal denaturation is absent, a contaminating background of genomic DNA is not a concern. Specimens can be stored in NASBA lysis buffer at $-80°C$

until further processing. In addition, the NASBA technique requires only 100 μL of whole blood compared to 5 mL of blood for PCR.

To our knowledge, only one assay has been described so far for the detection of *Aspergillus* RNA (76). This protocol was compared to a previously published, well-defined real-time PCR assay amplifying a region of the *Aspergillus* 18S rRNA gene. NASBA showed a lower detection limit of 1 CFU and detected RNA from five different clinically relevant *Aspergillus* species, including *A. fumigatus*. All 77 blood samples tested by PCR and NASBA showed identical results in both assays. Results with the NASBA technique were obtained within six hours.

Pyrosequencing Assay

The Pyrosequencing technology (Biotage, Uppsala, Sweden) is a non-electrophoretic, bioluminometric DNA sequencing method. The method employs a cascade of four coupled enzymatic reactions followed by Genbank/BLAST analysis. Only one protocol has been described so far for the identification of fungal DNA (77). The assay was performed on amplicons derived from the 18S rRNA gene using universal primers for the amplification of DNA of nine strains of clinically relevant fungi (including *A. fumigatus*) and 12 clinical specimens from patients suffering from proven invasive fungal infections (including IA). All samples were PCR-amplified and analyzed by gel electrophoresis, PCR-enzyme-linked immunosorbent assay (ELISA), and the Pyrosequencing technology. All data obtained by the Pyrosequencing technology were in agreement with the results obtained by PCR-ELISA using species/genus-specific oligonucleotides and were in accordance with the culture results as well. The authors concluded that their Pyrosequencing method is a reproducible and reliable technique for the identification of fungal pathogens.

Single-Strand Conformational Polymorphism

Walsh et al. reported the application of single-strand conformational polymorphism (SSCP) to distinguish between fungal species and/or genera (78). They used a 197-bp fragment amplified from the 18S rRNA gene. The patterns obtained from *Candida* species differed markedly from those of the genus *Aspergillus*. The SSCP patterns permitted distinction between strains of *A. fumigatus* and *Aspergillus flavus*. There was consistency of the SSCP banding pattern among different strains of the same *Aspergillus* species. The SSCP patterns for other medically important opportunistic fungi, such as *Cryptococcus neoformans*, *Pseudallescheria boydii*, and *Rhizopus arrhizus*, were sufficiently unique to permit distinction from those of *C. albicans* and *A. fumigatus*. The authors concluded that the technique of PCR-SSCP provides a method by which to recognize and distinguish between medically important opportunistic fungi, thus having potential applications to molecular diagnosis, taxonomic classification, molecular epidemiology, and elucidation of mechanisms of antifungal drug resistance.

FUTURE PERSPECTIVES IN MOLECULAR DIAGNOSIS OF INVASIVE FUNGAL INFECTIONS

During the last decade, significant advances in the development of molecular assays for the diagnosis of invasive fungal infections have been achieved. The majority of these assays rely on PCR technology. Real-time PCR assays offer some theoretical advantages compared with conventional assays such as online quantification of the fungal load in clinical specimens, and these assays are much faster and thus easier applicable in the clinical routine. However, it is yet unknown whether quantitative assessment is of clinical significance in patient management. In the future, the development of commercial products will be essential for standardization and broader clinical evaluation of these assays.

REFERENCES

1. Saiki RK, Gelfand DH, Stoffel S, et al. Primer-directed enzymatic amplification of DNA with a thermostable DNA polymerase. Science 1988; 239:487–91.
2. Loeffler J, Hebart H, Brauchle U, Schumacher U, Einsele H. Comparison between plasma and whole blood specimens for detection of *Aspergillus* DNA by PCR. J Clin Microbiol 2000; 38:3830–3.
3. Bretagne S, Costa JM, Bart-Delabesse E, Dhedin N, Rieux C, Cordonnier C. Comparison of serum galactomannan antigen detection and competitive polymerase chain reaction for diagnosing invasive aspergillosis. Clin Infect Dis 1998; 26:1407–12.
4. Costa C, Costa JM, Desterke C, Botterel F, Cordonnier C, Bretagne S. Real-time PCR coupled with automated DNA extraction and detection of galactomannan antigen in serum by enzyme-linked immunosorbent assay for diagnosis of invasive aspergillosis. J Clin Microbiol 2002; 40:2224–7.
5. Kawazu M, Kanda Y, Nannya Y, et al. Prospective comparison of the diagnostic potential of real-time PCR, double-sandwich enzyme-linked immunosorbent assay for galactomannan, and a (1-3)-beta-D-glucan test in weekly screening for invasive aspergillosis in patients with hematological disorders. J Clin Microbiol 2004; 42:2733–4.
6. Challier S, Boyer S, Abachin E, Berche P. Development of a serum-based Taqman real-time PCR assay for diagnosis of invasive aspergillosis. J Clin Microbiol 2004; 42:844–6.
7. Williamson EC, Leeming JP, Palmer HM, et al. Diagnosis of invasive aspergillosis in bone marrow transplant recipients by polymerase chain reaction. Br J Haematol 2000; 108:132–9.
8. Yamakami Y, Hashimoto A, Yamagata E, et al. Evaluation of PCR for detection of DNA specific for *Aspergillus* species in sera of patients with various forms of pulmonary aspergillosis. J Clin Microbiol 1998; 36:3619–23.

9. Kawazu M, Kanda Y, Goyama S, et al. Rapid diagnosis of invasive pulmonary aspergillosis by quantitative polymerase chain reaction using bronchial lavage fluid. Am J Hematol 2003; 72:27–30.

10. Raad I, Hanna H, Huaringa A, Sumoza D, Hachem R, Albitar M. Diagnosis of invasive pulmonary aspergillosis using polymerase chain reaction-based detection of aspergillus in BAL. Chest 2002; 121:1171–6.

11. Buchheidt D, Baust C, Skladny H, Baldus M, Brauninger S, Hehlmann R. Clinical evaluation of a polymerase chain reaction assay to detect *Aspergillus* species in bronchoalveolar lavage samples of neutropenic patients. Br J Haematol 2002; 116:803–11.

12. Melchers WJ, Verweij PE, van den Hurk P, et al. General primer-mediated PCR for detection of *Aspergillus* species. J Clin Microbiol 1994; 32:1710–7.

13. Verweij PE, Brinkman K, Kremer HP, Kullberg BJ, Meis JF. Aspergillus meningitis: diagnosis by non-culture-based microbiological methods and management. J Clin Microbiol 1999; 37:1186–9.

14. Hendolin PH, Paulin L, Koukila-Kahkola P, et al. Panfungal PCR and multiplex liquid hybridization for detection of fungi in tissue specimens. J Clin Microbiol 2000; 38:4186–92.

15. Jaeger EE, Carroll NM, Choudhury S, et al. Rapid detection and identification of *Candida*, *Aspergillus*, and *Fusarium* species in ocular samples using nested PCR. J Clin Microbiol 2000; 38:2902–8.

16. Hope WW, Padwell A, Guiver M, Denning DW. Invasive pulmonary aspergillosis with spontaneous resolution and the diagnostic utility of PCR from tissue specimens. J Infect 2004; 49:136–40.

17. Grijalva M, Horvath R, Dendis M, Erny J, Benedik J. Molecular diagnosis of culture negative infective endocarditis: clinical validation in a group of surgically treated patients. Heart 2003; 89:263–8.

18. Tang CM, Holden DW, Aufauvre-Brown A, Cohen J. The detection of *Aspergillus* spp. by the polymerase chain reaction and its evaluation in bronchoalveolar lavage fluid. Am Rev Respir Dis 1993; 148:1313–7.

19. Scott J, Schekman R. Lyticase: endoglucanase and protease activities that act together in yeast cell lysis. J Bacteriol 1980; 142:414–23.

20. Loeffler J, Hebart H, Sepe S, Schumacher U, Klingebiel T, Einsele H. Detection of PCR-amplified fungal DNA by using a PCR-ELISA system. Med Mycol 1998; 36:275–9.

21. Hopfer RL, Walden P, Setterquist S, Highsmith WE. Detection and differentiation of fungi in clinical specimens using polymerase chain reaction (PCR) amplification and restriction enzyme analysis. J Med Ved Mycol 1993; 31:65–75.

22. Fujita S, Lasker BA, Lott TJ, Reiss E, Morrison CJ. Microtitre plate enzyme immunoassay to detect PCR-amplified DNA from *Candida* species in blood. J Clin Microbiol 1995; 33:962–7.

23. Velegraki A, Kambouris M, Kostourou A, Chalevelakis G, Legakis NJ. Rapid extraction of fungal DNA from clinical samples for PCR amplification. Med Mycol 1999; 37:69–73.

24. Van Burik JA, Myerson D, Schreckhise RW, Bowden RA. Panfungal PCR assay for the detection of fungal infection in human blood specimens. J Clin Microbiol 1998; 36:1169–75.

25. Maaroufi Y, Ahariz N, Husson M, Crokaert F. Comparison of different methods of isolation of DNA of commonly encountered *Candida* species and its quantitation by using a real-time PCR-based assay. J Clin Microbiol 2004; 42:3159–63.

26. Loeffler J, Schmidt K, Hebart H, Schumacher U, Einsele H. Automated extraction of genomic DNA from medically important yeast species and filamentous fungi by using the MagNA Pure LC system. J Clin Microbiol 2002; 40:2240–3.

27. Kappe R, Okeke CN, Fauser C, Maiwald M, Sonntag HG. Molecular probes for the detection of pathogenic fungi in the presence of human tissue. J Med Microbiol 1998; 47:811–20.

28. Fletcher HA, Barton RC, Verweij PE, Evans EG. Detection of *Aspergillus fumigatus* PCR products by a microtitre plate based DNA hybridisation assay. J Clin Pathol 1998; 51:617–20.

29. Willinger B, Obradovic A, Selitsch B, et al. Detection and identification of fungi from fungus balls of the maxillary sinus by molecular techniques. J Clin Microbiol 2003; 41:581–5.

30. Turenne CY, Sanche SE, Hoban DJ, Karlowsky JA, Kabani AM. Rapid identification of fungi by using the ITS2 genetic region and an automaited fluorescent capillary electrophoresis system. J Clin Microbiol 1999; 37:1846–51.

31. Meletiadis J, Melchers WJ, Meis JF, Van Den Hurk P, Jannes G, Verweij PE. Evaluation of a polymerase chain reaction reverse hybridization line probe assay for the detection and identification of medically important fungi in bronchoalveolar lavage fluids. Med Mycol 2003; 41:65–74.

32. Loeffler J, Henke N, Hebart H, et al. Quantification of fungal DNA by using fluorescence resonance energy transfer and the Light Cycler system. J Clin Microbiol 2000; 38:586–90.

33. Loeffler J, Kloepfer K, Hebart H, et al. Polymerase chain reaction detection of aspergillus DNA in experimental models of invasive aspergillosis. J Infect Dis 2002; 185:1203–6.

34. Spiess B, Buchheidt D, Baust C, et al. Development of a LightCycler PCR assay for detection and quantification of *Aspergillus fumigatus* DNA in clinical samples from neutropenic patients. J Clin Microbiol 2003; 41:1811–8.

35. Skladny H, Buchheidt D, Baust C, et al. Specific detection of *Aspergillus* species in blood and bronchoalveolar lavage samples of immunocompromised patients by two-step PCR. J Clin Microbiol 1999; 37:3865–71.

36. Bowman JC, Abruzzo GK, Anderson JW, et al. Quantitative PCR assay to measure *Aspergillus fumigatus* burden in a murine model of disseminated aspergillosis: demonstration of efficacy of caspofungin acetate. Antimicrob Agents Chemother 2001; 45:3474–81.

37. Costa C, Vidaud D, Olivi M, Bart-Delabasse E, Vidaud M, Bretagne S. Development of two real-time quantitative TaqMan PCR assays to detect circulating *Aspergillus fumigatus* DNA in serum. J Microbiol Methods 2001; 38:3478–80.

38. Pham AS, Tarrand JJ, May GS, Lee MS, Kontoyiannis DP, Han XY. Diagnosis of invasive mould infection by real-time quantitative PCR. Am J Clin Pathol 2003; 119:38–44.

39. Kami M, Fukui T, Ogawa S, et al. Use of real-time PCR on blood samples for diagnosis of invasive aspergillosis. Clin Infect Dis 2001; 33:1504–12.

40. Guiver M, Levi K, Oppenheim BA. Rapid identification of *Candida* species by TaqMan PCR. J Clin Pathol 2001; 54:362–6.

41. Loeffler J, Hagmeyer L, Hebart H, Henke N, Schumacher U, Einsele H. Rapid detection of point mutations by fluorescence resonance energy transfer and probe melting curves in *Candida* species. Clin Chem 2000; 46:631–5.

42. Selvarangan R, Bui U, Limaye AP, Cookson BT. Rapid identification of commonly encountered *Candida* species directly from blood culture bottles. J Clin Microbiol 2003; 41:5660–4.

43. Chau AS, Mendrick CA, Sabatelli FJ, Loebenberg D, McNicholas PM. Application of real-time quantitative PCR to molecular analysis of *Candida albicans* strains exhibiting reduced susceptibility to azoles. Antimicrob Agents Chemother 2004; 48:2124–31.

44. Loeffler J, Hebart H, Bialek R, et al. Contaminations occuring in fungal PCR assays. J Clin Microbiol 1999; 37:1200–2.

45. Kwok S, Higuchi R. Avoiding false positives with PCR. Nature 1989; 339:237–8.

46. Buchman TG, Rossier M, Merz WG, Charache P. Detection of surgical pathogens by in vitro DNA amplification. Part I. Rapid identification of *Candida albicans* by in vitro amplification of a fungus-specific gene. Surgery 1990; 108:338–46.

47. Burgener-Kairuz P, Zuber JP, Jaunin P, Buchman TG, Bille J, Rossier M. Rapid detection and identification of *Candida albicans* and Torulopsis (*Candida*) glabrata in clinical specimens by species-specific nested PCR amplification of a cytochrome P-450 lanosterol-alpha-demethylase (L1A1) gene fragment. J Clin Microbiol 1994; 32:1902–7.

48. Crampin AC, Matthews RC. Application of the polymerase chain reaction to the diagnosis of candidosis by amplification of an HSP 90 gene fragment. J Med Microbiol 1993; 39:233–8.

49. Kan VL. Polymerase chain reaction for the diagnosis of candidemia. J Infect Dis 1993; 168:779–83.

50. Miyakawa Y, Mabuchi T, Kagaya K, Fukazawa Y. Isolation and characterization of a species-specific DNA fragment for detection of *Candida albicans* by polymerase chain reaction. J Clin Microbiol 1992; 30:894–900.

51. van Deventer AJ, Goessens WH, van Belkum A, van Vliet HJ, van Etten EW, Verbrugh HA. Improved detection of *Candida albicans* by PCR in blood of neutropenic mice with systemic candidiasis. J Clin Microbiol 1995; 33:625–8.

52. Haynes KA, Westerneng TJ, Fell JW, Moens W. Rapid detection and identification of pathogenic fungi by polymerase chain reaction amplification of large subunit ribosomal DNA. J Med Vet Mycol 1995; 33:319–25.

53. Niesters HG, Goessens WH, Meis JF, Quint WG. Rapid, polymerase chain reaction-based identification assays for *Candida* species. J Clin Microbiol 1993; 31:904–10.

54. Hebart H, Loffler J, Reitze H, et al. Prospective screening by a panfungal polymerase chain reaction assay in patients at risk for fungal infections: implications for the management of febrile neutropenia. Br J Haematol 2000; 111:635–40.

55. Lin MT, Lu HC, Chen WL. Improving efficacy of antifungal therapy by polymerase chain reaction-based strategy among febrile patients with neutropenia and cancer. Clin Infect Dis 2001; 33:1621–7.

56. Kanbe T, Yamaki K, Kikuchi A. Identification of the pathogenic *Aspergillus* species by nested PCR using a mixture of specific primers to DNA topoisomerase II gene. Microbiol Immunol 2002; 46:841–8.

57. Einsele H, Hebart H, Roller G, et al. Detection and identification of fungal pathogens in blood by using molecular probes. J Clin Microbiol 1997; 35:1353–60.

58. Buchheidt D, Baust C, Skladny H, et al. Detection of *Aspergillus* species in blood and bronchoalveolar lavage samples from immunocompromised patients by means of 2-step polymerase chain reaction: clinical results. Clin Infect Dis 2001; 33:428–35.

59. Zhao J, Kong F, Li R, Wang X, Wan Z, Wang D. Identification of *Aspergillus fumigatus* and related species by nested PCR targeting ribosomal DNA internal transcribed spacer regions. J Clin Microbiol 2001; 39:2261–6.

60. Luo G, Mitchell TG. Rapid identification of pathogenic fungi directly from cultures by using multiplex PCR. J Clin Microbiol 2002; 40:2860–5.

61. Jones ME, Fox AJ, Barnes AJ, et al. PCR-ELISA for the early diagnosis of invasive pulmonary aspergillus infection in neutropenic patients. J Clin Pathol 1998; 51:652–6.

62. Raad I, Hanna H, Sumoza D, Albitar M. Polymerase chain reaction on blood for the diagnosis of invasive pulmonary aspergillosis in cancer patients. Cancer 2002; 94:1032–6.

63. Hebart H, Loffler J, Meisner C, et al. Early detection of aspergillus infection after allogeneic stem cell transplantation by polymerase chain reaction screening. J Infect Dis 2000; 181:1713–9.

64. Lass-Florl C, Aigner J, Gunsilius E, et al. Screening for *Aspergillus* spp. using polymerase chain reaction of whole blood samples from patients with haematological malignancies. Br J Haematol 2001; 113:180–4.

65. Einsele H, Quabeck K, Muller KD, et al. Prediction of invasive pulmonary aspergillosis from colonisation of lower respiratory tract before marrow transplantation. Lancet 1998; 352:1443.

66. Ferns RB, Fletcher H, Bradley S, Mackinnon S, Hunt C, Tedder RS. The prospective evaluation of a nested polymerase chain reaction assay for the early detection of *Aspergillus* infection in patients with leukaemia or undergoing allograft treatment. Br J Haematol 2002; 119:720–5.

67. de Aguirre L, Hurst SF, Choi JS, Shin JH, Hinrikson HP, Morrison CJ. Rapid differentiation of *Aspergillus* species from other medically important opportunistic molds and yeasts by PCR-enzyme immunoassay. J Clin Microbiol 2004; 42:3495–504.

68. Voigt K, Cigelnik E, O'donnell K. Phylogeny and PCR identification of clinically important Zygomycetes based on nuclear ribosomal-DNA sequence data. J Clin Microbiol 1999; 37:3957–64.

69. Wedde M, Muller D, Tintelnot K, De Hoog GS, Stahl U. PCR-based identification of clinically relevant Pseudallescheria/Scedosporium strains. Med Mycol 1998; 36:61–7.

70. Haugland RA, Varma M, Wymer LJ, Vesper SJ. Quantitative PCR analysis of selected *Aspergillus*, *Penicillium* and *Paecilomyces* species. Syst Appl Microbiol 2004; 27:198–210.

71. Williamson EC, Speers D, Arthur IH, Harnett G, Ryan G, Inglis TJ. Molecular epidemiology of Scedosporium apiospermum infection determined by PCR amplification of ribosomal intergenic spacer sequences in patients with chronic lung disease. J Clin Microbiol 2001; 39:47–50.

72. Gaudio PA, Gopinathan U, Sangwan V, Hughes TE. Polymerase chain reaction based detection of fungi in infected corneas. Br J Ophthalmol 2002; 86:755–60.

73. Martagon-Villamil J, Shrestha N, Sholtis M, et al. Identification of *Histoplasma capsulatum* from culture extracts by real-time PCR. J Clin Microbiol 2003; 41:1295–8.
74. Guedes HL, Guimaraes AJ, Muniz Mde M, et al. PCR assay for identification of *Histoplasma capsulatum* based on the nucleotide sequence of the M antigen. J Clin Microbiol 2003; 41:535–9.
75. Lindsley MD, Hurst SF, Iqbal NJ, Morrison CJ. Rapid identification of dimorphic and yeast-like fungal pathogens using specific DNA probes. J Clin Microbiol 2001; 39:3505–11.
76. Loeffler J, Hebart H, Cox P, Flues N, Schumacher U, Einsele H. Nucleic acid sequence-based amplification of *Aspergillus* RNA in blood samples. J Clin Microbiol 2001; 39:1626–9.
77. Gharizadeh B, Norberg E, Loffler J, et al. Identification of medically important fungi by the Pyrosequencing technology. Mycoses 2004; 47:29–33.
78. Walsh TJ, Francesconi A, Kasai M, Chanock SJ. PCR and single-strand conformational polymorphism for recognition of medically important opportunistic fungi. J Clin Microbiol 1995; 33:3216–20.

7

Superficial and Mucosal Fungal Infections

Peter G. Pappas

Division of Infectious Diseases, University of Alabama at Birmingham, Birmingham, Alabama, U.S.A.

Bethany Bergamo

Department of Dermatology, University of Alabama at Birmingham, Birmingham, Alabama, U.S.A.

INTRODUCTION

Superficial and mucosal fungal infections are among the most common infections in man, and are caused by a variety of dermatophytes, *Candida* spp., and less commonly, other fungi. These infections occur in all age groups and are recognized among both normal and immunocompromised hosts. Because of the high frequency of these infections, most diagnoses are based on clinical grounds alone; as such, misdiagnosis is not uncommon. A specific diagnosis for any of these infections require histopathologic, cytologic, and/or culture confirmation.

In this chapter, we describe the more common superficial and mucosal fungal infections, with an emphasis on clinical and laboratory diagnosis. Therapy for these disorders is not discussed, and the reader is referred to several excellent resources for detailed therapeutic information (1–3).

CANDIDIASIS

Oropharyngeal Candidiasis

Oropharyngeal candidiasis (OPC) is a superficial infection of the oral mucosa that is most prevalent in infants, the elderly, and immunocompromised patients.

Common predisposing conditions include diabetes mellitus, hematologic and solid organ neoplasia, glucocorticosteroids and other immunosuppressive agents, antibacterial therapy, radiation therapy, and advanced HIV disease (4,5). Among non-HIV infected patients, those at greatest risk of developing OPC include those receiving glucocorticosteroids and those with prolonged neutropenia who have oropharyngeal colonization with a *Candida* spp. (6). Among HIV-infected individuals, up to 90% will develop OPC at some stage of their disease in the absence of antiretroviral therapy or antifungal prophylaxis (7,8).

Candida albicans is responsible for up to 80% to 90% of cases of OPC (9), reflecting the ability of *C. albicans* to adhere to buccal epithelial cells better than non-albicans *Candida* spp. In the normal host, low numbers of colonizing organisms are the result of effective host defenses present in the oral cavity. However, local factors, such as low salivary flow rates, can result in higher prevalence of *Candida* colonization. Studies comparing *Candida* strains between HIV-infected patients and otherwise healthy individuals have not demonstrated any significant strain variability among the two groups, suggesting that *Candida* spp. causing OPC are not more virulent in HIV-infected patients, but rather reflect defects in host defense (2,10). In contrast, the clinical course and natural history of OPC in these two groups can be quite dissimilar. For example, non-albicans *Candida* spp. are much more common among HIV-infected patients, response to therapy is generally slower, and recurrent disease in the absence of prophylaxis is the rule (8,11,12).

The clinical symptoms of OPC are variable. Some patients report only a mild distortion of taste, while others complain of more severe symptoms such as soreness, painful mouth, burning tongue, and dysphagia (8). Some patients with relatively severe OPC are surprisingly symptom-free. Physical findings associated with OPC include diffuse erythema with discrete white patches on the buccal mucosa, hard and soft palate, gingiva, and tongue. The whitish lesions can be removed with gentle scraping, often revealing an erythematous or bleeding base (Fig. 1A). Oral hairy leukoplakia (OHL), an Epstein–Barr virus-associated condition characterized by confluent whitish patches on the lateral aspects of the tongue, is often mistaken for OPC. In contrast to OPC, the lesions of OHL cannot be removed with gentle scraping or rubbing (2).

Exudative OPC

This is one of the most common forms of OPC, typically seen in HIV-positive individuals and characterized by thick white to yellowish curd-like exudate on oral mucosal surfaces (Fig. 1B). Lesions may be discrete or confluent and are comprised of necrotic material including epithelial cells, yeast cells with penetrating hyphae, and few inflammatory cells. Histologically, there is superficial invasion into the stratum corneum (13).

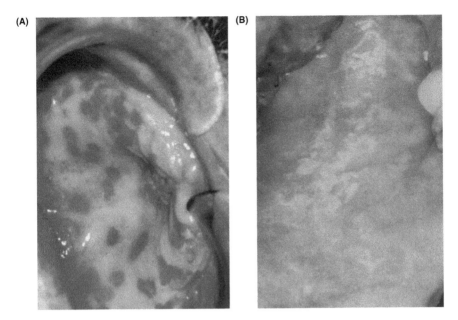

Figure 1 Oropharyngeal candidiasis. (**A**) Erythematous involvement of the hard palate. (**B**) Exudative involvement of the buccal mucosa.

Chronic Atrophic Stomatitis (Denture Stomatitis)

This variety of OPC may be associated with soreness and burning in the mouth, but is often asymptomatic. Diffuse erythema of the palate corresponding to the contact site with upper dentures is characteristic, and has been reported in up to 60% of denture wearers (Fig. 2). It is more common in females than males (14). *Candida* spp. can be isolated in the vast majority of symptomatic patients, but it is a common colonizer among asymptomatic denture wearers (15).

Angular Cheilitis

Angular cheilitis (cheilosis) is associated with soreness and fissuring at the corners of the mouth and may be associated with exudative OPC, denture stomatitis, or in isolation. It is important to distinguish this condition from angular cheilitis associated with vitamin and/or iron deficiency (16).

Diagnosis of OPC

Physical findings associated with OPC are easily recognized, but may be insufficient to allow for a reliable diagnosis. Oral lesions resembling candidiasis can be seen in neutropenic patients with severe mucositis or among patients with certain viral and bacterial infections. Moreover, severe mucositis due to cytotoxic agents and/or herpes simplex virus can be complicated by candidiasis.

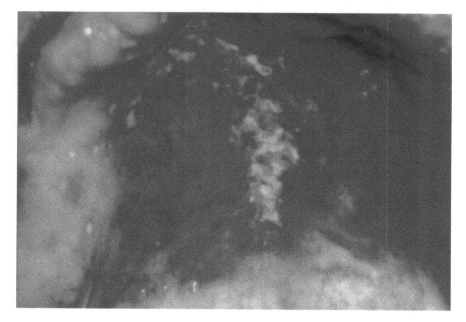

Figure 2 Chronic atrophic (denture-associated) oropharyngeal candidiasis with mixed erythematous and exudative findings.

Thus, a firm diagnosis of OPC requires mycologic confirmation. This can be accomplished by microscopic examination of wet mount specimens using 10–20% potassium hydroxide (KOH) or saline, and taken from scrapings of involved oral mucosal sites to confirm the presence of yeast cells with or without hyphae. Cultures are of limited value in the absence of cytologic confirmation, and culture alone does not distinguish between colonization and infection (17).

Esophageal Candidiasis

A relatively uncommon infection prior to the AIDS pandemic, esophageal candidiasis (EC) has become inextricably linked with advanced HIV disease (9). In addition to patients with AIDS, other individuals at risk include solid organ and hematopoietic stem cell transplant recipients, patients receiving immuno-suppressive therapy, patients with solid organ and hematologic neoplasia, and those who have undergone radiation therapy. *Candida* spp. are commonly isolated from the esophageal cultures, but rarely lead to invasion in the absence of one of these predisposing factors (18). Little is known about he pathogenesis of EC, but it is clear from the high prevalence of EC in patients with AIDS that cell-mediated immunity is important in preventing this complication. EC in an HIV-positive patient is an AIDS-defining illness, and is particularly prevalent in the developing world (9).

Common clinical symptoms associated with EC include dysphasia, odynophagia, and retrosternal pain. Weight loss and volume depletion associated with diminished oral intake are frequent concomitants of extensive EC. Systemic symptoms including fever and night sweats are much less common, and patients with AIDS and extensive EC may occasionally be asymptomatic (19).

Diagnosis of EC

A clinical diagnosis of EC is suspected among at risk patients with the triad of dysphasia, odynophagia, and retrosternal pain, with or without fever or concomitant OPC. In about two-thirds of patients, EC occurs in the absence of OPC and occurs more commonly in the distal two-thirds compared to the proximal one-third of the esophagus. EC is clinically classified on the basis of its endoscopic appearance (Fig. 3): Type I, few plaques up to 2 mm in diameter; Type II, numerous plaques larger than 2 mm, Type III, confluent linear and nodular elevated plaques with hyperemia and frank ulceration; Type IV, similar to Type III, but with worse mucosal friability and narrowing of the lumen (20). Rarely, esophageal perforation and extensive mucosal necrosis can occur; however, bacteremia and candidemia complicating EC are seen almost exclusively among neutropenic patients.

Laboratory diagnosis of EC can only be established reliably on the basis of histopathologic and mycologic evidence in tissue specimens. Specifically, yeast forms must be seen invading the mucosa to firmly establish this diagnosis. The isolation of yeast forms on smear or culture alone is a very sensitive but non-specific measurement, and does not distinguish readily between a commensal versus an invasive pathogen.

Before the widespread use of endoscopy for the diagnosis of EC, the barium swallow was the standard diagnostic tool. This modality is less useful today due to its low sensitivity and specificity. Currently, barium swallow is used among patients with suspected EC in whom endoscopy is not available or contraindicated (18).

Other disorders that may mimic EC symptomatically and/or endoscopically include esophagitis due to cytomegalovirus, herpes simplex virus, *Histoplasma capsulatum*, *Mycobacterium tuberculosis*, *Mycobacterium avium intracellulare*, and severe reflux esophagitis. Radiation esophagitis must also be considered among patients at risk. Polymicrobial esophagitis, especially among patients with AIDS, is not uncommon and should be considered in any patient and whom treatment for *Candida* esophagitis is not associated with a significant clinical response within 7 to 10 days.

Vulvovaginal Candidiasis

Vaginitis due to *Candida* spp. is the second most common cause of vaginitis in the developed world following non-specific vaginitis (bacterial vaginosis). Most women will experience at least one episode of vulvovaginal candidiasis (VVC)

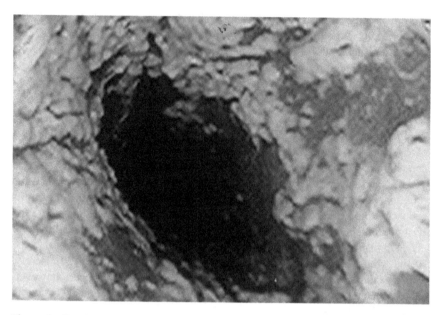

Figure 3 Esophageal candidiasis, Type III. Note the confluent linear and nodular plaques with erythema and friability. *Source*: Courtesy of C. Mel Wilcox, MD.

during their lifetime (21). *Candida* spp. are normal flora in the female genital tract and can be isolated from up to 20% of asymptomatic healthy women of childbearing age. Similar to the pathogenesis of OPC, *C. albicans* adheres to vaginal epithelial cells in significantly greater numbers when compared to non-albicans *Candida* spp. (22).

Several clinical conditions are associated with increased vaginal colonization with *Candida* spp. and symptomatic *Candida* vaginitis. These include pregnancy, oral contraceptives with high estrogen content, poorly controlled diabetes mellitus, systemic glucocorticosteroids, systemic antibacterial therapy, intra-uterine devices, and high frequency of coitus (23). Vulvovaginal candidiasis during pregnancy is most common during the third trimester, but may occur anytime throughout pregnancy. Symptomatic VVC associated with exposure to systemic broad-spectrum antibacterial agents is believed to result from the elimination of normal protective vaginal bacterial flora, such as *Lactobacillus*. Local conditions that may predispose to *Candida* vaginitis include tight, poorly ventilated undergarments and hypersensitivity dermatitis due to topical chemical agents. VVC is probably more common however among patients with AIDS; however, compelling data supporting this are lacking (5).

Vulvovaginal pruritis is the most common symptom of VVC. Vaginal discharge is typical but may be absent, and odor is usually absent. The discharge associated with VVC is often described as "cottage cheese-like" but may be thin and watery, or thick and homogenous. Vaginal irritation with vulvar burning, dyspareunia, and external dysuria are commonly seen. Symptoms are frequently exacerbated in the week prior to menses, and the onset of menstruation often provides some relief (24).

Diagnosis of VVC

The clinical diagnosis of VVC is usually straightforward, but can be challenging, particularly in the presence of mixed infection. A typical history coupled with the findings of erythema and swelling of the labia and vulva with discrete satellite lesions is common. On vaginal examination, the cervix usually appears normal and there is often a whitish exudate adherent to the vaginal mucosa. Systemic symptoms due to VVC are rare (5,24).

The laboratory diagnosis of VVC is based on microscopic examination of vaginal secretions. A wet mount of vaginal secretions with either saline or 10% KOH is the most useful means of identifying the presence of yeast cells. Vaginal pH is 4.0 to 4.5 among patients with VVC in the absence of co-infections due to trichomoniasis or bacterial vaginosis. Vaginal culture is usually unnecessary for making a diagnosis of VVC. Although cultures for *Candida* are quite sensitive, they are not useful in distinguishing routine colonization versus a true pathogen in the absence of microscopic data (5,24).

Cutaneous Candidiasis

Candida spp. can cause superficial infection of the skin, hair, and nails. *C. albicans* and *C. tropicalis* are the most common species associated with of cutaneous candidiasis and onychomycosis. Local conditions that favor growth of *Candida* include warm moist areas such as skin folds and intertriginous regions in obese persons. Cutaneous candidiasis occurs with greater frequency in HIV-positive and diabetic patients, and can be exacerbated by occlusive clothing, excessive moisture, use of broad-spectrum antibacterials, or pharmacologic immunosuppression. Dry, intact skin is a potent barrier to fungal invasion due to *Candida*.

Intertrigo

Intertrigo is one of the most common skin infections associated with *Candida* spp., affecting areas where skin sites are in close proximity or apposition in the context of a moist environment. Skin underlying the breasts, intra-axillary region, and abdominal-inguinal creases are especially vulnerable. A vesicular or pustular enlarging rash is typical, and this rash frequently progresses to maceration with erythema. Satellite lesions are frequent and ay coalesce into large lesions.

Generalized Cutaneous Candidiasis

This rare syndrome manifests as a diffuse eruption over the trunk, thorax, and proximal extremities. Patients experience pruritus and worsening rash in the intertriginal areas including the hands and feet. On examination, individuals manifest a widespread vesicular rash that may become confluent into larger lesions (25,26).

Paronychia and Onychomycosis

Nail plate infections are generally due to dermatophytes; however, *Candida* spp. can rarely cause paronychia and onychomycosis. These complications are usually seen among diabetic and among those with prolonged water emersion. *Candida* paronychia is a chronic infection and may present as a painful and erythematous area adjacent to or underneath the nail and nail fold. There is usually painful inflammation with erythema and expressible purulence in the periungual area. In its chronic form, the nail bed becomes thick with ridging, discoloration, and can be associated with nail loss not unlike onychomycosis due to a dermatophyte infection (27).

Diagnosis of Cutaneous Candidiasis and Onychomycosis

The diagnosis of a superficial cutaneous *Candida* infection is usually based on clinical findings alone. A more specific diagnosis is based on the ability to visualize the organism on microscopic examination of wet mount specimen (usually 10% KOH) taken from an affected area. Cultures are of less utility, with the exception of *Candida* onychomycosis, where the isolation of *Candida* spp. from nail clippings can be diagnostic.

DERMATOPHYTES

Dermatophytes are fungal organisms that are able to exist within the keratinous elements of living skin and which belong to one of 3 genera, *Epidermophyton*, *Microsporum*, and *Trichophyton*. Collectively, cutaneous infections caused by these organisms are lumped together as "tinea" together with the Latin designation describing the affected part of the body (3). Dermatophytoses occur in all populations worldwide, but are generally more common among immunocompromised patients (26,28).

Tineas

Tinea Corporis

Tinea corporis is a dermatophytosis of the glabrous (hairless) skin and may involve the face, trunk, and limbs. Other names for tinea corporis include ringworm, tinea circinata, and tinea glabrosa (29).

Tinea corporis is a very common disease worldwide, but especially among patients living in warm and humid climates (Fig. 4A–C). The infections occur in patients of all ages and with no particular predisposition according to sex, race, or ethnicity. Patients with significant underlying disorders affecting immune function including diabetes mellitus, HIV, and those receiving

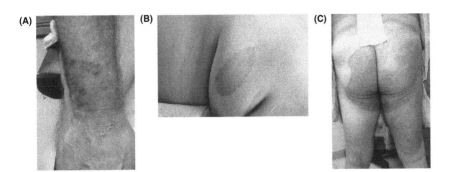

Figure 4 Tinea corporis. (**A**) Well demarcated, annular, erythematous plaque with scale at the leading edge. (**B**) Annular, erythematous plaque with scale. A few papules and pustules are also present, representing follicular invasion of the dermatophyte. (**C**) Large, well-demarcated, annular plaque present for several years. Potassium hydroxide preparation demonstrated numerous hyphae. *Source*: **B** and **C** Courtesy of Lauren Hughey, MD.

immunosuppressive agents are predisposed to this infection (28). Other risk factors include outdoor activity and animal husbandry. *Trichophyton rubrum* is the most common pathogen causing tinea corporis, although *T. tonsurans*, *T. mentagrophytes*, and *M. canis* can be associated with this disorder.

Skin lesions of tinea corporis vary between non-inflammatory scaly plaques to inflammatory pustules, and may vary according to the infecting organism. The invasion of hair follicles often results in perifollicular pustules resembling bacterial folliculitis, which may progress to granuloma formation (Majocchi's granuloma). A severe manifestation of this disorder is tinea profunda, a severe but rare presentation seen among patients with disorders associated with underlying cell-mediated immune dysfunction. In these patients, the lesions of tinea profunda are proliferative and verrucous and may resemble those of blastomycosis (29).

Tinea Barbae

Tinea barbae is defined as dermatophytosis of the beard area in men. Historically, it is linked to contaminated razors at barbershops, and it has become much less common in the last few decades. The two most common organisms responsible for tinea barbae, *T. mentagrophytes* and *T. versicolor*, produce an inflammatory reaction associated with elevated nodules, draining pustules, and sinus tracts. The hair in affected areas may be distorted or even absent. The chin and neck are usually involved and the upper lip is rarely affected. Untreated, it can result in significant scar formation. Clinically, tinea barbae can be easily confused with bacterial folliculitis, acne vulgaris, and contact dermatitis.

Tinea Cruris

Tinea cruris involves the medial upper thighs and the inguinal, pubic, perineal, and perianal area. Other names include jock itch, ringworm of the groin, and tinea inguinalis. Tinea cruris has a worldwide distribution, though more common in warm and moist environments. *T. rubrum* is the most common pathogen, although *E. folliculosum* and *T. mentagrophytes* are also important causes.

Clinically, tinea cruris presents with itching, erythema, and burning in affected areas. Vesicles or papules may appear on the leading edge of these lesions. Lesions are frequently bilateral and symmetric, although unilateral involvement can occur. Tinea cruris should be distinguished from other causes of intertrigo including candidiasis, erythrasma (secondary to *Corynebacterium minutissimum*), and psoriasis.

Tinea Pedis and Manuum

Tinea pedis and tinea manuum are dermatophytoses of the plantar and palmar surfaces of the hands and feet, respectively, and may involve the interdigital spaces. Tinea pedis is also called athlete's foot and ringworm of the feet. Tinea pedis is probably the most common dermatophytosis, affecting more than 70% of adult males. Chronic disease may result in onychomycosis of the toenails and/or fingernails. The most common etiologies of tinea pedis and tinea manuum include *T. rubrum* and *T. mentagrophytes*; *E. folliculosum* is a less common cause. The clinical presentation of tinea pedis is highly variable: *hyperkeratotic* or "moccasin" presentation is common and most typical of infection due to *T. rubrum*; *interdigital* tinea pedis is associated with maceration, scaling, and fissuring; *inflammatory* or *vesicular* tinea pedis is associated with vesicles and bulli involving the plantar surface of the feet; and *ulcerative* tinea pedis is probably the result of secondary bacterial infection complicating interdigital tinea pedis. The differential diagnosis of tinea pedis and tinea manuum include contact dermatitis, psoriasis, eczema, and keratodermas such as keratoderma blennorrhagica.

Tinea Capitis

Tinea capitis is a dermatophytosis of the scalp hair follicle also known as ringworm of the scalp. It is most commonly seen in prepubescent children. The most common etiology worldwide is *M. canis,* but in the United States, *T. tonsurans* is the most common pathogen. The clinical manifestations of tinea capitis may vary according to the specific dermatophyte. Lesions may be scaly patches of alopecia or inflammatory pustules. As with other superficial mycoses, the diagnosis of tinea capitis is based on a combination of clinical and mycologic findings. Clinical evidence supporting a diagnosis of tinea capitis includes scaling patches of scalp alopecia associated with broken hairs, with or without inflammatory lesions. These lesions can mimic superficial bacterial infections. The most direct method of distinguishing between fungal and bacterial infections includes the use of the Wood's light examination, direct microscopic examination of the hair, and fungal cultures (30).

The differential diagnosis of tinea capitis is extensive and includes primary dermatologic conditions such as alopecia areata, discoid lupus erythematosus, lichen planus, psoriasis, and seborrheic dermatitis. In addition, systemic lupus erythematosus, secondary syphilis, and impetigo can also produce a clinical picture that is easily confused with tinea capitis.

Tinea Unguium (Onychomycosis)

Onychomycosis refers to a fungal infection of the fingernails or toenails and is usually secondary to a dermatophyte. The term 'tinea unguium' refers specifically to infection of the fingernails or toenails secondary to a dermatophyte. It is estimated that between 3% and 13% of the population has onychomycosis and that the prevalence increases with advancing age. Over 90% of cases of onychomycosis are due to dermatophytes, most commonly *T. rubrum*, *T. mentagrophytes*, and *E. floccosom*. Other less common pathogens causing onychomycosis include *C. albicans*, *Scytalidium* spp, *Scopulariopsis brevicaulis*, *Aspergillus* spp., and *Fusarium* spp (31,32).

The clinical presentation of onychomycosis is highly variable. The most common early manifestations findings include onychomycosis and subungual thickening together with yellowish brown discoloration of the nail plate (Fig. 5). Well delineated opaque "white islands" on the nail plate are seen with "white superficial" onychomycosis. Diffusely thickened hyperkeratotic and dystrophic nails are the end result of these earlier manifestations of onychomycosis (Fig. 6) (33).

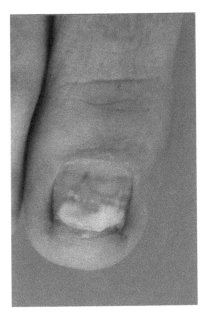

Figure 5 White superficial onychomycosis is characterized by a white opaque discoloration of the nail plate.

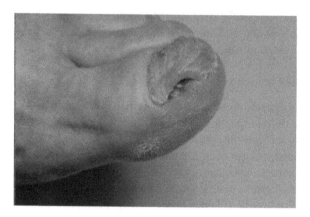

Figure 6 Distal subungual onychomycosis characterized by yellow-brown discoloration of the nail plate with subungual hyperkeratosis and onycholysis. Nail plate growth is affected, resulting in significant curvature. *Source*: Courtesy of Lauren Hughey, MD.

Diagnosis of Tineas and Onychomycosis

The laboratory diagnosis of tinea rests on identification of an organism by microscopic examination of skin or nail scrapings with 10% to 20% KOH on wet mount examination. The demonstration of fungal elements with this preparation confirms a diagnosis of a superficial fungal infection (Fig. 7). In tinea capitis, direct examination is performed by collecting the affected hairs (including the root) and examining these microscopically following preparation with 10% KOH and/or calcifluor white with the demonstration of endothrix or ectothrix spores (Fig. 8). Hairs, pustules, or skin scrapings from affected areas are all suitable for culture. Culture is required for more specific etiologic diagnosis for any of the tineas, and is generally not recommended unless the diagnosis is in question or disease is persistent or recurrent despite antifungal therapy. In certain situations, especially with suspected tinea barbae, fungal cultures may be warranted since bacterial folliculitis can mimic this condition. The use of a Wood's light examination with

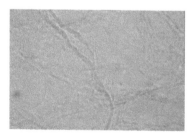

Figure 7 Potassium hydroxide preparation of a dermatophyte, demonstrating branching hyphae in a patient with tinea pedis.

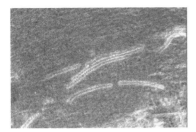

Figure 8 Tinea capitis. Septate hypha elements are identified on the surface of a hair shaft (ectothrix infection) in a patient with scaly patches of alopecia associated with posterior cervical lymphadenopathy. *Source*: Courtesy of Judy Warner.

the tineas is generally unrevealing except for tinea capitis and in cases of suspected erythrasma due to *C. minutissimum*. In tinea capitis, the Wood's light may elicit a yellow-green fluorescence, especially among patients with *M. canis* infection, whereas in erythrasma the examination reveals a deep red or coral fluorescence.

A specific diagnosis of onychomycosis is suspected on the basis of clinical findings of subungual hyperkeratosis, onycholysis, and yellow brown discoloration, and can be more challenging than for other superficial mycoses. While only approximately 50% of dystrophic nails are due to fungal infections, it is important to consider onychomycosis as a cause of nail dystrophy and to obtain fungal cultures and direct microscopy to confirm the diagnosis. In obtaining nail specimens for culture, the nail should be clipped as proximately as possible through its entire thickness. If the nail dystrophy is more proximal, then a scraping of the affected site may be more fruitful. Because fungal elements may not be numerous, adequate sampling is important for both direct microscopy (with 10% KOH or calcifluor white) and culture (34).

NON-DERMATOPHYTE MOLDS

Several molds demonstrate an ability to invade keratinous tissue and cause conditions resembling dermatophytosis. These include *Scytalidium dimidiatum* and *S. hyalinum*; a third agent, *S. brevicaulis* only causes onychomycosis (31,32). All of these agents are found in the soil and are generally found in a worldwide distribution. The infections caused by these three organisms are clinically indistinguishable from those due to dermatophytes, and fungal cultures are required to identify these organisms specifically.

Malassezioses

Malassezia spp. are the cause of tinea versicolor, a superficial cutaneous infection *characterized* by hypo- or hyperpigmented macules or slightly scaly patches on the upper trunk, neck, and arms. Seborrheic dermatitis and dandruff are also associated with *Malassezia* spp., typically *M. restricta*. The *Malassezia* spp. are part of normal skin flora and can be isolated from the skin of 97% of healthy adults (35,36).

Tinea Nigra

This is a condition caused by *Hortaea werneckii*, a dematiaceous fungus that is not a true dermatophyte. Tinea nigra is characterized by brown to dark patches on the palms and soles of young adults. These coin-sized lesions are usually asymptomatic and non-scaly (37).

Black Piedra

Black piedra is a superficial infection of hair shafts due to the organism *Piedra hortae*. This infection results in stone-like concretions on the scalp and facial hair, resulting in hair breaks at the site of the infection. Alopecia is uncommon with black piedra (3).

White Piedra

White piedra is a superficial infection of the hair shaft caused by *Trichosporon ovoides*. This infection leads to concretions that are white or tan and are typically found on facial, axillary, and pubic hair. As with black piedra, hairs become brittle and break at the site of infection (3).

Diagnosis of Non-Dermatophyte Fungi

The diagnosis of malassezioses is usually based on clinical findings supported by microscopic examination of skin scrapings prepared with 10% KOH. Microscopically, short, septate, branching filaments and clusters of small unicellular oval or round budding yeast are seen. This classic finding is often referred to as "spaghetti and meatballs" (Fig. 9). The organisms most commonly responsible for this include *M. furfur* complex and *M. pachydermatis*. Culture from skin

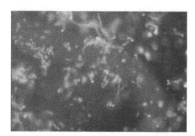

Figure 9 Tinea versicolor. Microscopic appearance of *Malassezia furfur* by KOH and calcifluor stain. Both yeast and hyphal forms are identified. *Source*: Courtesy of Judy Warner.

scrapings is usually unnecessary if confirmation can be made on the basis of direct examination of skin scrapings (35,36).

The diagnosis of tinea nigra can be made by microscopic examination of KOH prepared skin scrapings, demonstrating brownish pigmented hyphae and budding yeast. On culture, *H. werneckii* produces a black colony that is easily distinguished on Saborroud's media (37). The diagnosis of black piedra is made on the basis of microscopic examination of hairs with visible nodules that have been treated with KOH. Once crushed, examination reveals findings of septate brown hyphae and characteristic fusiform ascospores. Culture is usually not necessary to establish the diagnosis of black piedra. The diagnosis of white piedra is established by direct microscopic examination of hairs with nodules that have been treated with KOH and revealing masses of septate hyphae with numerous blastoconidia and arthroconidia (3).

SUMMARY

Compared with the invasive mycoses, the diagnosis of superficial and mucosal fungal infections rely more heavily on clinical findings and less on laboratory support, and a specific fungal etiology is often not pursued or considered clinically relevant. Nonetheless, it is important to recognize and there are selected laboratory tools available to the clinician that are useful in establishing a specific diagnosis when clinically indicated. It is noteworthy that these tools are not necessarily 'high-tech,' but rather based on traditional mycology and histo-pathology, and with the exception of dermatophyte cultures, can be performed in most hospital and office laboratories.

REFERENCES

1. Pappas PG, Rex JH, Sobel JD, et al. Guidelines for treatment of candidiasis. Clin Infect Dis 2004; 38:161–89.
2. Vazquez JA, Sobel JD. Candidiasis. In: Dismukes WE, Pappas PG, Sobel JD, eds. Clinical Mycology. New York: Oxford University Press, 2003:143–87.
3. Weeks J, Moser SA, Elewski BE. Superficial cutaneous fungal infections. In: Dismukes WE, Pappas PG, Sobel JD, eds. Clinical Mycology. New York: Oxford University Press, 2003:367–89.
4. Silverman S, Luangjarmekorn E, Greenspan D. Occurrence of oral *Candida* in irradiated head and neck cancer patients. J Oral Med 1984; 39:194–6.
5. Sobel JD, Vazquez JA. Gastrointestinal and hepatic infections. In: Surawicz CM, Owen RL, eds. Fungal Infections of the Gastrointestinal Tract. Philadelphia: W.B. Saunders, 1995:219–46.
6. Yeo E, Alvarado T, Fainstein V, Bodey GP. Prophylaxis or oropharyngeal candidiasis with clotrimazole. J Clin Oncol 1985; 3:1668–71.

7. Feigal DW, Katz MH, Greenspan D, et al. The prevalence of oral lesions in HIV-infected homosexual and bisexual men: three San Francisco epidemiological cohorts. AIDS 1991; 5:519–25.

8. Vazquez JA. Therapeutic options for the management of oropharyngeal and esophageal candidiasis in HIV/AIDS patients. HIV Clin Trials 2000; 1:47–59.

9. Coleman DC, Bennett DE, Sullivan DJ, et al. Oral *Candida* in HIV infection and AIDS: new perspective/new approaches. Crit Rev Microbiol 1993; 19:61–82.

10. Whelan WL, Delga JM, Wadsworth E, et al. Isolation and characterization of cell surface mutans of *Candida albicans*. Infect Immune 1990; 58:1552–7.

11. Barchiesi F, Morbiducci V, Ancarani F, Scalise G. Emergence of oropharyngeal candidiasis caused by non-*albicans* species of *Candida* in HIV-infected patients (letter). Eur J Epidemiol 1993; 9:455–6.

12. Darouiche RO. Oropharyngeal and esophageal candidiasis in immunocompromised patients: treatment issues. Clin Infect Dis 1998; 26:259–72.

13. Letiner T. Oral thrush or acute pseudomembranous candidiasis; a clinical-pathologic study of 44 cases. Oral Surg 1964; 18:27–37.

14. Budtz-Jorgensen E, Stenderup A, Grabowski M. An epidemiological study of yeasts in elderly denture wearers. Community Dent Oral Epidemiol 1975; 3:115–9.

15. Daniluk T, Tokajuk G, Stokowska W, et al. Occurrence rate of oral *Candida albicans* in denture wearer patients. Adv Med Sci 2006; Suppl 1:77–80.

16. Russotto SB. The role of *Candida albicans* in the pathogenesis of angular cheilosis. J Prosthet Dent 1980; 44:243–6.

17. Smith JM, Meech RJ. The polymicrobial nature of oropharyngeal thrush. N Z Med J 1984; 97:335–6.

18. Wheeler RR, Peacock JE, Cruz JM, Richter JE. Esophagitis in the immunocompromised host: role of esophagoscopy in diagnosis. Rev Infect Dis 1987; 9:88–96.

19. Clotet B, Grifol M, Parra O, et al. Asymptomatic esophageal candidiasis in the acquire-immunodeficiency-syndrome-related complex. Ann Intern Med 1986; 105:145.

20. Kodsi BE, Wickremesinghe C, Kozinn PJ, Iswara K, Goldberg PK. *Candida* esophagitis: a prospective study of 27 cases. Gastroenterol 1976; 71:715–9.

21. Hurley R, De Louvois J. *Candida* vaginitis. Postgrad Med J 1979; 55:645–7.

22. Sobel JD. Epidemiology and pathogenesis of recurrent vulvovaginal candidiasis. Am J Obstet Gynecol 1985; 152:924–35.

23. Reed BD. Risk factors for *Candida* vulvovaginitis. Obstet Gynecol Surv 1992; 47:551–9.

24. Sobel JD, Faro S, Force RW, et al. Vulvovaginal candidiasis: epidemiologic, diagnostic, and therapeutic considerations. Am J Obstet Gynecol 1998; 178:203–11.

25. Alteras I, Feuerman EJ, David M, Shohat B, Livni E. Widely disseminated cutaneous candidosis in adults. Sabouraudia 1979; 17:383–8.

26. Elewski BE, Hazen PG. The superficial mycoses and the dermatophytes. J Am Acad Dermatol 1989; 21:655–73.

27. Summerbell RC. Epidemiology and ecology of onychomycosis. Dermatology 1997; 194(Suppl. 1):32–6.

28. Aly R, Berger T. Common superficial fungal infections in patients with AIDS. Clin Infect Dis 1996; 22:S128–32.

29. Demis DJ, ed. Fungus infections. In: Clinical Dermatology. 26th ed., Section 17. Philadelphia: Lippincott Williams and Wilkins, 1999:1–23.
30. Elewski BE. Tinea capitis: a current perspective. J Am Acad Dermatol 2000; 42:1–20.
31. Ellis DH, Marley JE, Watson AB, Williams TG. Non-dermatophytes in onychomycosis of the toenails. Br J Dermatol 1997; 136:490–3.
32. Gupta AK, Elewski BE. Nondermatophyte causes of onychomycosis and superficial mycoses. Curr Topics Med Mycol 1996; 7:87–97.
33. Richardson M, Elewski BE. Tinea Unguium (Onychomycosis). In: Superficial Fungal Infections. Oxford: Health Press, 2000:36–7.
34. Zaias N, Glick B, Rebell G. Diagnosing and treating onychomycosis. J Fam Prac 1996; 42:513–8.
35. Hoeprich PD, Jordan MC, Ronald AR. Superficial fungal infections of the skin. In: Infectious Diseases. 5th ed. Philadelphia: J.B. Lippincott, 1994:1029–49.
36. Gemmer CM, De Angelis YM, Theelen B, Boekhour T, Dawson TL. Fast non-invasive method for molecular detection and differentiation of *Malassezia* yeast species in human skin and application of the method do dandruff microbiology. J Clin Microbiol 2002; 40:3350–7.
37. Kwon-Chung KJ, Bennett JE. Tinea nigra. In: Medical Mycology. Philadelphia: Lea & Febiger, 1992:191–7.

8

Invasive Mold Infections

Fernanda P. Silveira

Division of Infectious Diseases, Department of Medicine, University of Pittsburgh, Pittsburgh, Pennsylvania, U.S.A.

Flavio Queiroz-Telles

Department of Communitarian Health, Hospital de Clínicas, Universidade Federal do Paraná, Curitiba, Paraná, Brazil

Marcio Nucci

Department of Internal Medicine, Hospital Universitário Clementino Fraga Filho, Universidade Federal do Rio de Janeiro, Rio de Janeiro, Brazil

INTRODUCTION

Over the past 20 years, the incidence of invasive mold infections has increased substantially. These infections are considered opportunistic because they occur almost exclusively in immunocompromised individuals. Indeed, the increased incidence of invasive mold infections paralleled the increase in the population of immunosuppressed individuals, including patients with hematological malignancies, transplant recipients, acquired immunodeficiency syndrome (AIDS) patients, and those receiving broad-spectrum antibiotics or high-dose corticosteroids. The emergence of invasive mold infections has created a great challenge to microbiologists because most of these fungi were frequently considered as contaminants in the laboratory instead of true pathogens. The diagnosis of these opportunistic infections is supported by microbiologic documentation, including direct mycological examination, culture, and histopathology. Non-microbiologic tests such antigen and antibody detection are also relevant, but the current challenge is to develop rapid and accurate non-microbiologic based methods that may lead to the prompt institution of specific therapy (1). Furthermore, the spectrum and clinical presentation of infections caused by molds may overlap: different molds may cause a similar clinical picture and, depending on the host, different clinical presentations may occur with a single mold. Therefore, a comprehension of the epidemiology and clinical scenario where these infections develop is essential to interpret the results of laboratory tests and the growth of these molds in different biological materials, and consequently to make a correct diagnosis.

The classification of infections caused by molds is based on the genus or class of the fungus causing the infection (e.g., aspergillosis, fusariosis, scedosporiosis, zygomycosis), and when there is only histopathologic evidence of mycosis, it is based on the appearance of the hyphae in tissue (e.g., hyalohyphomycosis for hyaline hyphae, phaeohyphomycosis for darkly pigmented hyphae or zygomycosis for coenocytic/poor septate tortuous hyphae). Since *Aspergillus* spp. is by far the most frequent mold causing invasive infection, in this chapter a greater emphasis is devoted to the diagnosis of invasive aspergillosis (IA).

EPIDEMIOLOGY OF INVASIVE MOLD INFECTIONS

Among the invasive mold infections, *Aspergillus* spp. are the most frequent agents, accounting for 75% of mold infections in patients with hematological malignancies (2) and almost 85% in hematopoietic stem cell transplant recipients (3). In the latter population of patients, *Aspergillus* spp. are now the leading cause of invasive mycosis (4,5). An incidence of 12.4 cases of aspergillosis per million per year was estimated in a population-based active laboratory surveillance for invasive mycoses, and aspergillosis was the fourth most common fungal infection (6).

IA occurs in the setting of a variety of underlying conditions. In a series of 621 cases, underlying diseases such as alcoholism, chronic bronchitis, hepatitis, prematurity, and burns were present in some cases. However, the large majority of cases (72.6%) occurred in patients with hematological malignancies, especially acute leukemia (31.1%), chronic leukemia (12.2%), and lymphoma (9%). Thirty-six percent of the patients had undergone stem cell transplantation and 10% were recipients of solid organ transplants. Among transplant recipients, the incidence was higher in allogeneic stem cell transplants (12.8%), followed by heart-lung transplants (11.1%) and small bowel/liver-small bowel transplants (10.7%). Human immunodeficiency virus (HIV) infection (9%), solid tumors (2%), and chronic immunologic diseases (2%) completed the list of underlying diseases (7).

In a recent epidemiologic study, the incidence of IA was estimated in 4621 hematopoietic stem cell transplants and 4,110 solid organ transplants performed in 19 North American centers (8). The cumulative incidence at 12 months was 0.5% after autologous transplantation, 2.3% after allogeneic transplantation from a human leukocyte antigen (HLA)-matched related donor, and 3.9% after transplantation from an unrelated donor. Among solid organ transplant recipients, the 12-month cumulative incidence was 0.1% after kidney transplantation, 0.3% after liver transplantation, 0.8% after heart transplantation, and 2.4% after lung transplantation.

Major risk factors for IA include prolonged and profound neutropenia and the use of corticosteroids. This explains why patients with hematological malignancies are at greater risk for developing aspergillosis. In recent years, changes in the epidemiology of aspergillosis have been reported (Table 1). In hematopoietic stem cell transplant recipients, IA has a bimodal distribution, with the first peak in the early post-engraftment period and the second peak at a median of 100 days after transplant (9). Recent epidemiologic data showed that the incidence of early aspergillosis is decreasing, whereas that of late aspergillosis is increasing. These trends may be related to the increased use of non-myeloablative transplants, as well as myeloablative transplants using the peripheral blood as source of stem cells rather than bone marrow. Peripheral blood stem cell transplants are associated with a shorter duration of neutropenia, thus reducing the risk for aspergillosis occurring in the pre-engraftment period (early aspergillosis). However, the risk for late (after engraftment) aspergillosis increases because the incidence of graft-versus-host disease (GVHD), which is a risk factor for aspergillosis, increases (10,11). In recent years, the incidence of infection due to non-*fumigatus* species has also increased (4). In a series of 40 cases of IA in patients with cancer from 1998 to 2001, 70% were caused by non-*fumigatus Aspergillus*. Infection due to *Aspergillus fumigatus* was the predominant cause of late onset aspergillosis in allogeneic stem cell transplant recipients, whereas non-*fumigatus* aspergilli were more frequent in neutropenic patients (12).

Similar to stem cell transplantation, IA in liver transplant recipients tends to occur later compared to previous series. This trend may be related to the fact that cytomegalovirus disease, a risk factor for aspergillosis, occurs later in these patients, due to the prophylactic use of gancyclovir (13). In AIDS patients,

Table 1 Changes in the Epidemiology of IA

Setting	Change	Reason
Allogeneic HSCT	Late (after engraftment) occurrence	↑ Frequency and severity of GVHD
	Non-fumigatus	Unclear
Autologous HSCT	↓ Incidence	↓ Duration of neutropenia
Liver transplant	Late occurrence	Unclear
	Less disseminated infection	Unclear
AIDS	↓ Incidence	Better control of HIV infection

Abbreviations: AIDS, acquired immunodeficiency syndrome; GVHD, graft-versus-host disease; HIV, human immunodeficiency virus; HSCT, hematopoietic stem cell transplant; IA, invasive aspergillosis.

a decrease in the incidence of IA has been observed, possibly due to the better control of AIDS with the use of highly active anti-retroviral treatment (7).

The annual incidence of infections caused by non-*Aspergillus* molds is much lower than of aspergillosis: 1.7 cases per million per year for zygomycosis, 1.2 cases per million per year for hyalohyphomycosis and one case per million per year for phaeohyphomycosis (6). However, similar to aspergillosis, the incidence of these infections has increased in patients with hematological diseases and transplant recipients (14). In a review of 259 cases of fusariosis, including immunocompromised and immunocompetent patients, 79% had a diagnosis of cancer (15). In a study in 83 patients with hematological malignancies, the infection occurred more frequently in patients with acute leukemia (56%), and most patients (83%) were neutropenic (16). In stem cell transplant recipients, fusariosis has a first peak of incidence in the early post-transplant period (during neutropenia), a second peak of occurrence at a median of 70 days after transplant (patients with GVHD receiving corticosteroids), and a third peak more than one year after transplant. Different from early cases, in late fusariosis, neutropenia is not a risk factor (17). While in stem cell transplant recipients the incidence of fusariosis seems to be increasing (3), in solid organ transplant recipients the infection is unusual (14).

The class *Zygomycetes* has two orders: *Mucorales* and *Entomophthorales*. Fungi belonging to the order *Mucorales* usually cause acute, angioinvasive infections in immunocompromised patients, whereas members of the order *Entomophthorales* cause chronic subcutaneous infections in immunocompetent patients. Invasive zygomycosis (mucormycosis) occurs especially in diabetic patients with or without ketoacidosis, patients with hematological malignancies, transplant recipients, and patients receiving deferoxamine therapy for iron or aluminum overload (18). In a review of 929 reported cases of zygomycosis, diabetes was the most frequent underlying disease (36%), followed by cancer (17%), solid organ transplantation (7%), and deferoxamine therapy (6%) (19).

The incidence of zygomycosis has increased over the past years. In a study in cancer patients, the incidence was eight cases per 100,000 admissions between 1989 and 1993 and 20 cases per 100,000 admissions between 1994 and 1998 (20). In another report from the same institution, zygomycosis was the second most common invasive mold infection, with an incidence per 1,000 patient-days of 0.095 cases, compared with 0.302 cases of IA, and 0.073 cases of fusariosis (21). A higher incidence of zygomycosis in hematopoietic stem cell transplant recipients has also been reported in other studies (3,22). More recently, breakthrough zygomycosis in patients receiving voriconazole has been reported (23–26), and a single-center case-control study identified the previous exposure to voriconazole as a significant risk factor for zygomycosis by multivariate analysis (21). Although the use of voriconazole may have contributed to the occurrence of zygomycosis, there are some data indicating that the incidence of zygomycosis was increasing before the introduction of voriconazole in clinical practice. Other factors likely associated with the recent increase include severity and type of immunosuppression (27).

The mortality of invasive mold infections is high. In a study, the case-fatality rate of IA was 58%, and was highest in stem cell transplant recipients (86.7%) and in patients with infection involving the central nervous system or disseminated to other organs (88.1%) (28). In fusariosis, the 90-day survival was 25% among patients with hematological malignancies (16) and 13% among hematopoietic stem cell transplant recipients (17). Similarly, the mortality rate of infections caused by other molds is usually high, and depends on the degree of immunosuppression and if the infection is localized or disseminated. Zygomycosis in diabetic patients has a particularly rapid and fatal course (18).

DIAGNOSIS OF INVASIVE ASPERGILLOSIS

Clinical Diagnosis

Aspergillus species are widely distributed in nature and they cause a broad spectrum of diseases, including mycotoxicosis, allergic pulmonary disease, superficial and cutaneous infections, intracavitary colonization, and invasive disease. IA usually occurs after the inhalation of conidia contained in the air. Rare cases of direct inoculation into the skin, operative wounds, cornea, and ear have been reported. In addition, a gastrointestinal origin of aspergillosis has been suggested (29). The clinical spectrum of IA varies from localized to disseminated infection, and the clinical presentation depends on the portal of entry and the status of the immune system. A striking characteristic of IA is the tendency of hyphae to invade blood vessels, causing thrombosis and infarction, and subsequent invasion of the necrotic tissue. Depending on the status of the immune system, dissemination may occur. The lungs and the sinuses are by far the most frequent organs involved ($\sim$90%), and the infection may be acute or chronic. The main determinant of the clinical form of pulmonary aspergillosis is the status of the immune system of the host. Acute invasive pulmonary aspergillosis occurs in patients with severe immunosuppression, notably hematopoietic stem cell transplant recipients and patients with acute leukemia. A subacute form occurs in a group of less-severely immunosuppressed patients, including AIDS, chronic granulomatous disease, diabetes, and alcoholism. A chronic form of disease has been recently characterized, with three entities: chronic necrotizing, cavitary, and fibrosing pulmonary aspergillosis. Finally, aspergilloma (fungus ball) occurs in immunocompetent patients with a pre-existing pulmonary cavity that becomes colonized by *Aspergillus*. The fungus ball is separated from the normal lung by a cap of fibrotic tissue, and there is no invasion of hyphae in the surrounding lung tissue. In addition, there is another clinical entity, allergic bronchopulmonary aspergillosis, that affects atopic individuals who develop asthma following inhalation of *Aspergillus* conidia. The two later entities are not true invasive diseases and are not discussed in this chapter. Comprehensive reviews on these topics have been published recently (30–32).

Acute Invasive Pulmonary Aspergillosis

Acute invasive lung aspergillosis occurs most commonly in neutropenic patients or in non-neutropenic patients receiving high doses of immunosuppressive agents (especially corticosteroids). A diagnosis of IA should be considered in any patient with profound ($<100/mm^3$) and prolonged (>14 days) neutropenia who is persistently febrile despite appropriate antibiotics. In these patients, the clinical picture is typically of a pulmonary infarction, with fever, dry cough, and pleuritic chest pain (33). However, symptoms may be absent at presentation. On the other hand, patients receiving corticosteroids may not present with fever. As the disease progresses, other manifestations appear, including hemoptysis and dyspnea.

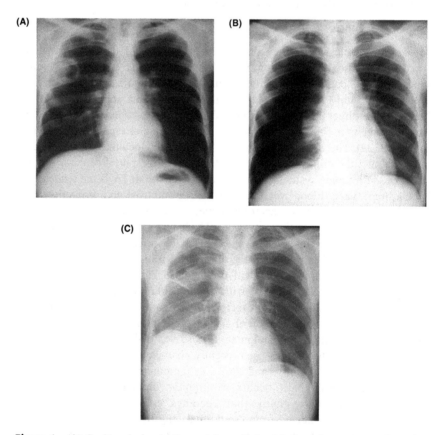

Figure 1 (**A**) Cavitary lesion in the periphery of the right lung in a neutropenic patient with acute lymphoid leukemia and prolonged fever. The X ray was performed on the day of neutrophils recovery. Five days later, the patient complained of excruciating thoracic pain. X ray showed pneumothorax in the right lung. (**B**) Before drainage and (**C**) after drainage.

Occasionally, spontaneous pneumothorax (Fig. 1) or pneumomediastinum may occur (34).

In the early stages of infection, the chest X ray is usually normal, or demonstrates non-specific images of patchy foci of airspace consolidation. However, the CT scan is a valuable diagnostic tool. The earliest radiological lesion is the halo sign (Fig. 2), a discrete zone or halo surrounding a pulmonary nodule with attenuation intermediate between the center of the lesion and the surrounding lung (35). The halo represents an area of hemorrhage, and may precede the development of cavitation by two to three weeks. Although the halo sign may be present in different diseases, its occurrence in the setting of a patient with profound and prolonged neutropenia with persistent fever is virtually diagnostic of pneumonia caused by a mold (*Aspergillus* spp. is by far the most frequent agent, but other fungi, such as Zygomycetes, *Fusarium* spp., and *Scedosporium apiospermum* may cause the same picture). The importance of the CT scan in the early diagnosis of IA has been demonstrated in a study that showed that the halo sign was present in 92% of cases when a CT scan was performed early and routinely in persistently febrile neutropenic patients, compared to 13% when CT scans were performed only after the appearance of signs and symptoms suggestive

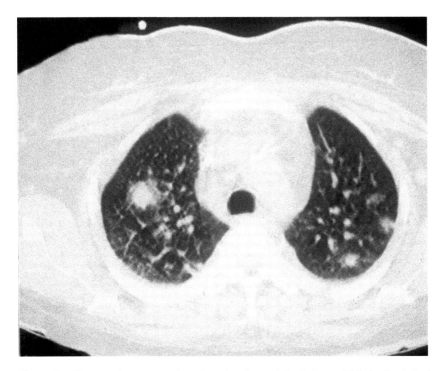

Figure 2 CT scan of a neutropenic patient showing nodular lesions with halo sign in both lungs.

of aspergillosis. More importantly, the early recognition of the halo sign allowed the early institution of appropriate antifungal therapy, with a significant reduction in the mortality rate (36). However, the duration of the halo sign is short, and after a few days it is substituted by non-specific infiltrates (Fig. 3) (37). Later in the course of the infection, another typical lesion appears, the air-crescent sign (Fig. 4), but its recognition has a much lower impact on the prognosis of IA, since it usually appears only when the patient is no longer neutropenic (38). By MRI, the earliest lesion appears as a "target" lesion, with a hypodense or isodense center, represented by cavitation or coagulative necrosis; a higher signal intensity in the periphery, corresponding to subacute hemorrhage or hemorrhagic infarction; and peripheral enhancement with gadolinium diethylenetriamine pentaacetic acid, which represents an area of inflammation and hyperemia (39). In the occasional patient who develops IA with neutrophil recovery, the whole sequence of images can be appreciated by X ray (Fig. 5).

In non-neutropenic patients, the clinical picture may be more insidious, and productive cough is more frequent. In patients with GVHD who are receiving corticosteroids, the presentation may be similar to a bacterial pneumonia, with the acute onset of high fever and productive cough. Indeed, in one study, bacterial pneumonia was frequently diagnosed concomitantly with aspergillosis. A clue to the diagnosis of aspergillosis in these patients was the presence of nodules, but they

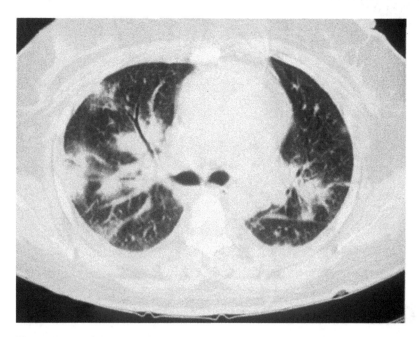

Figure 3 Multiple areas of non-specific alveolar consolidation in both lungs of a neutropenic patient with invasive aspergillosis.

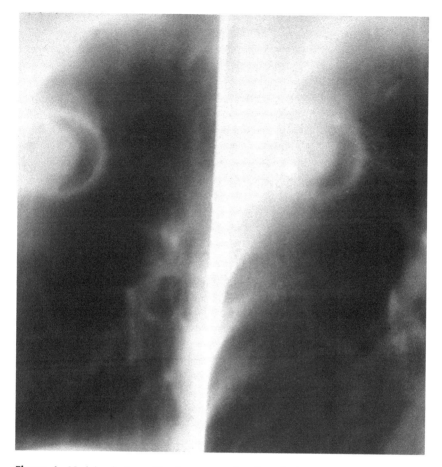

Figure 4 Nodular lesion with air-crescent sign in a leukemic patient with invasive aspergillosis.

were present in only 50% of the initial chest X ray, whereas subsequent CT scans were diagnostic in all cases, showing either nodules or cavitary lesions (40). The radiological picture (CT scan) of pulmonary IA occurring late in the course of hematopoietic stem cell transplantation was described in 27 patients. A total of 111 chest CT scans were reviewed and showed ill-defined consolidation in 13 CT scans, lesions with halo sign in 12, centrilobular nodules in 12, ground-glass attenuation in 8, pleural effusions in 7 and cavitary lesions in 4 (41).

In lung transplant recipients, 60% of patients with IA present with either cavitary or nodular lesions (42), whereas in a small series of pulmonary aspergillosis in cardiac transplantation, nodules were present in all patients (43). However, in other settings, the presence of nodules or cavities may not be frequent: in a series of 93 patients with AIDS and a diagnosis of invasive pulmonary

(A) (B)

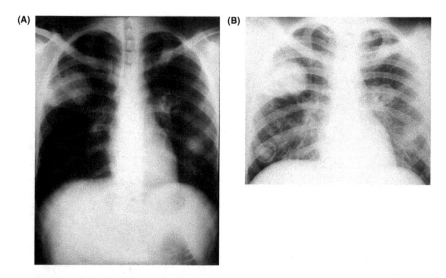

Figure 5 Invasive pulmonary aspergillosis in a patient with acute myeloid leukemia. On the day of bone marrow recovery the patient complained of dry cough and thoracic pain. X ray showed an alveolar consolidation in the right lung, and an ill-defined nodular lesion and a cavity in the left lung (**A**). X ray taken 2 days later showed multiple thin walled cavities with opacities in the interior (**B**).

aspergillosis, cavitary lesions and nodules were present in 31% and 14%, respectively, and the majority of patients (73%) had non-specific infiltrates (44). A comprehensive review of the radiological spectrum of pulmonary aspergillosis has been published recently (45).

Subacute and Chronic Invasive Pulmonary Aspergillosis

Subacute invasive pulmonary aspergillosis is much less frequent than acute pulmonary aspergillosis, and occurs in a variety of clinical conditions, such as chronic granulomatous disease, diabetes mellitus, alcoholism, AIDS, chronic use of corticosteroids, and sometimes no apparent underlying condition (29). The clinical picture is insidious, with productive cough, low-grade fever (may be absent), weight loss, and occasionally hemoptysis. The typical radiological pattern is one of a cavitary lesion that increases slowly over time, with lung consolidation surrounding the cavity (Fig. 6). The lesion may expand to affect the entire lung, and invade adjacent structures (chest wall, vertebral column).

Recently, three other clinical entities have been characterized: chronic necrotizing pulmonary aspergillosis, chronic cavitary pulmonary aspergillosis and chronic fibrosing pulmonary aspergillosis with or without pleural involvement. All entities have in common the chronic (> 3 months) duration of pulmonary symptoms and the radiological evidence of a progressive (over months or years)

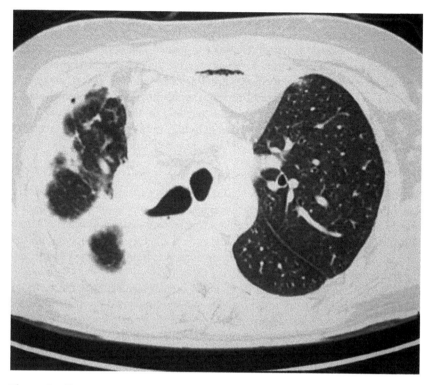

Figure 6 Chronic necrotizing aspergillosis in a patient with chronic obstructive lung disease. CT scan shows a fibrotic lesion in the upper lobe of the right lung with retraction and thickening of the pleura and alveolar opacities.

pulmonary lesion with surrounding inflammation. In a series of 18 cases, constitutional symptoms (weight loss, fatigue, malaise) were present in all patients. Chronic productive cough and hemoptysis were the most frequent pulmonary symptoms. A cavitary lesion in the lung was present in all patients, and frequently there was more than one lesion. Expansion of the size of the cavities and inflammation in the surrounding lung were remarkable findings (46).

Tracheobronchitis

Aspergillus tracheobronchitis occurs particularly in lung transplant recipients, although occasional cases have been reported in other diseases such as AIDS (47), lymphoma (48), lupus (49) and after hematopoietic stem cell transplantation (50–52). In lung transplant recipients, *Aspergillus* tracheobronchitis is the most frequent clinical form of IA, accounting for 37% of cases, followed by pulmonary aspergillosis (32%), bronchial anastomotic infection (21%), and disseminated infection (10%) (42).

The clinical manifestations of *Aspergillus* tracheobronchitis are non-specific, and consist of cough, dyspnea, wheezing, chest pain, hemoptysis, and fever (may be absent). If not diagnosed and treated appropriately, the disease progresses to respiratory failure due to obstructive lung disease. The chest X ray is usually normal early in the course of the disease, but the CT scan may show bronchial wall thickening, peribronchial consolidation, and centrilobular nodules. As the disease progresses, and depending on the immune status of the patient, extension to the lung parenchyma may occur, with alveolar consolidation.

Sinusitis

The clinical spectrum of *Aspergillus* sinusitis is similar to pulmonary aspergillosis: there is an acute invasive sinusitis that affects mainly neutropenic patients and hematopoietic stem cell transplant recipients, a chronic invasive sinusitis that occurs in immunocompetent or less severely immunocompromised patients, and two non-invasive forms of sinus aspergillosis: fungus ball and allergic sinusitis.

The typical clinical scenario of acute invasive sinusitis is the same as invasive pulmonary aspergillosis: patients with profound and prolonged neutro-penia with persistent fever despite antibiotic therapy, or hematopoietic stem cell transplant recipients receiving high doses of corticosteroids for the treatment of GVHD. Fever is a prominent feature, occurring in virtually all cases. Periorbital swelling, nasal congestion, headache, cough, and epistaxis are frequent mani-festations, and nasal discharge occurs later in the course of the disease. Extension to the palate and orbit may occur.

Chronic *Aspergillus* sinusitis may occur in immunocompetent individuals, or in patients with different underlying conditions such as alcoholism, diabetes, and AIDS. Early in the course of the disease, the clinical picture of *Aspergillus* chronic invasive sinusitis and of allergic sinusitis may overlap, with symptoms of headache and nasal obstruction. However, in chronic invasive sinusitis, the disease may progress to involve adjacent structures and the patient may complain of visual symptoms and proptosis.

The radiological appearance of fungal sinusitis is variable. Often the findings are non-specific, with mucosal thickening and sinus opacification (Fig. 7). The CT scan is helpful to detect bony destruction and extension to surrounding areas, whereas the MRI is useful to demonstrate soft tissue involvement.

Cutaneous Aspergillosis

Cutaneous aspergillosis may occur as a primary infection or as a manifestation of disseminated disease (53). Primary cutaneous aspergillosis usually involves sites of skin injury, such as intravenous catheter exit sites or sites of adhesive dressings, burns, or surgical wounds (54). Secondary cutaneous aspergillosis develops either as a result of hematogenous spread, or from contiguous extension to the skin from infected structures. Primary cutaneous aspergillosis occurs more frequently in

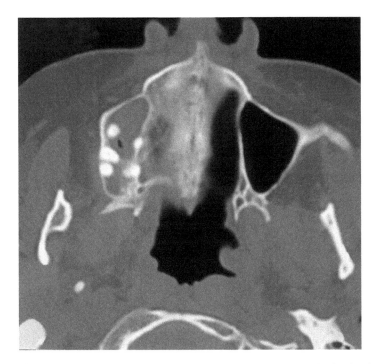

Figure 7 Sinus CT scan of a leukemic patient showing opacity in the right maxillary sinus and thickening of the mucosa.

three settings: neonates and neutropenic and burn patients. In neonates, most cases occur in premature infants who are receiving corticosteroids. A portal of entry is apparent in half of the cases (55,56). In neutropenic patients, the lesions appear at intravenous catheter exit sites, and are a result of contamination of adhesive dressings applied to the skin (57).

The lesions of cutaneous aspergillosis usually begin as macules, papules, nodules, or plaques. In neonates the lesions evolve to pustules and necrotic ulcers (56). Infections occurring in catheter exit sites usually begin with an erythematous lesion and those arising from occlusive dressings may have the appearance of a hemorrhagic bulla (58). Secondary lesions usually occur in the setting of disseminated aspergillosis. They may be single or multiple, papular or nodular, and are well circumscribed. The lesions may be painful and eventually develop central necrosis, taking the appearance of an ecthyma gangrenosum-like lesion.

Central Nervous System Aspergillosis

Aspergillosis in the central nervous system occurs almost exclusively in immuno-suppressed individuals, as a consequence of dissemination from a remote focus (usually the lungs), with vascular thrombosis and cerebral infarction (Fig. 8). It occurs in about 10% of cases of IA, and most cases occur in neutropenic patients with hematological malignancies. Other populations at risk include solid organ transplant recipients, patients receiving corticosteroids, burn patients, and patients with hepatic failure. Most of the infections involve the brain, with rare cases of myelitis and meningitis (59). Occasionally aspergillosis in the central nervous system arises as an extension from a sinusitis (60) or from traumatic inoculation (61).

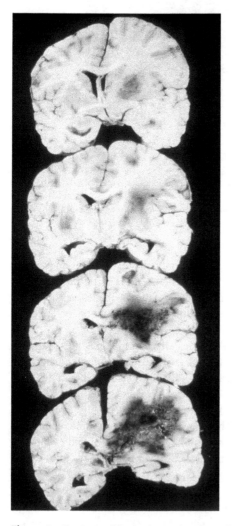

Figure 8 Sections of brain tissue showing a large area of hemorrhagic infarction in the right hemisphere. A smaller lesion is present in the left hemisphere.

In neutropenic patients, the sudden appearance of a paresis, confusion, behavior changes, or reduced consciousness should alert the clinician to the possible diagnosis of cerebral aspergillosis. Usually, highly immunosuppressed patients present with non-specific findings, such as alteration in mental status and seizures, whereas patients with less severe immunosuppression present with focal signs and headache.

The radiological appearance of cerebral aspergillosis is variable, depending on the degree of immunosuppression. Three radiological patterns of cerebral aspergillosis have been described: infarctions, abscesses, and dural enhancement (62). When the patient is neutropenic, multiple areas of cortical and subcortical hypodensity on CT and hyperintensity on MRI are consistent with infarction (Fig. 9). If the infarctions become hemorrhagic (which is frequent), they exhibit increased density on CT and increased T1 signal on MRI. As the neutrophil count increases, the lesions evolve to form abscesses, with ring-enhancing lesions (Fig. 10). Abscesses may be present at the gray-white matter junction. The third pattern, dural enhancement, occurs when aspergillosis arises as an extension of paranasal sinusitis.

Other Forms of Invasive Aspergillosis

IA may affect any organ. In the majority of cases, the clinical picture has no distinctive characteristics, and the diagnosis is made by biopsy and/or culture. This is the case of spinal osteomyelitis, which may occur both in immunocompromised

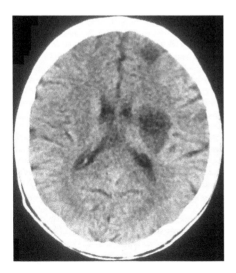

Figure 9   Invasive brain aspergillosis in a neutropenic patient with acute lymphoid leukemia. A diagnosis of pulmonary aspergillosis was performed 3 days before the sudden onset of left hemiparesis. Brain CT scan showed 2 areas of hypodensity in the left hemisphere.

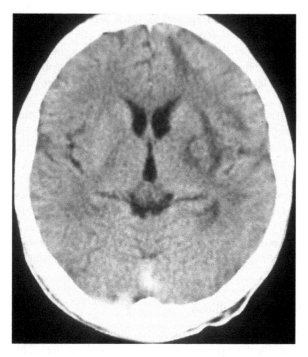

Figure 10 CT scan of the same patient as in Figure 9, 10 days later, showing a marked reduction in the edema and the appearance of a ring-enhancing lesion.

and immunocompetent patients (63), mediastinitis and prosthetic vascular graft infections, which occur as a result of contamination in the operative room (64,65), and stomatitis in patients with acute leukemia (66).

Culture-Based Diagnosis

The genus *Aspergillus* comprises several hundred of species, and 38 have been reported to cause disease in humans (67). However, most infections are caused by five species: *A. fumigatus* (~90% of cases), *Aspergillus flavus*, *Aspergillus niger*, *Aspergillus terreus*, and *Aspergillus nidulans*. A distinguishing characteristic of pathogenic *Aspergillus* species is their ability to grow at 35°C to 37°C. *Aspergillus* species grow easily in different media, including conventional agar media. The most useful media are Sabouraud's agar and malt extract agar. Colonies of *Aspergillus* grow rapidly and have a powdery appearance. They may be white, green, yellow, red, brown, or black, depending on the color of the hyphae and conidial heads. After 48 to 72 hours, conidial structures characteristic of each species are formed. However, in some circumstances, it may take days or weeks for spores to appear. The use of potato dextrose, potato flake, malt extract, or inhibitory mold agar as primary isolation media for *Aspergillus* spp. may speed growth rate and the production of conidia. Although most species of *Aspergillus* grow rapidly, there are variations in the rate of growth among some species. On direct microscopic examination, *Aspergillus* hyphae are easily found as branching, hyaline hyphae (Fig. 11). The hyphae may be present as small fragments, or in cases of cavitary aspergillosis, as long strands of hyphae. On rare occasions, conidial structures are visible by direct examination. The genus is easily recognized by its conidiophores terminating in an apical vesicle and in a basal foot cell inserted into the hyphae.

The identification of species is based on differences in morphological and cultural characteristics. In addition, biochemical and molecular approaches may be useful (68,69). The morphological identification of species is based on various aspects of the shape, color, and size of the different structures (conidial heads, conidiophores, vesicles, phialides, conidia, etc.) of *Aspergillus*. Although the appearance of the species may be appreciated in Sabouraud's agar, Czapek–Dox agar is very useful to better delineate its morphology. Table 2 shows the most important morphological characteristics of the five most frequent *Aspergillus* species. The colonies of *A. fumigatus* are downy to powdery, blue-green or gray-green, with a pale or yellowish reverse. The conidial head has a long columnar shape, the conidiophores are smooth walled, colorless or greenish, and the phialides are uniseriate, and concentrated on the upper pole of the vesicle. The conidia are round, disposed in chains and green. Unlike most other pathogenic

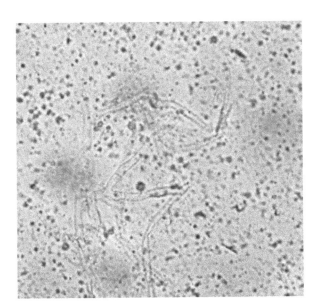

Figure 11 Wet mount of sputum from a patient with cavitary aspergillosis showing several hyaline septate hyphae with acute-angle branching. KOH.

Table 2 Morphological Characteristics of *Aspergillus* Species

Characteristic	A. fumigatus	A. flavus	A. niger	A. terreus	A. nidulans
Appearance of the colony	Downy to powdery	Downy to powdery	Downy to powdery	Powdery	Downy to powdery
Color of the colony	Blue-green or gray-green	Yellow-green	Begin white or yellow and become black or brown	Yellowish-brown or cinnamon-brown	Dark green or dark olive
Color of the reverse	Pale or yellowish	Pale or yellowish	Pale yellow or uncolored	Pale yellow to brown	Purple olive
Shape of the conidial head	Long column	Radiated	Radiated	Compact columns	Short compact columns
Conidiophores	Smooth walls, colorless or green	Rough walls	Smooth walls	Smooth and hyaline walls	Brown
Phialides	Uniseriate, in the upper surface of the vesicle	Uni- and biseriate	Biseriate, covering the entire surface of the vesicle	Biseriate, upper part of the vesicle surface	Biseriate
Conidia	Green, round, in chains	Round, in chains	Brown, round, in chains	Chains, round, brown	Round, green, in chains
Comments	Grows at 48°C			Aleurioconidia	Hüle cells

species of *Aspergillus*, *A. fumigatus* grows well at 48°C. The colonies of *A. flavus* grow rapidly, have a downy or powdery texture, and are yellow-green on the surface, with a pale or yellowish reverse. Unlike *A. fumigatus*, the conidial heads radiate, and conidiogenous cells are uni- and biseriate. Conidiophores are rough walled, and the conidia are round and in chains. *A. niger* produces downy or powdery colonies that begin as white or yellow and become black or brown on the surface, with a pale yellow or uncolored reverse. Similar to *A. flavus*, the conidial heads radiate, but the conidiophores are smooth-walled, the phialides are biseriate, and cover the entire surface of the vesicle. The conidia are brown, round, and in chains. *A. terreus* produces yellowish-brown or cinnamon-brown downy or powdery colonies with a reverse pale yellow to brown. The conidial heads are in the form of compact columns; the conidiophores are hyaline and smooth walled. The phialides are biseriate, and limited mainly to the upper part of the vesicle surface. The conidia are in chains, round, smooth-walled, and brown. A second and less conspicuous yeast-like type of conidia (aleurioconidia) is formed on the submerged hyphae. *A. nidulans* produces downy to powdery colonies that grow moderately rapidly. They have a dark green or dark olive color on the surface and a purple or olive reverse. Conidial heads appear as short, compact columns, conidiophores are brown and sinuous, and conidiogenous cells are biseriate. Conidia are round, green, and in chains. *A. nidulans* produces rounded hüle cells. Keys for the tentative identification of *Aspergillus* species are found in other texts (70).

Since pathogenic aspergilli are ubiquitous in the air, contamination of plates and biological material sent to the laboratory may occur. Therefore, it is important to be cautious in examining culture plates. The isolation of several colonies from the same specimen or the same fungus from different specimens is highly suggestive of a true growth, whereas the isolation of a single colony from only one biological sample should raise the question of contamination. When interpreting the result of a mycological examination, a positive direct examination of the biological material in addition to isolation of *Aspergillus* species in culture provides a more reliable diagnosis. However, the sensitivity of detection by smear examination is low. Therefore, the clinical significance of a single positive culture with a negative direct smear is difficult to determine. Potassium-hydroxide concentrated smears prepared from sedimented remains of clinical specimens may be useful to differentiate between contamination and infection (71).

In addition to technical aspects of direct examination and culture, the interpretation of the growth of *Aspergillus* species from different biological materials depends on the clinical context. Various studies have shown that the isolation of *Aspergillus* species from non-sterile fluids may have different yields, depending on the underlying disease. In general, allogeneic hematopoietic stem cell transplant recipients and neutropenic patients with hematological malignancies are in the higher-risk category. In these patients, the predictive value of a culture positive for *Aspergillus* from respiratory secretions is between 60% and

80% (72–74). Conversely, there is a low-risk group of non-immunocompromised patients, in which the growth of *Aspergillus* species almost always represents colonization or contamination instead of disease. The diagnosis of IA on the basis of a positive culture for *Aspergillus* species from a non-sterile fluid is more problematic in the intermediate group (patients with AIDS, solid organ transplant, malnutrition, diabetes), because the predictive value is 10% to 30% (74–76). In this category, the definition of infection must be based on other diagnostic tools such as histopathology, radiology, polymerase chain reaction (PCR), and serology. The difficulty in interpreting the results of respiratory cultures may be further exemplified by a study of 222 autopsies in intensive care unit patients. Five cases of IA were diagnosed in patients with chronic obstructive lung disease who had received corticosteroids. Sputum cultures had been positive for *A. fumigatus* before death in all cases, but were interpreted as colonization (77). Although sputum cultures may be helpful in the diagnosis of IA, material from a bronchoalveolar lavage is more reliable.

The growth of *Aspergillus* species from sinus aspirate or biopsy in a clinical scenario of acute sinusitis in severely immunocompromised patients must be interpreted as diagnostic of sinus aspergillosis until proven otherwise. Confirmation of the diagnosis is made by histopathology. A positive culture from nasal swabs must be interpreted with caution. Positive cultures are relatively frequent, even in neutropenic patients, and the value of a positive nose culture for *Aspergillus* is controversial (78). In chronic sinusitis, the growth of *Aspergillus* species from aspirate or biopsy is indicative of aspergillosis, but the distinction between chronic IA and allergic sinusitis requires histopathologic analysis.

Blood culture is a limited diagnostic tool for IA because *Aspergillus* fungemia is rarely encountered, even in disseminated disease. In a series of 36 cancer patients with positive blood cultures for *Aspergillus* species, 24 were classified as pseudo-fungemias, 5 were probable, and 7 were true aspergillemias. Aspergillemia occurred exclusively in patients with acute leukemia and *A. terreus* was the most frequent species (79). In another series of 10 aspergillemias in patients with hematological malignancies, the most frequent species was *A. fumigatus*. A positive blood culture was not associated with dissemination (80). Therefore, outside the setting of neutropenic patients, a positive blood culture for *Aspergillus* species must be considered contamination. Even in neutropenic patients, the clinical significance of this finding is uncertain.

The growth of *Aspergillus* species from other biological materials such as urine, cerebrospinal fluid, pleural effusion, and ascites is rare, and must be interpreted with caution. Although contamination is the most likely possibility, one must keep in mind the possibility of some unusual clinical form of IA (65). Results of isolation of *Aspergillus* species from surgically removed material are significant only if the biopsy of the same material shows tissue invasion by hyphae.

Non–Culture-Based

Histopathology

The typical hyphae of *Aspergillus* have parallel contours, measure 3 to 6 μm in diameter, and are hyaline and septated, with branches in acute angles. Although the hyphae may be visible with hematoxylin and eosin, sometimes they are only apparent with other stains such as periodic acid-Schiff (PAS) and Gomori methenamine silver. The hallmark of IA is the demonstration of tissue invasion by the fungus (Fig. 12). However, although it is absolutely specific for fungal infection, it does not allow us to make the diagnosis of aspergillosis, since a large number of other molds have the same appearance as *Aspergillus* species in tissue. When there is tissue invasion by hyaline hyphae and cultures are negative or not available, a diagnosis of hyalohyphomycosis is made (mycoses caused by hyaline fungi). The list of fungi that have the same appearance as *Aspergillus* in tissue is broad, and includes *Fusarium* spp., *S. apiospermum*, *Acremonium* spp., *Paecilomyces lilacinus*, and others. Therefore, the combination of the demonstration of tissue invasion and the growth of *Aspergillus* species in culture of the same tissue is the cornerstone of the diagnosis of IA.

Aspergillus grows only in the hyphal form in tissue. The histopathologic pattern depends on the form of disease. In acute IA in neutropenic patients, the lesions contain hyphae within blood vessels that exhibit thrombosis. The tissue

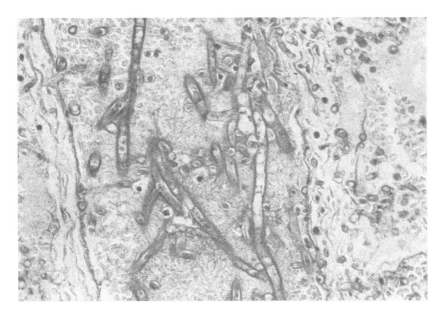

Figure 12 Periodic acid-Schiff staining of lung tissue showing septate acute-branching hyphae of *Aspergillus* spp. inside a blood vessel.

presents with edema, hemorrhage and infarction, with minimal inflammatory response. Hyphae are numerous, disposed in parallel or radial arrays, and invade necrotic tissue (Fig. 13). As the neutrophils appear in the blood, the lesions become more circumscribed. In patients with chronic forms of IA, no vascular invasion is apparent. Few hyphae are surrounded by large amounts of inflammation, with epithelioid cells, multinucleated giant cells, and lymphocytes. In this form of aspergillosis, non-branching short segments of hyphae or dichotomous branching hyphae may be apparent.

As mentioned before, in the absence of tissue culture growing *Aspergillus* species, the finding of tissue invasion by hyphae with an aspect similar to *Aspergillus* species is diagnostic of hyalohyphomycosis. In this case, unless other tools such as PCR, in situ hybridization, and immunohistochemical analysis are used on paraffin-embedded sections, the diagnosis of aspergillosis cannot be made. These techniques have been applied in relatively small number of samples, but the results are promising (81). In a study of 26 tissue specimens, morphologic examination with PAS and Gomori methenamine silver showed a sensitivity of 100% in detecting fungi, compared to 84.6% with in situ hybridization. However, DNA probes allowed definitive identification of organisms in all cases in which DNA was detected in the tissue sample, with a 100% positive predictive value and no cross-reactivity with other fungi (82). In another study, a commercially

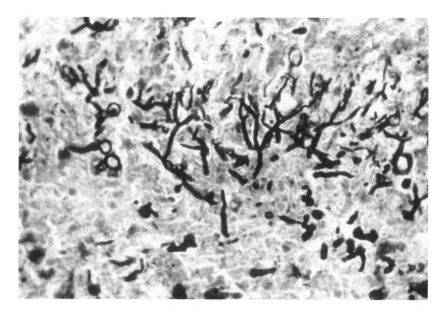

Figure 13 Radiate orientation of hyphal strands, with dichotomous branching, and several hyphae oriented in the same direction, with a brush-like appearance. Gomori methenamine silver stain.

available monoclonal antibody, Mab-WF-AF-1, was applied on paraffin-embedded sections from 16 pediatric cases with IA, with good performance (83).

Serology and Antigen Detection

IA is associated with a very high mortality. One of the most important factors contributing to its poor outcome is the late initiation of appropriate antifungal therapy. The clinical presentation is often non-specific, the yield of cultures is poor, and histopathologic diagnosis is often not feasible because of the critical condition of the patient and often severe thrombocytopenia. Therefore, in the past years there has been a growing interest in the development of surrogate markers of fungal infections, such as antibodies, fungal DNA fragments, and fungal cell wall components, such as galactomannan (GM) and (1-3)-β-D-glucan. These markers are potentially novel tools for rapid, specific, and non-invasive diagnosis of IA.

Antibody tests for *Aspergillus* are commercially available. However, they lack enough specificity and sensitivity: a positive result does not distinguish between past and active infection, or between colonization and invasive disease. Furthermore, a negative result does not rule out invasive disease, since the majority of patients at risk are unable to mount an effective antibody response. Antibody tests are, however, useful in the diagnosis of allergic bronchopulmonary aspergillosis and aspergilloma.

GM is a polysaccharide cell-wall component that is released by growing *Aspergillus* hyphae. Initial studies used a latex agglutination (LA) test for the detection of GM. In the early 1990s, an *Aspergillus* GM double-sandwich enzyme-linked immunosorbent assay (ELISA), known as Platelia$^{\circledR}$ *Aspergillus*, was developed (Bio-Rad, Marnes-la-Coquette, France) (84). It has been available in Europe for over five years and in 2003 it was approved for clinical use in the United States. The GM ELISA utilizes an anti-GM rat monoclonal antibody EB-A2, which recognizes GM epitopes. The GM epitope is constituted by four β (1-5) galactofuranose residues. Each GM molecule contains at least 10 epitopes, making it possible for EB-A2 to act as both the capture and detector antibody. With the same antibody being employed as the captor and detector, the detection limit threshold is decreased significantly. The lower limit of detection for the LA test is 15 ng of GM per mL, while for the GM ELISA it is 0.5 to 1.0 ng/mL.

The impact of this difference in detection threshold has been shown in clinical studies (85,86). The sensitivity of the LA test is lower than that seen with the ELISA, and a sensitivity of only 38% has been reported. Moreover, GM ELISA detected GM in serum up to five days earlier than the LA test. In some patients, LA yielded positive results only during advanced stages of infection, not contributing to an earlier diagnosis and consequent earlier initiation of therapy. However, the improvement in sensitivity with ELISA is accompanied by a loss in specificity and greater occurrence of false-positive results. The results of the ELISA test are reported as an optical density index (OD): a ratio of the OD of the test specimen relative to a control serum containing 0.5 ng/mL of GM.

Upon initial clinical utilization of the test, an OD index of 1.5 was recommended as diagnostic cut-off, and several of the earlier studies were based on these values. It was later observed that by reducing the cut-off value to 1.0, 0.7, or even 0.5, there was significant gain in sensitivity without considerable loss in specificity (87). However, considerable debate exists on the cut-off level to be used in clinical practice.

Several studies have assessed the detection of serum antigenemia by GM ELISA test in the diagnosis of IA. Most of these studies were performed in patients with hematologic malignancies, patients with chemotherapy-induced neutropenia, or those receiving allogeneic stem-cell transplantation. Serial monitoring of antigenemia in these patients has shown a sensitivity ranging from 50% to greater than 90%. Table 3 summarizes a few of the recent studies (90).

Table 3   Summary of Studies Evaluating the Performance of Double-Sandwich ELISA in the Detection of Galactomannan Antigenemia

Reference	Type of study	Sensitivity	Specificity
84	Retrospective, analysis of serum and urine, leukemic patients with proven or suggested IA. Cut-off ≥ 0.79	100%	92%
88	Prospective, HSCT recipients, weekly sampling. Cut-off ≥ 0.5	80%	80%
89	Prospective, children with hematological malignancies, adults after HSCT. Biweekly. Cut-off ≥ 1.5	90.6%	94%
90	Prospective, patients at risk for IA, 1–2 samples/week. Cut-off ≥ 1.0	50%	99.6%
91	Consecutive patients undergoing lung transplant. Biweekly. Cut-off ≥ 0.5	30%	93%
92	Prospective, prolonged neutropenia and/or steroid-treated with hematological disorders. Biweekly. Cut-off ≥ 1.0	92.6%	95.4%
86	Retrospective, chemotherapy-induced neutropenia. Cut-off ≥ 1.0	90%	84%
93	Neutropenic and HSCT. Cut-off ≥ 1.5	Definite 64.5% Probable 16.4% Possible 25.5%	94.8%
94	Prospective, allogeneic HSCT recipients	94.4%	98.8%
95	Retrospective, case-control study of IA in liver transplant recipients	55.6%	93.9%
96	Prospective, liver transplant recipients, cut-off ≥ 0.5	—	87%

Abbreviations: ELISA, enzyme-linked immunosorbent assay; HSCT, hematopoietic stem cell transplant; IA, invasive aspergillosis.

The performance of the GM ELISA test depends on several factors, such as the fungal burden, the rate of growth of *Aspergillus*, the degree of angioinvasion and the presence or absence of anti-*Aspergillus* antibodies. For example, in a study in lung transplant recipients (91), the sensitivity of the GM assay was only 30%. The lower sensitivity in this patient population could be due to the frequent use of antifungal prophylaxis, absence of neutropenia (which could be associated with a lower fungal burden), and occurrence of *Aspergillus* tracheobronchitis, which would represent a localized form of disease, without significant angioinvasion.

In a meta-analysis that included 27 studies and approximately 4000 patients, the overall sensitivity of the GM assay was 71% and the specificity was 89% for proven cases of IA. The test was shown to be more useful in patients with hematological malignancies or who underwent hematopoietic stem cell transplantation than in solid-organ transplant recipients. For solid-organ transplant recipients the overall sensitivity was 22% and the specificity was 84%. The positive and negative predictive values for cases of proven or probable IA were 31% and 98%, respectively, when the prevalence of IA was 5%, and 69% and 91%, respectively, when the prevalence was 20%. Therefore, the GM assay seems to be better at ruling out rather than confirming the diagnosis of IA (97).

Twice-weekly monitoring of antigenemia in patients at risk for IA facilitates early diagnosis. In more than 2/3 of patients, antigenemia precedes radiological and microbiologic findings by at least a week (17,89,94). The specificity of the test has ranged from 80% to 100%. Some of the variables affecting the specificity are the cut-off used to define positivity and the requirement for demonstration of at least two consecutive positive results. False-positive results have been documented in about 8% to 10% of cases, with some studies showing a false-positive rate as high as 44% in children (92,93,98). A possible explanation for the high false-positive rate among children is the presence of GM in milk, protein-rich foods, and cereals. In adults, a high rate of false-positive results has also been observed during the first month after bone marrow transplantation (99) or within the first two weeks after cytoreductive therapy. A postulated explanation for these observations is that fungal translocation occurs frequently in these patients while they are neutropenic, resulting in transient antigenemia. Fungal organisms would be spontaneously cleared once neutrophil recovery is achieved. Reports have also shown an association between the use of beta-lactams, especially piperacillin/ tazobactam and amoxicillin/clavulanic acid and false-positive results (100–102). Piperacillin and tazobactam are drugs derived from compounds produced by molds of the *Penicillium* genus, and the monoclonal antibody EB-A2 recognizes constituents of molds from other genera, including *Penicillium* spp. The administration of beta-lactams containing GM may cause false-positive results up to five days after the cessation of the drug (102,103). Other potential reasons for false-positive results include cyclophosphamide and GVHD. It was suggested that paraproteins or auto-reactive antibodies, sometimes present in patients with GVHD, might react with the assay (104).

False-negative results are also encountered. Factors that decrease the amount of GM include use of antifungal drugs, with reduction in mycelial growth and decrease in the expression of cell-wall components, and the presence of specific anti-*Aspergillus* antibodies. Patients with chronic granulomatous disease, who are frequently challenged by recurrent *Aspergillus* infections, have been noted to have false-negative antigenemia. In these patients, the infection follows a more subacute course and it is possible that encapsulation of the infectious process occurs, causing a lesser degree of angioinvasion and preventing leakage of antigens to body fluids.

The GM antigen has also been detected in body fluids other than serum. In urine, GM can be detected by the GM ELISA assay but the test has a lower sensitivity than antigenemia for several reasons: (*i*) GM is not detected in the urine of all patients with IA who have antigenemia; (*ii*) the amount of antigen is found to be lower in the urine than in the serum; and (*iii*) detection of antigen in the serum always precedes detection in the urine.

Antigen detection in broncho-alveolar lavage (BAL) has been studied and compared to antigenemia (105). Antigen was detected in the BAL of all patients with invasive pulmonary aspergillosis, while in serum samples the sensitivity was only 47%. Limitations to the use of GM in BAL include negativation of the test after a few days of antifungal therapy and fungal airway colonization possibly yielding false-positive results. More recently, the usefulness of GM in BAL was assessed in lung transplant recipients. A total of 116 consecutive patients presenting for bronchoscopy were prospectively evaluated. The incidence of IA was 5.2%. Using a cut-off of 0.5, the sensitivity and specificity of the GM in the BAL were 60% and 98%, respectively. The specificity was increased to 98% by increasing the cut-off value to 1.0. High false-positive results (OD index ≥ 2.0) occurred in patients who had *Penicillium* colonization or were receiving concomitant piperacillin/tazobactam, but not in those with *Aspergillus* colonization (106).

A few studies have evaluated the use of GM detection in the cerebrospinal fluid (CSF) as a means to diagnose cerebral aspergillosis. It has been documented that in patients with cerebral aspergillosis, there is significant intrathecal production of GM. However, there is also crossing of GM through the blood–brain barrier (107). Therefore, the detection of CSF GM is diagnostic of cerebral aspergillosis in the appropriate clinical setting only when antigenemia is negative.

The clinician should be aware of the limitations of the test, keeping in mind that a negative GM antigenemia does not rule out IA and that a positive test alone does not confirm the diagnosis. A positive GM test result should always be confirmed by another positive test. If rising titers are observed in the appropriate clinical context, these results can be used as a guide to initiate specific antifungal therapy against *Aspergillus*. Whenever possible, antigenemia results should be combined with radiological and/or microbiological data. Persistently negative

Table 4 Indications for Use of Galactomannan Antigenemia Testing

Obtain supplemental supportive evidence in cases of suspected IA in patients with compatible clinical findings, preferably prior to initiation of antifungal drugs (to minimize false-negative results)
Biweekly surveillance for aspergillosis in patients experiencing acute severe immunosuppression
Monitoring response to antifungal therapy
Confirmation of initial positive results

Abbreviation: IA, invasive aspergillosis.

results should alert the clinicians to search for alternative diagnosis, including infections caused by non-*Aspergillus* molds.

Monitoring antigenemia is also useful in assessing response to therapy (108). Persistently positive or rising titers are associated with poor prognosis and should precipitate a switch to new antifungal drugs or combination therapy. On the other hand, conversion to negative antigenemia results is associated with good outcomes. Rebound antigenemia after suspension of therapy should prompt investigation for relapse and resumption of antifungals (Table 4). At the present moment, data regarding the performance of the GM ELISA cannot be applied to patients other than neutropenic patients with hematological malignancies, since the vast majority of studies have been conducted in that patient population. Therefore, its application in other settings such as solid organ transplant and congenital immunodeficiencies needs further studies.

The $(1-3)$-β-D-glucan is a major cell-wall component of yeasts and molds, except *Zygomycetes*. It can be detected in the blood and other body fluids by its ability to activate factor G of the horseshoe crab coagulation cascade. It has been shown to have high sensitivity and specificity for the diagnosis of invasive fungal infections. In a study with more than 200 febrile neutropenic patients, the sensitivity was 90% and the specificity was 100% (109). This assay has not yet been studied in organ transplant recipients. The use of antifungal prophylaxis does not seem to alter the performance of the test, and fungal colonization is not associated with increased $(1-3)$-β-D-glucan levels (110). The assay not only reacts with *Aspergillus* but also with *Candida, Trichosporon, Fusarium, Penicillium, Saccharomyces, Acremonium* and even *Pneumocystis jiroveci* (111). While its broad spectrum is an attractive characteristic for screening of fungal infections in immunocompromised patients, it is of limited value for the diagnosis of a specific infection such as aspergillosis.

DNA-Based Methods

In the past several years, different PCR assays have been developed with the intent to detect *Aspergillus* DNA in different clinical specimens. These assays have used different targets, which include limited copy genes (18 kDa IgE binding protein, alkaline protease), multiple copy genes (26S intergenic spacer genes, 18S rRNA genes, mitochondrial DNA), and panfungal targets (small subunit rRNA gene). They usually have a detection limit of 10 fg of *Aspergillus* DNA. Although promising and with sensitivities ranging from 55% to 100% and specificities from 65% to 100%, the use of PCR for the diagnosis of IA cannot yet be supported due to the lack of a consensual technique. Several discrepancies among studies exist, making comparison of results impossible. Studies have used different clinical specimens (whole blood, serum, BAL), different protocols for sample preparation and amplification, as well as different DNA targets, which will all affect the sensitivity and specificity of the PCR (112).

The choice of the clinical specimen, whether it is whole blood, plasma, or serum, has an impact on the sensitivity of DNA testing. A comparison between plasma and whole blood demonstrated greater sensitivity with the use of whole blood for qualitative PCR (113). When *Aspergillus* DNA is extracted from the whole blood, the loss of fungal particles entrapped in the red cell precipitate is avoided. Therefore, the frequency of false-negative results is lower. False-positive results are common, and are independent of the DNA target used.

Studies available have not shown that the use of PCR have any impact on patients' management or survival. Negative PCR results after the start of antifungal therapy do not correlate with clinical response (114,115). The *Aspergillus* PCR in the BAL of patients with pneumonia has a high negative predictive value (96–99%), and therefore could be a useful tool to rule out the diagnosis of aspergillosis (116). On the other hand, the positive predictive value is poor, with false-positive rates occurring in up to 25% of healthy control subjects (117–119). The use of *Aspergillus* PCR in BAL specimens is much less promising since it cannot distinguish between upper airway colonization and invasive disease. Conversely, the detection of *Aspergillus* DNA in the CSF may be useful in the diagnosis of CNS aspergillosis, with sensitivity and specificity of 100% (120).

The advent of real-time PCR and automated DNA extraction has brought hope to the molecular diagnosis of IA. This technique offers the advantages of a faster turnaround time, usually less than two hours, and significantly less opportunities for contamination. However, we still have to define the meaning of identifying fungal nucleic acid in a clinical sample.

Recently, studies have focused on comparing the performance of different non-culture based methods in the diagnosis of invasive pulmonary aspergillosis. Studies with animal models as well as prospective studies in humans have shown the superiority of GM ELISA over PCR and (1-3)-β-D-glucan (121,122).

In summary, the use of non-culture-based tests for the detection of *Aspergillus* infection is limited by the interpretation of the results in view of the clinical setting. As these tests continue to be developed and further improved, there is a potential for them to have a major role in the early diagnosis and management of IA.

HYALOHYPHOMYCOSES

Hyalohyphomycosis is a term used to designate invasive fungal infections caused by hyaline septated hyphae in tissue. This term is useful only when the causative agent is not recognized either by culture or by DNA-based methods in tissue (see previous section). When the causative organism is identified, it is better to designate the infection with the specific term, such as fusariosis or scedosporiosis (infection caused by *Fusarium* spp. or *Scedosporium* spp., respectively). Hyalohyphomycosis is caused by a large list of fungi, including *Fusarium* spp., *Scedosporium* spp., *Acremonium* spp., *Paecilomyces* spp., and *Penicillium* spp.

Fusariosis

Fusarium is a plant pathogen and a soil saprophyte that causes a broad spectrum of infections in humans, including superficial (such as keratitis and onychomycosis), locally invasive, and disseminated infection. The latter occurs almost exclusively in immunocompromised patients (15). The most frequent species causing infection in humans are *Fusarium solani*, *Fusarium oxysporum*, and *Fusarium moniliforme* (123). The usual portals of entry of *Fusarium* are the airways and the skin in areas of tissue breakdown. As in aspergillosis, the clinical form depends on the immune status of the host.

In immunocompetent individuals, invasive fusariosis occurs mostly in the skin of patients with tissue lesions, such as burns and wounds. In a review of skin lesions in fusariosis, 10 of 14 immunocompetent patients with fusarial skin involvement had a history of recent skin breakdown at the site of infection, as a result of trauma or of pre-existing onychomycosis (15). Cellulitis, necrotic lesions, chronic ulcers, plaques, and subcutaneous abscesses were the most frequent clinical presentations. Other infections in immunocompetent patients include pneumonia (124,125), arthritis (126,127), peritonitis in patients receiving peritoneal dialysis (128–130), sinusitis (131), fungemia (15,132), endophthalmitis (133,134), and osteomyelitis (135). The clinical presentation of such infections is indistinguishable from that caused by other pathogens.

In immunocompromised patients, the typical clinical form is disseminated fusariosis, with characteristic skin lesions. Although prolonged and profound neutropenia is a major risk factor for disseminated fusariosis, fusariosis occurring later than one year after hematopoietic stem cell transplantation is not associated with neutropenia (17). The most frequent skin lesions among patients with disseminated disease are multiple erythematous papular or nodular and painful lesions with or without central necrosis. Skin lesions with necrosis may have the appearance of ecthyma gangrenosum or an aspect of target lesions (a thin rim of erythema of 1–3 cm in diameter surrounding the papular or nodular lesions). The lesions evolve rapidly, usually over a few days. Lesions at different stages of evolution are frequent (Fig. 14). Although blood cultures are positive in up to 57% of patients with disseminated skin lesions, the skin is frequently the single source of diagnosis of fusariosis. Therefore, biopsy with culture and

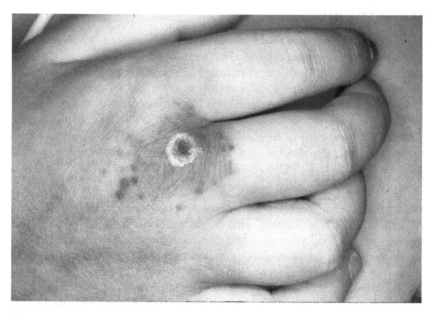

Figure 14 Skin lesions caused by *Fusarium* spp. in a patient with acute leukemia. The lesion has the appearance of ecthyma gangrenosum.

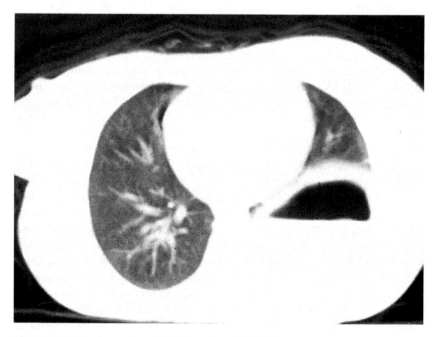

Figure 15 A large opacity with thick wall and air fluid level caused by *Fusarium* spp. in the left lung of a patient with acute lymphoid leukemia.

histopathology is an important diagnostic tool for the diagnosis of invasive fusariosis. These and other manifestations of disseminated fusariosis usually present in persistently febrile neutropenic patients. In a series of 83 patients with hematological malignancies and fusariosis, pneumonitis with lung infiltrates was present in 54% of cases and consisted of non-specific alveolar infiltrates (8 unilateral and 19 bilateral), nodules (3 unilateral and 6 bilateral), interstitial infiltrates (1 unilateral and 6 bilateral), and cavities (Fig. 15) (3). The radiologic pattern was not different among neutropenic and non-neutropenic patients. The pulmonary involvement by *Fusarium* spp. is similar to that of *Aspergillus* spp., with hemorrhagic infarction. Other manifestations included sinusitis (36%), blindness (8%), and central nervous system lesions similar to aspergillosis (6%). The infection was disseminated in 66 patients (16).

Fusarium species grow easily and rapidly in most media without cycloheximide. On potato dextrose agar, the colonies have a velvety or cottony surface, and are white, yellow, pink, purple, salmon, or gray on the surface, with a pale, red,

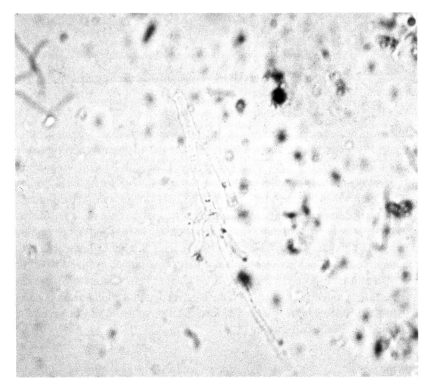

Figure 16 Direct examination of a tissue specimen from a skin lesion of a patient with disseminated fusariosis. The hyphae are hyaline, acute-branching, and septate, with parallel walls. KOH.

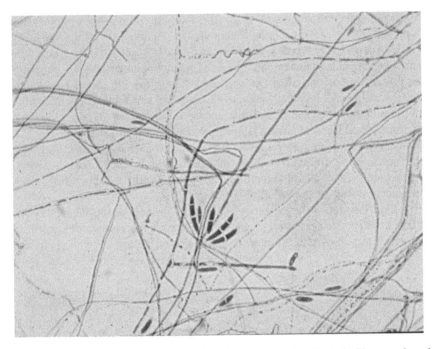

Figure 17 Microscopic appearance of *Fusarium* spp., showing the typical banana-shaped macroconidia.

violet, brown, or sometimes blue reverse. In tissue, the hyphae are similar to those of *Aspergillus* species, with hyaline and septate filaments that typically dichotomize in acute and right angles (Fig. 16). Like with *Aspergillus* species, in-situ hybridization in paraffin embedded tissue specimens may be useful to define the genus when cultures are negative (81,82). However, a marked difference of fusariosis in comparison with aspergillosis is that in the case of fusariosis the diagnosis is easier because of the high frequency of skin lesions and positive blood cultures. The phialides are cylindrical, short or long, simple or branched, with a collarette at the apex. Microconidia are usually unicellular, hyaline, ovoid, or ellipsoid, and it is disposed in slimy heads or chains. The hallmark of the genus *Fusarium* is the production of hyaline, banana-shaped, multicellular macroconidia with a foot cell at the base (Fig. 17). The identification of the *Fusarium* species is difficult and is described elsewhere (123).

Scedosporiosis

The genus *Scedosporium* contains two medically important species: *S. apiospermum* and *Scedosporium prolificans*. *S. apiospermum* has a sexual form called *Pseudallescheria boydii*, and genetic relatedness studies showed that the genus *Petriella* may be a sexual relative of *S. prolificans* (136). There is some controversy regarding the classification of *S. prolificans* as an agent of hyalohyphomycosis (137,138) or phaeohyphomycosis (139).

In normal hosts, *S. apiospermum* causes localized infection after penetrating trauma and pneumonia or disseminated infection after near drowning accidents. In North America, *S. apiospermum* is the most frequent cause of eumycotic mycetoma, a chronic fistulous suppurative infection of the subcutaneous tissue, fascia, and contiguous bones that arises after penetrating trauma. The lesion begins as a subcutaneous nodule that enlarges gradually. A characteristic feature of mycetoma is the drainage of grains.

In immunocompromised patients, *S. apiospermum* causes deeply invasive infections such as pneumonia, sinusitis, and brain abscess (137,140). The clinical presentation may be similar to aspergillosis, especially pneumonia. Neutropenia and organ transplantation represent the most frequent underlying conditions. Pulmonary involvement is common in hematopoietic stem cell transplant recipients: in a series of 10 cases, 9 had lung disease, frequently with sinusitis (6 cases). In another recently published series of 23 cases of *S. apiospermum* infection in solid organ transplant recipients between 1976 and 1999, there were eight cases of disseminated disease, three cases of cutaneous disease, four pneumonias, two brain abscesses, two cases of fungus ball (one in the lung and one in the sinuses), and one case each of endophthalmitis, meningitis, eye infection with brain abscess, and mycotic aneurysm (141). In another series, 11 additional cases of infection due to *S. apiospermum* were reported: 4 in hematopoietic stem cell transplant (HSCT) and 7 in solid organ transplantation (5 renal, 1 liver, and 1 heart) recipients. There were 6 cases of disseminated disease, 2 pulmonary infections, 2 cases of skin infection and 1 brain abscess (142).

S. prolificans causes localized infections in immunocompetent patients, usually after surgery or trauma. Bones and soft tissues are the most frequent sites. Neutropenia is a main risk factor among immunocompromised patients (139). In a review of 16 cases, 15 were neutropenic, and most developed disseminated infection with persistent fever, lung infiltrates, renal failure, and neurologic involvement. Skin lesions with central necrosis were present in four patients (143). Another frequent feature of disseminated infection that has important implications for the diagnosis is the high frequency of positive blood cultures. In a review of 26 cases in patients with cancer, a blood culture was positive in 20 (144).

S. apiospermum grows rapidly, forming wooly to cottony colonies that begin white and become brownish, with a pale reverse with brownish black zones. The conidiophores have simple or branched annellides, unicellular conidia with a pale brown color, truncated bases, formed singly or in small clusters at the end of conidiophores, or from annellidic necks that arise directly from the hyphae. The sexual form produces dark round sexual structures called cleistothecia. *S. prolificans* differs from *S. apiospermum* by its basally inflated annellides, its growth at 45°C, and its inhibition by cycloheximide.

INFECTIONS CAUSED BY DEMATIACEOUS FUNGI

Dematiaceous fungi comprise a group of darkly pigmented fungi. The pigment results from the production of melanin by the fungus. Dematiaceous fungi are widely distributed in the environment, and occasionally cause infection in humans. These fungi are considered to have a relatively low virulence, and the spectrum of disease is influenced mainly by host factors. The clinical spectrum of infection includes black grain mycetomas, chromoblastomycosis, sinusitis, and superficial, cutaneous, subcutaneous, and systemic phaeohyphomycosis (145). Recently, other conditions such as fungemia have been added to the spectrum of diseases caused by dematiaceous fungi (146). The clinical presentation of mycetoma was described in the previous session. The most frequent dematiaceous fungi causing mycetoma is *Madurella mycetomatis*. Chromoblastomycosis is an infection that involves the skin and subcutaneous tissues, and is a consequence of penetrating trauma to the skin, especially in the lower extremities. The infection has a chronic course, and different types of skin lesions may occur, including papules and nodules that increase over time to produce extensive lesions with different aspects, such as plaques and verrucous, cicatricial, and tumorous lesions (147). The diagnosis characteristic of chromoblastomycosis in tissue is the presence of sclerotic or muriform bodies, round fungal elements with horizontal and vertical septa. Phaeohyphomycosis is designated when there is invasive infection with darkly pigmented hyphae in tissue or abscesses. Several pigmented

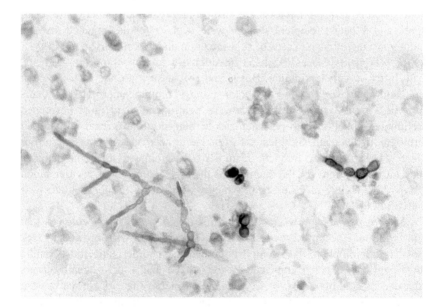

Figure 18 Cystic subcutaneous phaeohyphomycosis with different shapes of fungal structures. Catenulate or toruloid hyphae with vesicular budding are observed.

fungal structures, including septate hyphae, yeast cells, and vesicular bodies may be observed (Fig. 18). The hallmark of its diagnosis is the demonstration of tissue invasion by these pigmented elements. However, hyphal pigmentation may be difficult to detect by the most frequently used stains, unless the Masson–Fontana stain is used. Although it is not specific for these fungi (148), a positive staining with Masson–Fontana is virtually diagnostic of a phaeohyphomycosis.

Subcutaneous phaeohyphomycosis may occur either in immunocompetent or compromised hosts and present as polymorphic lesions (cysts, nodules, plaques, etc.) (Fig. 19). Localized infections occur in immunocompetent individuals (usually in the subcutaneous tissues), whereas invasive or disseminated

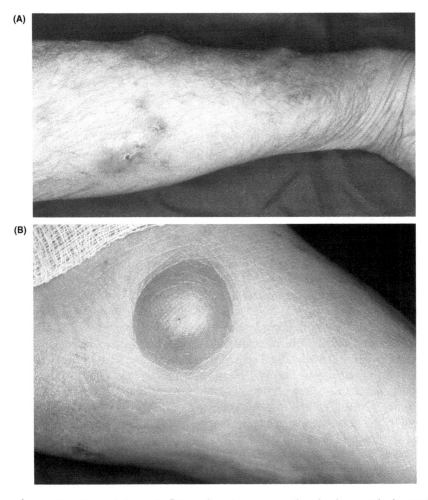

Figure 19 (**A**) Nodular and (**B**) cystic subcutaneous phaeohyphomycosis in renal transplant recipients.

infection occurs in immunocompromised patients (neutropenic patients, organ transplant recipients, patients receiving corticosteroids). The most common species causing phaeohyphomycosis are *Bipolaris spicifera* and *Exophiala jeanselmei*. Dematiaceous fungi are also a frequent cause of chronic invasive sinusitis, with clinical and radiological aspects indistinguishable from aspergillosis. Some agents of phaeohyphomycosis are neurotropic, and cause infection in the central nervous system, most in the form of intracerebral mass lesions (Fig. 20). This is the case of *Cladophialophora bantiana*, *Exophiala dermatitidis*, and *Dactylaria gallopavum*. Disseminated phaeohyphomycosis may involve any organ, but the lungs are frequently involved (139).

The colonies of *Exophiala* species are mucoid (yeast-like) in the beginning and with time become velvety. Other fungi, such as *Aureobasidium* species produce only yeast-like colonies, whereas the majority of dematiaceous fungi produce colonies composed of hyphae. Since the dematiaceous fungi comprise a large group of agents, a detailed description of the morphologic characteristics of each genus is beyond the scope of this chapter.

ZYGOMYCOSES

Infection caused by the order *Entomophthorales* usually occurs in immuno-competent patients from subtropical and tropical climates, in the form of a non-angioinvasive, chronic infection in the subcutaneous tissue localized in the thigh, buttock, or trunk (*Basidiobolus ranarum*), or in the face (*Conidiobolus* spp.). The portal of entry is the skin, and there is no apparent predisposing factor for the infection.

Infection caused by *Mucorales* occurs mostly in immunocompromised patients. The most frequent genera are *Mucor*, *Rhizopus*, *Rhizomucor*, *Absidia*, and *Cunninghamella*. The clinical forms of zygomycosis include a rhino-orbito-cerebral form, pulmonary, cutaneous, gastrointestinal, and disseminated infection (18). Rhino-cerebral zygomycosis is the most frequent clinical presentation, and occurs predominantly in diabetic patients (149). The clinical presentation is of an acute sinusitis, with fever, headache, and nasal discharge. The disease has a rapid clinical course, with extension to the orbits. Blindness, ophthalmoplegia, proptosis, ptosis, and periorbital cellulitis may occur. The lesions extend to the brain causing lethargy and coma. Necrosis of the palate may be observed. X ray examination shows signs of sinusitis with opacification and air-fluid levels. CT scan or MRI is helpful to define the extent of disease to surrounding tissues (Figs. 21 and 22). Rhino-cerebral zygomycosis differs from sinus aspergillosis by its occurrence in settings other than neutropenia or organ transplant, especially in diabetic patients, and by its very rapid clinical course.

Pulmonary zygomycosis is more frequent in leukemic patients with neutropenia. In neutropenic patients, its clinical presentation is indistinguishable from acute pulmonary aspergillosis. In a retrospective study, patients with pulmonary zygomycosis were more likely to have concomitant sinusitis, pleural

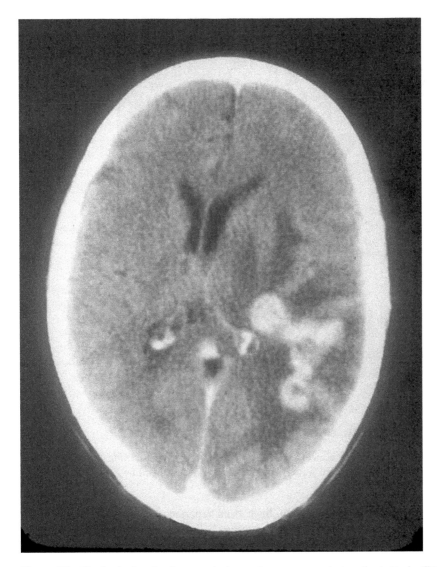

Figure 20 Cerebral phaeohyphomycosis in an immunocompetent patient. Brain CT shows a multi-lobular abscess with surrounding edema.

effusion, and >10 pulmonary nodules, compared to patients with IA (150). Pulmonary zygomycosis in diabetic patients usually present with endobronchial lesions, with hoarseness, hemoptysis, and post-obstructive pneumonia (151). Cutaneous zygomycosis usually occurs in patients without an underlying immunosuppression. Infection may follow breaks in skin's barrier from burns, trauma, surgery, contaminated adhesive tapes and bone fractures (Fig. 23).

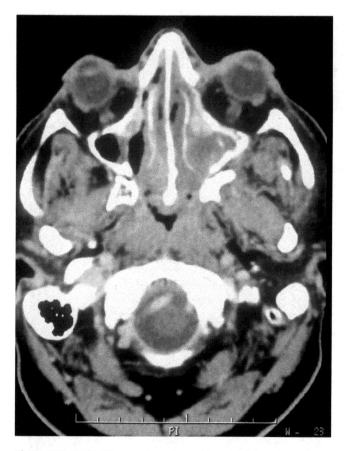

Figure 21 Sinus CT scan of a patient with multiple myeloma showing opacities and bone destruction in the medial wall of both maxillary sinuses caused by *Zygomycetes*.

Various clinical presentations have been reported, including nodules with or without central necrosis, necrotizing cellulitis, and pustules (152,153). Gastrointestinal zygomycosis occurs more frequently in neutropenic leukemic patients. Gastrointestinal bleeding is a prominent manifestation because of the angio-invasive nature of the infection. Gastric and colonic ulcers are visible by endoscopy (154).

The demonstration of hyphae of the Zygomycetes from cytologic preparations may be difficult. Fungal elements may be rare, and when evident, they appear in fragments. The characteristic hyphae are wide, and non-septated or poorly septated, and usually appear in middle of necrotic debris. Branching may be seen, with wide (90°) angles and cell walls are thin and non-parallel (Fig. 24) (155). The fungus grows well and very rapidly, with mycelia covering the entire plate in a few days. When plating tissue material, one should avoid homogenizing

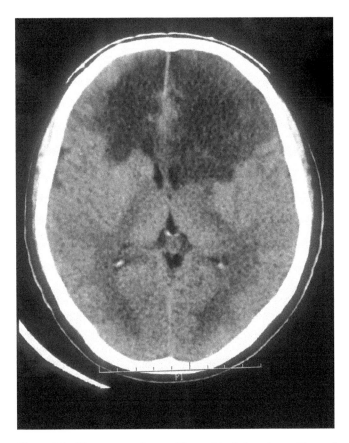

Figure 22 The same patient as Figure 21, 3 days later. The patient developed coma and brain CT scan showed large hypodense images in both frontal lobes. The lesions represented an extension of sinus zygomycosis.

the material because it may destroy hyphae and decrease the yield of culture. A piece of sterile bread placed on the surface of the agar plate can enhance the recovery of Zygomycetes. The order *Mucorales* has erect aerial mycelium, described as cotton candy-like. The colonies of *Mucor* are grayish to brown on the surface, with a pale reverse. The hyphae are broad, not or scarcely septated, with sporangia with columellas, and sporangiophores round to ellipsoidal. *Rhizopus* produces white colonies that become grey brown, with a pale reverse, and differs from *Mucor* by the presence of rhizoids and stolons (Fig. 25). The rhizoids are situated at the point where sporangiophores are attached to the stolons. *Rhizomucor* differs from *Mucor* by its high tolerance to temperatures higher than 54°C and by the occasional presence of rhizoids and stolons. However, the rhizoids are scarce and poorly developed. *Absidia* is distinguished from *Mucor, Rhizopus,*

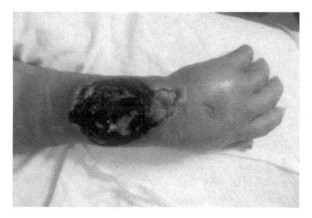

Figure 23 Large necrotic ulcer at the site of a previous venous puncture caused by *Rhizopus oryzae*.

and *Rhizomucor* by branched sporangiophores incorporating a funnel-shaped swelling (apophysis). *Cunninghamella* has branched sporangiophores that terminate in a vesicle (155). In histopathologic material, the hyphae are broad, irregularly branched, and rarely septated. Like *Aspergillus*, the hyphae are usually encountered in the blood vessels and surrounding structures. In chronic infection, including that caused by the order *Entomophthorales*, a chronic granulomatous process is formed, with a strong eosinophilic perihyphal reaction (Splendore-Hoeppli phenomenon).

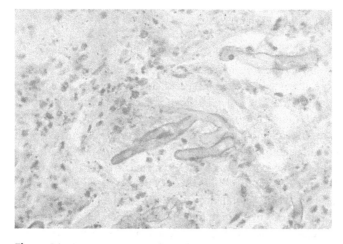

Figure 24 Large non-septate irregular hyphae in a patient with zygomycosis.

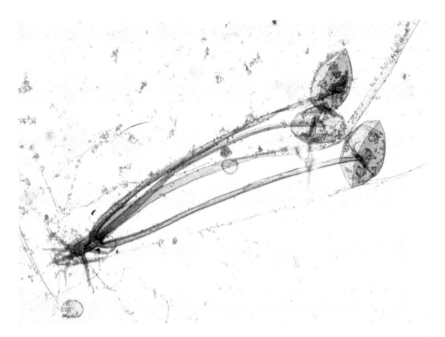

Figure 25 Microscopic aspect of *Rhizopus oryzae* in a case of cutaneous zygomycosis.

ACKNOWLEDGMENTS

We would like to thank Dr. Amarino de Oliveira Jr. for reviewing the radiological figures.

REFERENCES

1. O'Shaughnessy EM, Shea YM, Witebsky FG. Laboratory diagnosis of invasive mycoses. Infect Dis Clin North Am 2003; 17:135–58.
2. Pagano L, Girmenia C, Mele L, et al. Infections caused by filamentous fungi in patients with hematologic malignancies. A report of 391 cases by GIMEMA Infection Program. Haematologica 2001; 86:862–70.
3. Marr KA, Carter RA, Crippa F, Wald A, Corey L. Epidemiology and outcome of mould infections in hematopoietic stem cell transplant recipients. Clin Infect Dis 2002; 34:909–17.
4. Marr KA, Carter RA, Boeckh M, Martin P, Corey L. Invasive aspergillosis in allogeneic stem cell transplant recipients: changes in epidemiology and risk factors. Blood 2002; 100:4358–66.
5. Martino R, Subira M, Rovira M, et al. Invasive fungal infections after allogeneic peripheral blood stem cell transplantation: incidence and risk factors in 395 patients. Br J Haematol 2002; 116:475–82.
6. Rees JR, Pinner RW, Hajjeh RA, Brandt ME, Reingold AL. The epidemiological features of invasive mycotic infections in the San Francisco Bay area, 1992–1993:

results of population-based laboratory active surveillance. Clin Infect Dis 1998; 27:1138–47.

7. Cornet M, Fleury L, Maslo C, Bernard JF, Brucker G. Epidemiology of invasive aspergillosis in France: a six-year multicentric survey in the Greater Paris area. J Hosp Infect 2002; 51:288–96.

8. Morgan J, Wannemuehler KA, Marr KA, et al. Incidence of invasive aspergillosis following hematopoietic stem cell and solid organ transplantation: interim results of a prospective multicenter surveillance program. Med Mycol 2005; 43(Suppl. 1): S49–58.

9. Wald A, Leisenring W, Van Burik JA, Bowden RA. Epidemiology of *Aspergillus* infections in a large cohort of patients undergoing bone marrow transplantation. J Infect Dis 1997; 175:1459–66.

10. Champlin RE, Schmitz N, Horowitz MM, et al. Blood stem cells compared with bone marrow as a source of hematopoietic cells for allogeneic transplantation. IBMTR Histocompatibility and Stem Cell Sources Working Committee and the European Group for Blood and Marrow Transplantation (EBMT). Blood 2000; 95:3702–9.

11. Cutler C, Giri S, Jeyapalan S, Paniagua D, Viswanathan A, Antin JH. Acute and chronic graft-versus-host disease after allogeneic peripheral-blood stem-cell and bone marrow transplantation: a meta-analysis. J Clin Oncol 2001; 19:3685–91.

12. Torres HA, Rivero GA, Lewis RE, Hachem R, Raad II, Kontoyiannis DP. Aspergillosis caused by non-fumigatus *Aspergillus* species: risk factors and in vitro susceptibility compared with *Aspergillus fumigatus*. Diagn Microbiol Infect Dis 2003; 46:25–8.

13. Singh N, Avery RK, Munoz P, et al. Trends in risk profiles for and mortality associated with invasive aspergillosis among liver transplant recipients. Clin Infect Dis 2003; 36:46–52.

14. Nucci M. Emerging moulds: *Fusarium*, *Scedosporium* and *Zygomycetes* in transplant recipients. Curr Opin Infect Dis 2003; 16:607–12.

15. Nucci M, Anaissie E. Cutaneous infection by *Fusarium* species in healthy and immunocompromised hosts: implications for diagnosis and management. Clin Infect Dis 2002; 35:909–20.

16. Nucci M, Anaissie EJ, Queiroz-Telles F, et al. Outcome predictors of 84 patients with hematologic malignancies and Fusarium infection. Cancer 2003; 98:315–9.

17. Nucci M, Marr KA, Queiroz-Telles F, et al. Fusarium infection in hematopoietic stem cell transplant recipients. Clin Infect Dis 2004; 38:1237–42.

18. Prabhu RM, Patel R. Mucormycosis and entomophthoramycosis: a review of the clinical manifestations, diagnosis and treatment. Clin Microbiol Infect 2004; 10(Suppl. 1):31–47.

19. Roden MM, Zaoutis TE, Buchanan WL, et al. Epidemiology and outcome of zygomycosis: a review of 929 reported cases. Clin Infect Dis 2005; 41:634–53.

20. Kontoyiannis DP, Wessel VC, Bodey GP, Rolston KV. Zygomycosis in the 1990s in a tertiary-care cancer center. Clin Infect Dis 2000; 30:851–6.

21. Kontoyiannis DP, Lionakis MS, Lewis RE, et al. Zygomycosis in a tertiary-care cancer center in the era of Aspergillus-active antifungal therapy: a case-control observational study of 27 recent cases. J Infect Dis 2005; 191:1350–60.

22. Park BJ, Kontoyiannis DP, Pappas PG, et al. Comparison of zygomycosis and fusariosis to invasive aspergillosis among transplant recipients reporting to

TRANSNET [abstract M-666]. In: Program and abstracts of the 44th Interscience Conference on Antimicrobial Agents and Chemotherapy (Washington). Washington, DC: American Society for Microbiology, 2004:411.

23. Marty FM, Cosimi LA, Baden LR. Breakthrough zygomycosis after voriconazole treatment in recipients of hematopoietic stem-cell transplants. N Engl J Med 2004; 350:950–2.

24. Siwek GT, Dodgson KJ, Silverman MM, et al. Invasive zygomycosis in hematopoietic stem cell transplant recipients receiving voriconazole prophylaxis. Clin Infect Dis 2004; 39:584–7.

25. Imhof A, Balajee SA, Fredricks DN, Englund JA, Marr KA. Breakthrough fungal infections in stem cell transplant recipients receiving voriconazole. Clin Infect Dis 2004; 39:743–6.

26. Kobayashi M, Sonobe H, Ikezoe T, Hakoda E, Ohtsuki Y, Taguchi H. In situ detection of *Aspergillus* 18S ribosomal RNA in invasive pulmonary aspergillosis. Intern Med 1999; 38:563–9.

27. Nucci M, Marr KA. Emerging fungal diseases. Clin Infect Dis 2005; 41:521–6.

28. Lin SJ, Schranz J, Teutsch SM. Aspergillosis case-fatality rate: systematic review of the literature. Clin Infect Dis 2001; 32:358–66.

29. Denning DW. Invasive aspergillosis. Clin Infect Dis 1998; 26:781–803.

30. Greenberger PA. Allergic bronchopulmonary aspergillosis. J Allergy Clin Immunol 2002; 110:685–92.

31. Judson MA, Stevens DA. The treatment of pulmonary aspergilloma. Curr Opin Investig Drugs 2001; 2:1375–7.

32. Stevens DA, Moss RB, Kurup VP, et al. Allergic bronchopulmonary aspergillosis in cystic fibrosis—state of the art: Cystic Fibrosis Foundation Consensus Conference. Clin Infect Dis 2003; 37(Suppl. 3):S225–64.

33. Gerson SL, Talbot GH, Lusk E, Hurwitz S, Strom BL, Cassileth PA. Invasive pulmonary aspergillosis in adult acute leukemia: clinical clues to its diagnosis. J Clin Oncol 1985; 3:1109–16.

34. Martino P, Girmenia C, Venditti M, et al. Spontaneous pneumothorax complicating pulmonary mycetoma in patients with acute leukemia. Rev Infect Dis 1990; 12:611–7.

35. Kuhlman JE, Fishman EK, Siegelman SS. Invasive pulmonary aspergillosis in acute leukemia: characteristic findings on CT, the CT halo sign, and the role of CT in early diagnosis. Radiology 1985; 157:611–4.

36. Caillot D, Casasnovas O, Bernard A, et al. Improved management of invasive pulmonary aspergillosis in neutropenic patients using early thoracic computed tomographic scan and surgery. J Clin Oncol 1997; 15:139–47.

37. Caillot D, Couaillier JF, Bernard A, et al. Increasing volume and changing characteristics of invasive pulmonary aspergillosis on sequential thoracic computed tomography scans in patients with neutropenia. J Clin Oncol 2001; 19:253–9.

38. Gefter WB, Albelda SM, Talbot GH, Gerson SL, Cassileth PA, Miller WT. Invasive pulmonary aspergillosis and acute leukemia. Limitations in the diagnostic utility of the air crescent sign. Radiology 1985; 157:605–10.

39. Herold CJ, Kramer J, Sertl K, et al. Invasive pulmonary aspergillosis: evaluation with MR imaging. Radiology 1989; 173:717–21.

40. Alangaden GJ, Wahiduzzaman M, Chandrasekar PH. Aspergillosis: the most common community-acquired pneumonia with gram-negative Bacilli as copathogens

in stem cell transplant recipients with graft-versus-host disease. Clin Infect Dis 2002; 35:659–64.

41. Kojima R, Tateishi U, Kami M, et al. Chest computed tomography of late invasive aspergillosis after allogeneic hematopoietic stem cell transplantation. Biol Blood Marrow Transplant 2005; 11:506–11.

42. Singh N, Husain S. *Aspergillus* infections after lung transplantation: clinical differences in type of transplant and implications for management. J Heart Lung Transplant 2003; 22:258–66.

43. Montoya JG, Chaparro SV, Celis D, et al. Invasive aspergillosis in the setting of cardiac transplantation. Clin Infect Dis 2003; 37(Suppl. 3):S281–92.

44. Mylonakis E, Barlam TF, Flanigan T, Rich JD. Pulmonary aspergillosis and invasive disease in AIDS: review of 342 cases. Chest 1998; 114:251–62.

45. Greene R. The radiological spectrum of pulmonary aspergillosis. Med Mycol 2005; 43(Suppl. 1):S147–54.

46. Denning DW, Riniotis K, Dobrashian R, Sambatakou H. Chronic cavitary and fibrosing pulmonary and pleural aspergillosis: case series, proposed nomenclature change, and review. Clin Infect Dis 2003; 37(Suppl. 3):S265–80.

47. Kemper CA, Hostetler JS, Follansbee SE, et al. Ulcerative and plaque-like tracheobronchitis due to infection with Aspergillus in patients with AIDS. Clin Infect Dis 1993; 17:344–52.

48. Routsi C, Platsouka E, Prekates A, Rontogianni D, Paniara O, Roussos C. Aspergillus bronchitis causing atelectasis and acute respiratory failure in an immunocompromised patient. Infection 2001; 29:243–4.

49. Angelotti T, Krishna G, Scott J, Berry G, Weinacker A. Nodular invasive tracheobronchitis due to Aspergillus in a patient with systemic lupus erythematosus. Lupus 2002; 11:325–8.

50. Machida U, Kami M, Kanda Y, et al. Aspergillus tracheobronchitis after allogeneic bone marrow transplantation. Bone Marrow Transplant 1999; 24:1145–9.

51. van Assen S, Bootsma GP, Verweij PE, Donnelly JP, Raemakers JM. Aspergillus tracheobronchitis after allogeneic bone marrow transplantation. Bone Marrow Transplant 2000; 26:1131–2.

52. Koh LP, Goh YT, Linn YC, Hwang J, Tan P. Pseudomembranous tracheobronchitis caused by Aspergillus in a patient after peripheral blood stem cell transplantation. Ann Acad Med Singapore 2000; 29:531–3.

53. Van Burik JA, Colven R, Spach DH. Cutaneous aspergillosis. J Clin Microbiol 1998; 36:3115–21.

54. Allo MD, Miller J, Townsend T, Tan C. Primary cutaneous aspergillosis associated with Hickman intravenous catheters. N Engl J Med 1987; 317:1105–8.

55. Singh SA, Dutta S, Narang A, Vaiphei K. Cutaneous *Aspergillus flavus* infection in a neonate. Indian J Pediatr 2004; 71:351–2.

56. Woodruff CA, Hebert AA. Neonatal primary cutaneous aspergillosis: case report and review of the literature. Pediatr Dermatol 2002; 19:439–44.

57. Girmenia C, Gastaldi R, Martino P. Catheter-related cutaneous aspergillosis complicated by fungemia and fatal pulmonary infection in an HIV-positive patient with acute lymphocytic leukemia. Eur J Clin Microbiol Infect Dis 1995; 14:524–6.

58. Grossman ME, Fithian EC, Behrens C, Bissinger J, Fracaro M, Neu HC. Primary cutaneous aspergillosis in six leukemic children. J Am Acad Dermatol 1985; 12:313–8.

59. Kleinschmidt-DeMasters BK. Central nervous system aspergillosis: a 20-year retrospective series. Hum Pathol 2002; 33:116–24.

60. Robinson MR, Fine HF, Ross ML, et al. Sino-orbital-cerebral aspergillosis in immunocompromised pediatric patients. Pediatr Infect Dis J 2000; 19:1197–203.

61. Colombo AL, Rosas RC. Successful treatment of an Aspergillus brain abscess with caspofungin: case report of a diabetic patient intolerant of amphotericin B. Eur J Clin Microbiol Infect Dis 2003; 22:575–6.

62. Ashdown BC, Tien RD, Felsberg GJ. Aspergillosis of the brain and paranasal sinuses in immunocompromised patients: CT and MR imaging findings. AJR Am J Roentgenol 1994; 162:155–9.

63. Vinas FC, King PK, Diaz FG. Spinal aspergillus osteomyelitis. Clin Infect Dis 1999; 28:1223–9.

64. Vandecasteele SJ, Boelaert JR, Verrelst P, Graulus E, Gordts BZ. Diagnosis and treatment of *Aspergillus flavus* sternal wound infections after cardiac surgery. Clin Infect Dis 2002; 35:887–90.

65. Paterson DL. New clinical presentations of invasive aspergillosis in non-conventional hosts. Clin Microbiol Infect 2004; 10(Suppl. 1):24–30.

66. Myoken Y, Sugata T, Kyo T, et al. Invasive Aspergillus stomatitis in patients with acute leukemia: report of 12 cases. Clin Infect Dis 2001; 33:1975–80.

67. The Aspergillus Web Site. http://www.aspergillus.man.ac.uk. Last accessed June, 2007.

68. Rath PM, Ansorg R. Identification of medically important *Aspergillus* species by single strand conformational polymorphism (SSCP) of the PCR-amplified intergenic spacer region. Mycoses 2000; 43:381–6.

69. Henry T, Iwen PC, Hinrichs SH. Identification of *Aspergillus* species using internal transcribed spacer regions 1 and 2. J Clin Microbiol 2000; 38:1510–5.

70. de Hoog GS, Guarro J, Gené J, Figueiras MJ. Atlas of Clinical Fungi. Utrecht, The Netherlands/Reus, Spain: Centraalbureau voor Schimmelcultures and Universitat Rovira i Virgili, 2004:444–5.

71. Yuen KY, Woo PC, Ip MS, et al. Stage-specific manifestation of mold infections in bone marrow transplant recipients: risk factors and clinical significance of positive concentrated smears. Clin Infect Dis 1997; 25:37–42.

72. Yu VL, Muder RR, Poorsattar A. Significance of isolation of Aspergillus from the respiratory tract in diagnosis of invasive pulmonary aspergillosis. Results from a three-year prospective study. Am J Med 1986; 81:249–54.

73. Horvath JA, Dummer S. The use of respiratory-tract cultures in the diagnosis of invasive pulmonary aspergillosis. Am J Med 1996; 100:171–8.

74. Perfect JR, Cox GM, Lee JY, et al. The impact of culture isolation of *Aspergillus* species: a hospital-based survey of aspergillosis. Clin Infect Dis 2001; 33:1824–33.

75. Brown RS, Jr., Lake JR, Katzman BA, et al. Incidence and significance of Aspergillus cultures following liver and kidney transplantation. Transplantation 1996; 61:666–9.

76. Wallace JM, Lim R, Browdy BL, et al. Risk factors and outcomes associated with identification of Aspergillus in respiratory specimens from persons with HIV disease. Pulmonary Complications of HIV Infection Study Group. Chest 1998; 114:131–7.

77. Dimopoulos G, Piagnerelli M, Berre J, Eddafali B, Salmon I, Vincent JL. Disseminated aspergillosis in intensive care unit patients: an autopsy study. J Chemother 2003; 15:71–5.

78. Nucci M, Biasoli I, Barreiros G, et al. Predictive value of a positive nasal swab for *Aspergillus* spp. in the diagnosis of invasive aspergillosis in adult neutropenic cancer patients. Diagn Microbiol Infect Dis 1999; 35:193–6.

79. Kontoyiannis DP, Sumoza D, Tarrand J, Bodey GP, Storey R, Raad II. Significance of aspergillemia in patients with cancer: a 10-year study. Clin Infect Dis 2000; 31:188–9.

80. Girmenia C, Nucci M, Martino P. Clinical significance of *Aspergillus fungaemia* in patients with haematological malignancies and invasive aspergillosis. Br J Haematol 2001; 114:93–8.

81. Kaufman L, Standard PG, Jalbert M, Kraft DE. Immunohistologic identification of *Aspergillus* spp. and other hyaline fungi by using polyclonal fluorescent antibodies. J Clin Microbiol 1997; 35:2206–9.

82. Hayden RT, Isotalo PA, Parrett T, et al. In situ hybridization for the differentiation of *Aspergillus*, *Fusarium*, and *Pseudallescheria* species in tissue section. Diagn Mol Pathol 2003; 12:21–6.

83. Choi JK, Mauger J, McGowan KL. Immunohistochemical detection of *Aspergillus* species in pediatric tissue samples. Am J Clin Pathol 2004; 121:18–25.

84. Stynen D, Goris A, Sarfati J, Latge JP. A new sensitive sandwich enzyme-linked immunosorbent assay to detect galactofuran in patients with invasive aspergillosis. J Clin Microbiol 1995; 33:497–500.

85. Machetti M, Feasi M, Mordini N, et al. Comparison of an enzyme immunoassay and a latex agglutination system for the diagnosis of invasive aspergillosis in bone marrow transplant recipients. Bone Marrow Transplant 1998; 21:917–21.

86. Verweij PE, Stynen D, Rijs AJ, de Pauw BE, Hoogkamp-Korstanje JA, Meis JF. Sandwich enzyme-linked immunosorbent assay compared with Pastorex latex agglutination test for diagnosing invasive aspergillosis in immunocompromised patients. J Clin Microbiol 1995; 33:1912–4.

87. Mennink-Kersten MA, Donnelly JP, Verweij PE. Detection of circulating galacto-mannan for the diagnosis and management of invasive aspergillosis. Lancet Infect Dis 2004; 4:349–57.

88. Marr KA, Balajee SA, McLaughlin L, Tabouret M, Bentsen C, Walsh TJ. Detection of galactomannan antigenemia by enzyme immunoassay for the diagnosis of invasive aspergillosis: variables that affect performance. J Infect Dis 2004; 190:641–9.

89. Sulahian A, Boutboul F, Ribaud P, Leblanc T, Lacroix C, Derouin F. Value of antigen detection using an enzyme immunoassay in the diagnosis and prediction of invasive aspergillosis in two adult and pediatric hematology units during a 4-year prospective study. Cancer 2001; 91:311–8.

90. Pinel C, Fricker-Hidalgo H, Lebeau B, et al. Detection of circulating *Aspergillus fumigatus* galactomannan: value and limits of the Platelia test for diagnosing invasive aspergillosis. J Clin Microbiol 2003; 41:2184–6.

91. Husain S, Kwak EJ, Obman A, et al. Prospective assessment of Platelia trade mark Aspergillus galactomannan antigen for the diagnosis of invasive Aspergillosis in lung transplant recipients. Am J Transplant 2004; 4:796–802.

92. Maertens J, Verhaegen J, Demuynck H, et al. Autopsy-controlled prospective evaluation of serial screening for circulating galactomannan by a sandwich enzyme-linked immunosorbent assay for hematological patients at risk for invasive Aspergillosis. J Clin Microbiol 1999; 37:3223–8.

93. Herbrecht R, Letscher-Bru V, Oprea C, et al. Aspergillus galactomannan detection in the diagnosis of invasive aspergillosis in cancer patients. J Clin Oncol 2002; 20:1898–906.

94. Maertens J, Van Eldere J, Verhaegen J, Verbeken E, Verschakelen J, Boogaerts M. Use of circulating galactomannan screening for early diagnosis of invasive aspergillosis in allogeneic stem cell transplant recipients. J Infect Dis 2002; 186:1297–306.

95. Fortun J, Martin-Davila P, Alvarez ME, et al. Aspergillus antigenemia sandwich-enzyme immunoassay test as a serodiagnostic method for invasive aspergillosis in liver transplant recipients. Transplantation 2001; 71:145–9.

96. Kwak EJ, Husain S, Obman A, et al. Efficacy of galactomannan antigen in the Platelia Aspergillus enzyme immunoassay for diagnosis of invasive aspergillosis in liver transplant recipients. J Clin Microbiol 2004; 42:435–8.

97. Pfeiffer CD, Fine JP, Safdar N. Diagnosis of invasive aspergillosis using a galactomannan assay: a meta-analysis. Clin Infect Dis 2006; 42:1417–727.

98. Maertens J, Verhaegen J, Lagrou K, Van Eldere J, Boogaerts M. Screening for circulating galactomannan as a noninvasive diagnostic tool for invasive aspergillosis in prolonged neutropenic patients and stem cell transplantation recipients: a prospective validation. Blood 2001; 97:1604–10.

99. Kami M, Tanaka Y, Ogawa S, et al. The limitation of circulating Aspergillus antigen detection methods for BMT recipients. Bone Marrow Transplant 1998; 22:832–3.

100. Adam O, Auperin A, Wilquin F, Bourhis JH, Gachot B, Chachaty E. Treatment with piperacillin–tazobactam and false-positive Aspergillus galactomannan antigen test results for patients with hematological malignancies. Clin Infect Dis 2004; 38:917–20.

101. Tanriover MD, Metan G, Altun B, Hascelik G, Uzun O. False positivity for Aspergillus antigenemia related to the administration of piperacillin/tazobactam. Eur J Intern Med 2005; 16:489–91.

102. Bart-Delabesse E, Basile M, Al Jijakli A, et al. Detection of Aspergillus galactomannan antigenemia to determine biological and clinical implications of beta-lactam treatments. J Clin Microbiol 2005; 43:5214–20.

103. Aubry A, Porcher R, Bottero J, et al. Occurrence and kinetics of false-positive Aspergillus galactomannan test results following treatment with beta-lactam antibiotics in patients with hematological disorders. J Clin Microbiol 2006; 44:389–94.

104. Hamaki T, Kami M, Kanda Y, et al. False-positive results of Aspergillus enzyme-linked immunosorbent assay in a patient with chronic graft-versus-host disease after allogeneic bone marrow transplantation. Bone Marrow Transplant 2001; 28:633–4.

105. Becker MJ, Lugtenburg EJ, Cornelissen JJ, Van Der SC, Hoogsteden HC, de Marie S. Galactomannan detection in computerized tomography-based broncho-alveolar lavage fluid and serum in haematological patients at risk for invasive pulmonary aspergillosis. Br J Haematol 2003; 121:448–57.

106. Husain S, Paterson DL, Studer S, et al. Prospective assessment of Platelia™ *Aspergillus* EIA in the bronchoalveolar lavage fluid for the early diagnosis of invasive aspergillosis (IA) in lung transplant recipients. Boston, MA: World Transplant Congress, 2006 (Abstract 2741).

107. Viscoli C, Machetti M, Gazzola P, et al. Aspergillus galactomannan antigen in the cerebrospinal fluid of bone marrow transplant recipients with probable cerebral aspergillosis. J Clin Microbiol 2002; 40:1496–9.

108. Boutboul F, Alberti C, Leblanc T, et al. Invasive aspergillosis in allogeneic stem cell transplant recipients: increasing antigenemia is associated with progressive disease. Clin Infect Dis 2002; 34:939–43.

109. Obayashi T, Yoshida M, Mori T, et al. Plasma (1->3)-beta-D-glucan measurement in diagnosis of invasive deep mycosis and fungal febrile episodes. Lancet 1995; 345:17–20.

110. Odabasi Z, Mattiuzzi G, Estey E, et al. Beta-D-Glucan as a diagnostic adjunct for invasive fungal infections: validation, cutoff development, and performance in patients with acute myelogenous leukemia and myelodysplastic syndrome. Clin Infect Dis 2004; 39:199–205.

111. Yoshida M, Obayashi T, Iwama A, et al. Detection of plasma (1->3)-beta-D-glucan in patients with *Fusarium, Trichosporon, Saccharomyces* and *Acremonium* fungaemias. J Med Vet Mycol 1997; 35:371–4.

112. Bretagne S, Costa JM. Towards a molecular diagnosis of invasive aspergillosis and disseminated candidosis. FEMS Immunol Med Microbiol 2005; 45:361–8.

113. Loeffler J, Hebart H, Brauchle U, Schumacher U, Einsele H. Comparison between plasma and whole blood specimens for detection of Aspergillus DNA by PCR. J Clin Microbiol 2000; 38:3830–3.

114. Lass-Florl C, Aigner J, Gunsilius E, et al. Screening for *Aspergillus* spp. using polymerase chain reaction of whole blood samples from patients with haematological malignancies. Br J Haematol 2001; 113:180–4.

115. Yamakami Y, Hashimoto A, Yamagata E, et al. Evaluation of PCR for detection of DNA specific for *Aspergillus* species in sera of patients with various forms of pulmonary aspergillosis. J Clin Microbiol 1998; 36:3619–23.

116. Raad I, Hanna H, Huaringa A, Sumoza D, Hachem R, Albitar M. Diagnosis of invasive pulmonary aspergillosis using polymerase chain reaction-based detection of *Aspergillus* in BAL. Chest 2002; 121:1171–6.

117. Kawazu M, Kanda Y, Goyama S, et al. Rapid diagnosis of invasive pulmonary aspergillosis by quantitative polymerase chain reaction using bronchial lavage fluid. Am J Hematol 2003; 72:27–30.

118. Buchheidt D, Baust C, Skladny H, Baldus M, Brauninger S, Hehlmann R. Clinical evaluation of a polymerase chain reaction assay to detect *Aspergillus* species in bronchoalveolar lavage samples of neutropenic patients. Br J Haematol 2002; 116:803–11.

119. Bretagne S, Costa JM, Marmorat-Khuong A, et al. Detection of *Aspergillus* species DNA in bronchoalveolar lavage samples by competitive PCR. J Clin Microbiol 1995; 33:1164–8.

120. Kami M, Ogawa S, Kanda Y, et al. Early diagnosis of central nervous system aspergillosis using polymerase chain reaction, latex agglutination test, and enzyme-linked immunosorbent assay. Br J Haematol 1999; 106:536–7.

121. Becker MJ, de Marie S, Willemse D, Verbrugh HA, Bakker-Woudenberg IA. Quantitative galactomannan detection is superior to PCR in diagnosing and monitoring invasive pulmonary aspergillosis in an experimental rat model. J Clin Microbiol 2000; 38:1434–8.

122. Kawazu M, Kanda Y, Nannya Y, et al. Prospective comparison of the diagnostic potential of real-time PCR, double-sandwich enzyme-linked immunosorbent assay for galactomannan, and a (1->3)-beta-D-glucan test in weekly screening for invasive aspergillosis in patients with hematological disorders. J Clin Microbiol 2004; 42:2733–41.

123. Nelson PE, Dignani MC, Anaissie EJ. Taxonomy, biology, and clinical aspects of *Fusarium* species. Clin Microbiol Rev 1994; 7:479–504.

124. Madhavan M, Ratnakar C, Veliath AJ, Kanungo R, Smile SR, Bhat S. Primary disseminated fusarial infection. Postgrad Med J 1992; 68:143–4.

125. Sander A, Beyer U, Amberg R. Systemic *Fusarium oxysporum* infection in an immunocompetent patient with an adult respiratory distress syndrome (ARDS) and extracorporal membrane oxygenation (ECMO). Mycoses 1998; 41:109–11.

126. Jakle C, Leek JC, Olson DA, Robbins DL. Septic arthritis due to *Fusarium solani*. J Rheumatol 1983; 10:151–3.

127. Gradon JD, Lerman A, Lutwick LI. Septic arthritis due to *Fusarium moniliforme*. Rev Infect Dis 1990; 12:716–7.

128. Rippon JW, Larson RA, Rosenthal DM, Clayman J. Disseminated cutaneous and peritoneal hyalohyphomycosis caused by *Fusarium* species: three cases and review of the literature. Mycopathologia 1988; 101:105–11.

129. Kerr CM, Perfect JR, Craven PC, et al. Fungal peritonitis in patients on continuous ambulatory peritoneal dialysis. Ann Intern Med 1983; 99:334–6.

130. Flynn JT, Meislich D, Kaiser BA, Polinsky MS, Baluarte HJ. Fusarium peritonitis in a child on peritoneal dialysis: case report and review of the literature. Perit Dial Int 1996; 16:52–7.

131. Kurien M, Anandi V, Raman R, Brahmadathan KN. Maxillary sinus fusariosis in immunocompetent hosts. J Laryngol Otol 1992; 106:733–6.

132. Sturm AW, Grave W, Kwee WS. Disseminated *Fusarium oxysporum* infection in patient with heatstroke. Lancet 1989; 1:968.

133. Pflugfelder SC, Flynn HW, Jr., Zwickey TA, et al. Exogenous fungal endophthalmitis. Ophthalmology 1988; 95:19–30.

134. Gabriele P, Hutchins RK. Fusarium endophthalmitis in an intravenous drug abuser. Am J Ophthalmol 1996; 122:119–21.

135. Bourguignon RL, Walsh AF, Flynn JC, Baro C, Spinos E. *Fusarium* species osteomyelitis. Case report. J Bone Joint Surg Am 1976; 58:722–3.

136. Issakainen J, Jalava J, Eerola E, Campbell CK. Relatedness of *Pseudallescheria*, *Scedosporium* and Graphium pro parte based on SSU rDNA sequences. J Med Vet Mycol 1997; 35:389–98.

137. Walsh TJ, Groll A, Hiemenz J, Fleming R, Roilides E, Anaissie E. Infections due to emerging and uncommon medically important fungal pathogens. Clin Microbiol Infect 2004; 10(Suppl. 1):48–66.

138. Dignani MC, Niwan EN, Anaissie EJ. Hyalohyphomycoses. In: Anaissie EJ, McGinnis MR, Pfaller MA, eds. Clinical Mycology. New York/Edingurgh/London/Philadelphia: Churchill Livingstone, 2003:309–24.

139. Revankar SG, Patterson JE, Sutton DA, Pullen R, Rinaldi MG. Disseminated phaeohyphomycosis: review of an emerging mycosis. Clin Infect Dis 2002; 34:467–76.

140. Bouza E, Munoz P. Invasive infections caused by Blastoschizomyces capitatus and *Scedosporium* spp. Clin Microbiol Infect 2004; 10(Suppl. 1):76–85.

141. Castiglioni B, Sutton DA, Rinaldi MG, Fung J, Kusne S. *Pseudallescheria boydii* (Anamorph *Scedosporium apiospermum*). Infection in solid organ transplant recipients in a tertiary medical center and review of the literature. Medicine (Baltimore) 2002; 81:333–48.

142. Montejo M, Muniz ML, Zarraga S, et al. Case Reports. Infection due to *Scedosporium apiospermum* in renal transplant recipients: a report of two cases and literature review of central nervous system and cutaneous infections by *Pseudallescheria boydii/S. apiospermum*. Mycoses 2002; 45:418–27.

143. Berenguer J, Rodriguez-Tudela JL, Richard C, et al. Deep infections caused by *Scedosporium prolificans*. A report on 16 cases in Spain and a review of the literature. *Scedosporium Prolificans* Spanish Study Group. Medicine (Baltimore) 1997; 76:256–65.

144. Maertens J, Lagrou K, Deweerdt H, et al. Disseminated infection by *Scedosporium prolificans*: an emerging fatality among haematology patients. Case report and review. Ann Hematol 2000; 79:340–4.

145. Silveira F, Nucci M. Emergence of black moulds in fungal disease: epidemiology and therapy. Curr Opin Infect Dis 2001; 14:679–84.

146. Nucci M, Akiti T, Barreiros G, et al. Nosocomial fungemia due to *Exophiala jeanselmei* var. *jeanselmei* and a *Rhinocladiella* species: newly described causes of bloodstream infection. J Clin Microbiol 2001; 39:514–8.

147. Queiroz-Telles F, McGinnis MR, Salkin I, Graybill JR. Subcutaneous mycoses. Infect Dis Clin North Am 2003; 17:59–85 (see also viii).

148. Kimura M, McGinnis MR. Fontana–Masson-stained tissue from culture-proven mycoses. Arch Pathol Lab Med 1998; 122:1107–11.

149. Dokmetas HS, Canbay E, Yilmaz S, et al. Diabetic ketoacidosis and rhino-orbital mucormycosis. Diabetes Res Clin Pract 2002; 57:139–42.

150. Chamilos G, Marom EM, Lewis RE, Lionakis MS, Kontoyiannis DP. Predictors of pulmonary zygomycosis versus invasive pulmonary aspergillosis in patients with cancer. Clin Infect Dis 2005; 41:60–6.

151. Donohue JF, Scott RJ, Walker DH, Bromberg PA. Phycomycosis: a cause of bronchial obstruction. South Med J 1980; 73:734–6.

152. Hata TR, Johnson RA, Barnhill R, Dover JS. Ecthymalike lesions on the leg of an immunocompromised patient. Primary cutaneous mucormycosis. Arch Dermatol 1995; 131:833–7.

153. Cocanour CS, Miller-Crotchett P, Reed RL, Johnson PC, Fischer RP. Mucormycosis in trauma patients. J Trauma 1992; 32:12–5.

154. Lawson HH, Schmaman A. Gastric phycomycosis. Br J Surg 1974; 61:743–6.

155. Ribes JA, Vanover-Sams CL, Baker DJ. *Zygomycetes* in human disease. Clin Microbiol Rev 2000; 13:236–301.

9

Invasive Yeast Infections

Luis Ostrosky-Zeichner

University of Texas Health Science Center at Houston,
Houston, Texas, U.S.A.

INTRODUCTION

The incidence of invasive fungal infections has been steadily on the rise for the past three decades (1,2). Of particular importance are invasive yeast infections since they account for the vast majority of these serious infections both in immunocompromised and "non-immunocompromised" patients (3–6). This book chapter concentrates on *Candida*, by far the most prevalent invasive yeast pathogen, and for which the most diagnostic methods have been developed. Other emerging yeasts, such as *Trichosporon*, *Saccharomyces*, *Malassezia*, and *Rhodotorula*, of increasing prevalence in immunocompromised patients (4), will be discussed towards the end of the chapter. A list of the most relevant invasive yeast pathogens for humans (excluding *Cryptococcus neoformans*) is shown in Table 1.

Despite the prevalence and impact of these infections, experience with the current diagnostic methods for their causative agents has been very disappointing, lagging many years behind bacterial, viral, and even other fungal diagnostic methods (7). Recent and exciting developments in the field will not only improve the diagnostic performance themselves, but will allow clinicians to use them as tools for prophylaxis or pre-emptive therapy and as prognostic or treatment response markers.

CANDIDA

Epidemiology

Candidemia is the 4th most common hospital-acquired bloodstream infection in the United States, with similar trends being reported in epidemiological studies

Table 1 Most Common Causative Agents
for Invasive Yeast Infections in Humans[a]

Candida spp.
   C. albicans
   C. glabrata
   C. krusei
   C. tropicalis
   C. parapsilosis
   C. lusitaniae
Trichosporon spp.
Saccharomyces spp.
Malassezia spp.
Rhodotorula spp.
Blastoschizomyces spp.
Sporobolomyces spp.
Hansenula spp.

---

[a] Excluding *Cryptococcus neoformans*.

worldwide (6,8–10). This infection has a high societal impact, having an attributable mortality in excess of 30%, despite significant advancements in patient management, critical care, and the development and availability of highly active antifungal agents (11–13). An episode of candidemia is also estimated to add ~ $40,000 in excess health care costs (14). The risk factors for this infection have been described extensively. The most common ones are: use of central venous catheters, use of broad-spectrum antibiotics, total parenteral nutrition, diabetes mellitus, intravenous drug use, high severity of illness, prolonged stay in the intensive care unit, hemodialysis, abdominal surgery (particularly of the upper gastrointestinal tract), severe pancreatitis, and prematurity in neonates (9,15–22). Knowledge of these risk factors is important since current diagnostic techniques are imperfect and clinicians often use them as surrogates when making empirical therapy decisions.

Clinical Features and Diagnostic Clues

The clinical manifestations of candidemia and other forms of invasive candidiasis are non-specific and cannot distinguish the disease from other infections (23–25), except for cases of deep organ involvement, such as endophthalmitis and hepatosplenic candidiasis (26). Endophthalmitis usually occurs as a consequence of disseminated candidiasis, and although less than 3% of patients with candidemia have eye involvement, it is recommended for all patients with this disease to have a dilated eye exam by an ophthalmologist to exclude this condition, which often requires a surgical approach and prolonged local and systemic antifungals (27–30). Hepato-splenic candidiasis is a well-defined pathological entity that occurs only in neutropenic patients. It often presents as chronic fever with characteristic nodular lesions in the liver and spleen by ultrasound and CT scan, requiring prolonged systemic antifungals (26,31,32). Pulmonary candidiasis is incredibly rare, and with few exceptions (mainly severely immunocompromised hosts with histopathological demonstration) recovery of *Candida* from the sputum should be considered colonization (33). The same applies for urinary candidiasis, where unless the patient has repeatedly positive cultures, symptoms, urinalysis abnormalities, and other infections have been excluded, the recovery of yeast from the urine should be considered colonization (34–38).

Clinical signs and symptoms of candidemia and disseminated candidiasis include fever or hypothermia and hypotension. Occasionally it may present as septic shock, although its course is usually slow and insidious (13,25,39). Laboratory abnormalities usually include leukocytosis. Thrombocytopenia is frequently cited, particularly in the pediatric literature (3,23,40). With the exception of hepatosplenic candidiasis (where hyperechoic lesions in the liver are seen by ultrasound and hyperdense lesions are seen by CT scan), there are no radiological abnormalities that are characteristic to these diseases (31).

As discussed above, these clinical manifestations are largely non-specific, and clinicians often face this disease with suboptimal diagnostic methods, so in many instances the diagnosis is made by excluding other infections and noninfectious causes of fever, and by therapeutic trials in patients that have multiple risk factors (41–43).

Diagnostic Modalities

The diagnostic gold standards for invasive candidiasis are, as in most mycoses, histopathological evidence of infection and culturing of the organism from a normally sterile site or body fluid. Unfortunately, histopathology is not readily available in the patient populations that are at the highest risk of the disease (due to coagulopathies, thrombocytopenia, hemodynamic instability, etc.), and cultures have less than optimal performance, as discussed below. These diagnostic difficulties have prompted the development of alternative diagnostic methods such as antibody and antigen detection, and most recently genetic material detection methods. Current evidence and recent advances in the field are discussed below. Table 2 presents a summary of the most common diagnostic modalities for invasive candidiasis.

Histopathology and Traditional Microbiological Methods

Candida cells are readily found in both direct microscopy of body fluids, swabs from infected surfaces (such as the oral mucosa), and in biopsy specimens. The microscopic appearance of *Candida* is that of budding yeast cells with hyphae or pseudohyphae present. They appear as Gram positive organisms in the Gram stain, and in histopathological slides they are best visualized with the silver-methenamine and periodic acid Schiff stains (44–46).

Candida can be cultured from any body fluid, but as mentioned above, recovery from non-sterile body sites, such as sputum, mucosal surfaces, and even

Table 2 Diagnostic Methods for Invasive Candidiasis

Method	Typical performance	Advantages	Disadvantages
Blood cultures	50–70% sensitivity	Readily available in all clinical microbiology laboratories. Relatively inexpensive	Many false negatives. Several days to have results. Advanced culture and detection methods required for optimal performance
Antibody and antigen detection	Sensitivity 30–80%, variable specificity	Many commercially available kits. Relatively inexpensive and easy to set up in clinical laboratories	Poor performance to date, particularly in immunocompromised hosts
Fungal metabolite detection	Sensitivity and specificity ~90%	Excellent performance	Many require advanced biochemical assays that are not easily translated into clinical laboratories
Fungal cell wall component detection	Sensitivity and specificity >90%	Excellent performance even in immunocompromised hosts and in the setting of antifungal prophylaxis. Easy to set up in the clinical laboratory	Potential for contamination from environmental sources (false positives). More experience needed
Genetic amplification and detection	Sensitivity and specificity >90%	Very high sensitivity, potential for rapid detection of a variety of fungi from primary clinical specimens	Investigational. Relatively expensive. No consensus on primers or techniques. Difficult translation into clinical laboratories

urine is hard to interpret due to the ubiquitous presence of this organism at those sites and contamination with normal flora. Recovery from blood cultures is usually challenging. Candidemia is characteristically a disease of low organism burden, so blood cultures using traditional techniques have been reported to have sensitivity as low as 50%. Cell-centrifugation blood cultures techniques have been reported to increase the sensitivity to 70% (47,48), so it is easy to conclude that blood cultures, although currently the best diagnostic methods, offer poor diagnostic performance, since a negative blood culture does not exclude the diagnosis. Using automated methods, a positive culture is usually detected in two to four days, depending on the degree of fungemia and the *Candida* species growing [non-*albicans* species usually grow more slowly (45)]. When *Candida* species are suspected, the microbiology laboratory should be advised, so that the cultures are incubated longer.

Initial isolation and identification of *Candida* spp. is typically done in antibiotic-supplemented Sabouraud's agar with incubation at 35°C, although they can grow well on other basic media such as blood agar. Colonies are usually cream colored and optimal growth occurs at three to five days. Identification to the species level is usually accomplished by incubation in cornmeal agar to identify species specific blastoconidia and formation of hyphae or pseudohyphae, as well as commercial carbohydrate metabolism-based methods such as API20 or API32 (45,46). Recent advances in differentiation media provide a faster identification to the species level from primary cultures. Most relevantly, CHROMagar facilitates presumptive identification of *Candida albicans*, by the color and appearance of the colonies (49–51). Another test that facilitates the presumptive identification of *C. albicans* versus non-albicans species is the germ tube test (production of germ tubes by incubation of cells on serum at 37°C), which is easy to set up in any microbiology laboratory (44,52). Newer selective media are becoming more widely spread in the market and they provide faster identification to the species level from the primary isolation (53–55).

Serological Methods

Difficulties and the poor performance of cultures and histopathology prompted intense research since the late 1960s in serological methods for the diagnosis of this infection. Researched focused initially in immunological methods of antibody and antigen detection, later evolving to the detection of fungal metabolites and fungal cell wall components (7,56,57). This area of research unfortunately suffers from the lack of large multi-center clinical trials and from a lack of standardized definitions of disease when most of the limited studies were carried out. Recently, immunological methods are resurfacing, and the increased incidence of these diseases has promoted a prioritization of this area. Although far from ideal at this time, these methods represent important advances in the field, and will occupy a prominent role in the future.

Antibody assays: Antibody detection methods have focused on the detection of naturally produced antibodies against a variety of fungal targets, the most successful being mannan, enolase, and hsp90 (7,58). Methods range from basic hemagglutination essays to the more reliable ELISA-based tests. Sensitivities have historically ranged from 30% to 80% with false negatives frequently seen in immunocompromised patients (56,59–62). Another problem with these tests is the high prevalence of false positives associated with the frequency of previous exposure to *Candida* antigens, resulting in a serious problem in differentiating between active disease and previous infection or colonization (58,63–65). Experience with some of the most recent kits, such as *Candida* Platelia® (BioRad Laboratories, Marnes-La Coquette, France) and Syscan3® (Rockeby Biomed, Ltd., West Perth, Australia) is encouraging (66–68).

Antigen assays: When researchers realized there were serious problems with false negatives and positives in antibody detection, research concentrated on detection of *Candida* antigens. The two most promising antigens are *Candida* mannan and enolase (69–73). The currently available kit for detection of mannan is the Cand-Tec™ kit (Ramco Laboratories, Stafford, Texas, U.S.A.), which is a hemagglutination-based method that has had variable performance in smaller studies. A recent improvement in the kit has shown sensitivity of 100% and specificity of 80% in a small study (73). Enolase detection had a sensitivity of 54% in a small study as well, with improved performance in serial sampling, which is an attractive surveillance strategy for pre-emptive therapy in high risk hosts (74,75). Research is currently concentrating on simultaneous testing of antibodies and antigens for improved performance, particularly of the Platelia system (66,67).

Fungal metabolite assays: The major fungal metabolite used for diagnosis is D-arabinitol (76–78). Although initially hampered by the human endogenous production of L-arabinitol in the face of non-specific assays and by its renal elimination (and subsequent accumulation in renal failure), detection methods for this agent improved and were further refined by exploring the ratios of D-arabinitol to L-arabinitol and creatinine-adjusted D-arabinitol levels (56,79–81). Sensitivity and specificity have been reported to be as high as 88% and 91%, respectively, when using D-arabinitol/L-arabinitol ratios in serial sampling (81). When using it as a surveillance tool, this method also offers positive results several days before the clinical or microbiological diagnosis is made, and studies have shown usefulness in a variety of populations and correlation with clinical outcomes (82–84). Unfortunately, this test has not made it into the clinical laboratory due to its dependence on complex assay techniques, such as high-performance liquid chromatography. Recent research has focused on alternative assay methods more easy to implement in the clinical laboratory (78,85,86).

Fungal cell wall component assays: Beyond other cellular antigens, and using non-immunological methods, detection of fungal cell wall components has emerged as the newest trend in fungal diagnostics (7). β-D-glucan has been investigated for this purpose since the 1980s (87). Although it is a panfungal marker, when detected on the appropriate epidemiological context it has sensitivities and specificities that have been reported to be >80% for *Candida*, in a variety of patient populations, including immunocompromised hosts and in patients on antifungal prophylaxis, with serial and single sample testing (61,88–91). Head-to-head comparison with other serological methods has demonstrated superior performance (74,92,93). Detection is based on a chemical reaction to clotting blood components of the horseshoe crabs *Tachypleus* and *Limulus* (94–97). The *Tachypleus*-based kit has increased affinity to β-D-glucan, resulting into a lower cut-off for results [20 pg/mL vs. 60 pg/mL for *Limulus*-based testing (91)]. The assay is commercially available in Japan and the United States. False-positives occur in patients exposed to other sources of glucan, such as found in hemodialysis filters and surgical gauze (98–101). Further research is required to acquire more experience with these assays, as well as more head-to-head comparison with other contemporary methods.

Genetic Material Detection Methods

Genetic material detection methods have three basic areas of interest for this organism: (*i*) identification to the species level from cultures, (*ii*) taxonomical and epidemiological studies, and (*iii*) rapid and reliable diagnosis from primary clinical specimens, such as blood cultures (6,102,103). The first two areas have enjoyed the most attention so far, having multiple commercially available restriction enzymes and species-specific primers available for almost any fungal species to be used for blotting, amplification, or in situ hybridization. Although costly and restricted to reference laboratories, these methods contribute significantly to the identification of difficult or less frequent *Candida* spp. and to the study of outbreaks and transmission of particular strains (11,15,102).

Assays using in situ hybridization from positive blood cultures have recently been introduced into the market and have shown significant advantages in rapid identification of the *Candida* species, allowing for switches in antifungal therapy with economic advantages (104–106).

Although many polymerase chain reaction (PCR) primers and molecular techniques have been developed for the detection of *Candida* from primary clinical specimens, there is still lack of consensus on which are the most sensitive, specific, and most importantly, the most readily translatable into the clinical setting. Recently investigated methods (mostly real-time and quantitative PCR) have shown detection thresholds as low as 3 cells/mL of blood, and sensitivities in the 80% to 100% range in a wide variety of populations including immunocompromised hosts, adults, and children (3,107–112). As is true with most highly sensitive genetic assays, specificity problems have often been reported.

OTHER INVASIVE YEAST INFECTIONS

As discussed in the introduction, the vast majority of invasive yeast infections are caused by *Candida* spp. Nevertheless, non-Candida yeasts are starting to surface as emerging yeast pathogens, seen almost exclusively in clinical settings with a large immunocompromised patient base (4,113). Although many tools are available for the genetic identification of these organisms for taxonomical or epidemiological purposes, or at reference laboratories, the relatively low frequency of these organisms has resulted in a reduced priority for the development of advanced diagnostics at the clinical level; thus, we still rely on traditional microbiological and histopathological methods. These methods have been extensively described (44–46) and are summarized for each agent in this section. It is important to consider, though, that many of these pathogens can be identified by panfungal genetic primers (110,114–116), and when detection techniques based on them make it into the clinical setting, the true incidence of theses agents will be better understood. This section covers some of the most salient clinical and epidemiological features of the most common of these agents, as well as key microbiological findings.

Trichosporon spp.

Trichosporon spp. are the causative agents of both superficial skin infections (white piedra) and invasive or disseminated disease (117–120). This yeast is one of the leading emerging fungal pathogens in highly immunocompromised hosts. Risk factors include: hematological malignancy, systemic steroids, bone marrow transplant, neutropenia, exposure to the intensive care setting (both in adults and premature infants), burns, and renal transplant. This agent can be a well-recognized cause of breakthrough fungemia during treatment with amphotericin B or fluconazole (121–123).

Histopathological appearance includes pleomorphic yeast-like organisms and septate hyphae. In the microbiology laboratory, this organism can be identified by its rapid growing colonies, wrinkled in appearance with characteristic central heaping. Biochemically, this organism is known to produce urease. Microscopically these organisms are characterized by the production of arthroconidia (45,46).

Saccharomyces spp.

While this yeast had been "domesticated" for the production of a variety of human foods and beverages, and extensively used as a "probiotic," it is also considered an emerging fungal pathogen for immunocompromised hosts (122,124–126). Major risk factors for infection with this organism include: leukemia and neutropenia, bone marrow transplant, AIDS, burns, rheumatoid arthritis, prolonged hospitalization, and broad-spectrum antibiotics. Its spectrum of clinical presentations has significant overlap with infection by *Candida* spp. (4,127).

The histopathological appearance is characterized by evidence of budding yeasts, and the microbiological characteristics include rapidly growing flat colonies and the ability to metabolize a wide variety of carbohydrates. Microscopically, this organism is characterized by blastoconidia formation, and media-dependent ascospore production (45,46).

Malassezia

The most common species for this genus, *Malassezia furfur*, is a common colonizer in humans and animals. Its spectrum of disease includes characteristic superficial skin infections (such as pityriasis versicolor, seborrheic dermatitis, and sebaceous miliaria) mostly in immunocompetent hosts, and severe folliculitis with potential for dissemination in immunocompromised patients (122,128–130). Nevertheless, most cases of disseminated disease occur in immunocompromised patients with central venous lines and have been strongly associated with lipid infusions. Risk factors include: diabetes, corticosteroid use, broad spectrum antibiotics, bone marrow transplant, hematological malignancy, and solid organ transplant as well (131–133).

Malassezia grows best at 37°C, and colonies are initially smooth, evolving to a dried, wrinkled colony over time. Yeasts in this genus are characteristically Lipophilic, and medium may be supplemented with oils to enhance growth when this yeast is suspected. The microscopic appearance is of globose cells with few hyphal elements. These have been classically described as having the "spaghetti and meatballs" appearance (45,46) described in more detail in Chapter 7.

Rhodotorula

Rhodotorula spp. are ubiquitous in the environment and are associated with fungemia and occasional deep organ infections (134–136). The most common species is *Rhodotorula mucilaginosa* (formerly known as *Rhodotorula rubra*). Frequently described risk factors include neutropenia, broad-spectrum antibiotics, burns, and other causes of immunosuppression. Its clinical presentation is undistinguishable from other bloodstream infections and other causes of fungemia (119,122).

The *Rhodotorula* genus is characterized by the production of carotenoid pigments. Colonies often grow fast and are very colorful. Urease production is a key identification factor, and the microscopic appearance is that of globose (and often encapsulated) blastoconidia with the absence of hyphae and pseudohyphae (45,46).

BEYOND DIAGNOSIS AND THE FUTURE

As discussed extensively in this book chapter, there is an urgent need to develop diagnostic methods for these infections that are fast, accurate, practical, and easily translated into the clinical setting. The development of clinical versions of diagnostics based on gene chip and gene array technologies is just one of the exciting diagnostic modalities we may look forward to (137,138). Once these and other methods and markers are available, clinicians will be able to move from a simple diagnostic approach to other more aggressive interventions, such as surveillance and pre-emptive therapy (139,140). Having more reliable markers that diagnose infection before non-specific clinical signs and symptoms are present is bound to have a positive effect in patient outcomes, since early therapy has already been associated with increased treatment success (141,142).

These diagnostic methods will also need to be explored in relationship to clinical outcomes, prognosis, and as tools to assess response to therapy, a vastly unexplored area in medical mycology (7,114,143,144).

Undoubtedly the future will bring accurate and reliable tools that will increase our understanding of these diseases and improve patient outcomes.

REFERENCES

1. McNeil MM, Nash SL, Hajjeh RA, et al. Trends in mortality due to invasive mycotic diseases in the United States, 1980–1997. Clin Infect Dis 2001; 33(5):641–7.
2. Dixon DM, McNeil MM, Cohen ML, Gellin BG, La Montagne JR. Fungal infections: a growing threat. Public Health Rep 1996; 111(3):226–35.
3. Kaufman D. Fungal infection in the very low birthweight infant. Curr Opin Infect Dis 2004; 17(3):253–9.
4. Walsh TJ, Groll A, Hiemenz J, Fleming R, Roilides E, Anaissie E. Infections due to emerging and uncommon medically important fungal pathogens. Clin Microbiol Infect 2004; 10(Suppl. 1):48–66.
5. Eggimann P, Garbino J, Pittet D. Epidemiology of *Candida* species infections in critically ill non-immunosuppressed patients. Lancet Infect Dis 2003; 3(11):685–702.
6. Ellis D, Marriott D, Hajjeh RA, Warnock D, Meyer W, Barton R. Epidemiology: surveillance of fungal infections. Med Mycol 2000; 38(Suppl. 1):173–82.
7. Alexander BD. Diagnosis of fungal infection: new technologies for the mycology laboratory. Transpl Infect Dis 2002; 4(Suppl. 3):32–7.
8. Wisplinghoff H, Bischoff T, Tallent SM, Seifert H, Wenzel RP, Edmond MB. Nosocomial bloodstream infections in U.S. hospitals: analysis of 24,179 cases from a prospective nationwide surveillance study. Clin Infect Dis 2004; 39(3):309–17.
9. Garbino J, Kolarova L, Rohner P, Lew D, Pichna P, Pittet D. Secular trends of candidemia over 12 years in adult patients at a tertiary care hospital. Medicine (Baltimore) 2002; 81(6):425–33.
10. Pfaller MA, Jones RN, Messer SA, Edmond MB, Wenzel RP. National surveillance of nosocomial blood stream infection due to *Candida albicans*: frequency of occurrence and antifungal susceptibility in the SCOPE Program. Diagn Microbiol Infect Dis 1998; 31(1):327–32.
11. Diekema DJ, Messer SA, Brueggemann AB, et al. Epidemiology of candidemia: 3-year results from the emerging infections and the epidemiology of Iowa organisms study. J Clin Microbiol 2002; 40(4):1298–302.

12. Gudlaugsson O, Gillespie S, Lee K, et al. Attributable mortality of nosocomial candidemia, revisited. Clin Infect Dis 2003; 37(9):1172–7.
13. Pappas PG, Rex JH, Lee J, et al. A prospective observational study of candidemia: epidemiology, therapy, and influences on mortality in hospitalized adult and pediatric patients. Clin Infect Dis 2003; 37(5):634–43.
14. Rentz AM, Halpern MT, Bowden R. The impact of candidemia on length of hospital stay, outcome, and overall cost of illness. Clin Infect Dis 1998; 27(4):781–8.
15. Blumberg HM, Jarvis WR, Soucie JM, et al. Risk factors for candidal bloodstream infections in surgical intensive care unit patients: the NEMIS prospective multicenter study. The National Epidemiology of Mycosis Survey. Clin Infect Dis 2001; 33(2):177–86.
16. De Waele JJ, Vogelaers D, Blot S, Colardyn F. Fungal infections in patients with severe acute pancreatitis and the use of prophylactic therapy. Clin Infect Dis 2003; 37(2):208–13.
17. Jarvis WR. Epidemiology of nosocomial fungal infections, with emphasis on *Candida* species. Clin Infect Dis 1995; 20(6):1526–30.
18. Nucci M, Anaissie E. Should vascular catheters be removed from all patients with candidemia? An evidence-based review. Clin Infect Dis 2002; 34(5):591–9.
19. Nucci M, Colombo AL, Silveira F, et al. Risk factors for death in patients with candidemia. Infect Control Hosp Epidemiol 1998; 19(11):846–50.
20. Pappas PG, Rex JH, Sobel JD, et al. Guidelines for treatment of candidiasis. Clin Infect Dis 2004; 38(2):161–89.
21. Pittet D, Monod M, Suter PM, Frenk E, Auckenthaler R. Candida colonization and subsequent infections in critically ill surgical patients. Ann Surg 1994; 220(6):751–8.
22. Rangel-Frausto MS, Wiblin T, Blumberg HM, et al. National epidemiology of mycoses survey (NEMIS): variations in rates of bloodstream infections due to *Candida* species in seven surgical intensive care units and six neonatal intensive care units. Clin Infect Dis 1999; 29(2):253–8.
23. Fairchild KD, Tomkoria S, Sharp EC, Mena FV. Neonatal *Candida glabrata* sepsis: clinical and laboratory features compared with other *Candida* species. Pediatr Infect Dis J 2002; 21(1):39–43.
24. Benjamin DK, Jr., Ross K, McKinney RE, Jr., Benjamin DK, Auten R, Fisher RG. When to suspect fungal infection in neonates: a clinical comparison of *Candida albicans* and *Candida parapsilosis* fungemia with coagulase-negative staphylococcal bacteremia. Pediatrics 2000; 106(4):712–8.
25. Goodrich JM, Reed EC, Mori M, et al. Clinical features and analysis of risk factors for invasive candidal infection after marrow transplantation. J Infect Dis 1991; 164(4):731–40.
26. Pagano L, Mele L, Fianchi L, et al. Chronic disseminated candidiasis in patients with hematologic malignancies. Clinical features and outcome of 29 episodes. Haematologica 2002; 87(5):535–41.
27. Fishman LS, Griffin JR, Sapico FL, Hecht R. Hematogenous *Candida endophthalmitis*—a complication of candidemia. N Engl J Med 1972; 286(13):675–81.
28. Weinstein AJ, Johnson EH, Moellering RC, Jr. *Candida endophthalmitis*. A complication of candidemia. Arch Intern Med 1973; 132(5):749–52.
29. Donahue SP. Intraocular candidiasis in patients with candidemia. Ophthalmology 1998; 105(5):759–60.

30. Edwards JE, Jr., Bodey GP, Bowden RA, et al. International Conference for the Development of a Consensus on the Management and Prevention of Severe Candidal Infections. Clin Infect Dis 1997; 25(1):43–59.
31. Kontoyiannis DP, Luna MA, Samuels BI, Bodey GP. Hepatosplenic candidiasis. A manifestation of chronic disseminated candidiasis. Infect Dis Clin North Am 2000; 14(3):721–39.
32. Pagano L, Antinori A, Ammassari A, et al. Retrospective study of candidemia in patients with hematological malignancies. Clinical features, risk factors and outcome of 76 episodes. Eur J Haematol 1999; 63(2):77–85.
33. Kontoyiannis DP, Reddy BT, Torres HA, et al. Pulmonary candidiasis in patients with cancer: an autopsy study. Clin Infect Dis 2002; 34(3):400–3.
34. Lundstrom T, Sobel J. Nosocomial candiduria: a review. Clin Infect Dis 2001; 32(11):1602–7.
35. Sobel JD, Lundstrom T. Management of candiduria. Curr Urol Rep 2001; 2(4):321–5.
36. Sobel JD, Kauffman CA, McKinsey D, et al. Candiduria: a randomized, double-blind study of treatment with fluconazole and placebo. The National Institute of Allergy and Infectious Diseases (NIAID) Mycoses Study Group. Clin Infect Dis 2000; 30(1):19–24.
37. Kauffman CA, Vazquez JA, Sobel JD, et al. Prospective multicenter surveillance study of funguria in hospitalized patients. The National Institute for Allergy and Infectious Diseases (NIAID) Mycoses Study Group. Clin Infect Dis 2000; 30(1):14–8.
38. Sobel JD. Management of asymptomatic candiduria. Int J Antimicrob Agents 1999; 11(3–4):285–8.
39. Ostrosky-Zeichner L, Rex JH, Bennett J, Kullberg BJ. Deeply invasive candidiasis. Infect Dis Clin North Am 2002; 16(4):821–35.
40. Benjamin DK, Jr., DeLong ER, Steinbach WJ, Cotton CM, Walsh TJ, Clark RH. Empirical therapy for neonatal candidemia in very low birth weight infants. Pediatrics 2003; 112(3 Pt 1):543–7.
41. Rex JH, Sobel JD. Preventing intra-abdominal candidiasis in surgical patients. Crit Care Med 1999; 27(6):1033–4.
42. Sobel JD, Rex JH. Invasive candidiasis: turning risk into a practical prevention policy? Clin Infect Dis 2001; 33(2):187–90.
43. Ostrosky-Zeichner L. New approaches to the risk of Candida in the intensive care unit. Curr Opin Infect Dis 2003; 16(6):533–7.
44. Freydiere AM, Guinet R, Boiron P. Yeast identification in the clinical microbiology laboratory: phenotypical methods. Med Mycol 2001; 39(1):9–33.
45. Sutton DA, Fothergill AW, Rinaldi MG. Guide to Clinically Significant Fungi. 1st ed. Baltimore, MD: Williams & Wilkins, 1998.
46. Larone DH. Medically Important Fungi—A Guide to Identification. 3rd ed. Washington, DC: ASM Press, 1995.
47. Berenguer J, Buck M, Witebsky F, Stock F, Pizzo PA, Walsh TJ. Lysis-centrifugation blood cultures in the detection of tissue-proven invasive candidiasis. Disseminated versus single-organ infection. Diagn Microbiol Infect Dis 1993; 17(2):103–9.
48. Whimbey E, Wong B, Kiehn TE, Armstrong D. Clinical correlations of serial quantitative blood cultures determined by lysis-centrifugation in patients with persistent septicemia. J Clin Microbiol 1984; 19(6):766–71.

49. Tornai-Lehoczki J, Peter G, Dlauchy D. CHROMagar Candida medium as a practical tool for the differentiation and presumptive identification of yeast species isolated from salads. Int J Food Microbiol 2003; 86(1–2):189–200.

50. Horvath LL, Hospenthal DR, Murray CK, Dooley DP. Direct isolation of *Candida* spp. from blood cultures on the chromogenic medium CHROMagar Candida. J Clin Microbiol 2003; 41(6):2629–32.

51. Ainscough S, Kibbler CC. An evaluation of the cost-effectiveness of using CHROMagar for yeast identification in a routine microbiology laboratory. J Med Microbiol 1998; 47(7):623–8.

52. Gow NA. Germ tube growth of *Candida albicans*. Curr Top Med Mycol 1997; 8(1–2):43–55.

53. Moore JE, McMullan R. Comparison of media for optimal recovery of *Candida albicans* and *Candida glabrata* from blood culture. Ir J Med Sci 2003; 172(2):60–2.

54. Letscher-Bru V, Meyer MH, Galoisy AC, Waller J, Candolfi E. Prospective evaluation of the new chromogenic medium Candida ID, in comparison with Candiselect, for isolation of molds and isolation and presumptive identification of yeast species. J Clin Microbiol 2002; 40(4):1508–10.

55. McDonald LC, Weinstein MP, Fune J, Mirrett S, Reimer LG, Reller LB. Controlled comparison of BacT/ALERT FAN aerobic medium and BATEC fungal blood culture medium for detection of fungemia. J Clin Microbiol 2001; 39(2):622–4.

56. de Repentigny L, Reiss E. Current trends in immunodiagnosis of candidiasis and aspergillosis. Rev Infect Dis 1984; 6(3):301–12.

57. Matthews RC, Burnie JP. New developments in the serological diagnosis of Candida infection. Mykosen Suppl 1988; 2:34–8.

58. Klingspor L. Candida antigen and antibody assays. Acta Paediatr 1995; 84(8):964.

59. Persat F, Topenot R, Piens MA, Thiebaut A, Dannaoui E, Picot S. Evaluation of different commercial ELISA methods for the serodiagnosis of systemic candidosis. Mycoses 2002; 45(11–12):455–60.

60. Porsius JC, van Vliet HJ, van Zeijl JH, Goessens WH, Michel MF. Detection of an antibody response in immunocompetent patients with systemic candidiasis or *Candida albicans* colonisation. Eur J Clin Microbiol Infect Dis 1990; 9(5):352–5.

61. Navarro D, Monzonis E, Lopez-Ribot JL, et al. Diagnosis of systemic candidiasis by enzyme immunoassay detection of specific antibodies to mycelial phase cell wall and cytoplasmic candidal antigens. Eur J Clin Microbiol Infect Dis 1993; 12(11):839–46.

62. Chakrabarti A, Roy P, Kumar D, Sharma BK, Chugh KS, Panigrahi D. Evaluation of three serological tests for detection of anti-candidal antibodies in diagnosis of invasive candidiasis. Mycopathologia 1994; 126(1):3–7.

63. van Deventer AJ, van Vliet HJ, Hop WC, Goessens WH. Diagnostic value of anti-Candida enolase antibodies. J Clin Microbiol 1994; 32(1):17–23.

64. Martinez JP, Gil ML, Lopez-Ribot JL, Chaffin WL. Serologic response to cell wall mannoproteins and proteins of *Candida albicans*. Clin Microbiol Rev 1998; 11(1):121–41.

65. Walsh TJ, Chanock SJ. Diagnosis of invasive fungal infections: advances in nonculture systems. Curr Clin Top Infect Dis 1998; 18:101–53.

66. Sendid B, Caillot D, Baccouch-Humbert B, et al. Contribution of the Platelia Candida-specific antibody and antigen tests to early diagnosis of systemic *Candida tropicalis* infection in neutropenic adults. J Clin Microbiol 2003; 41(10):4551–8.

67. Sendid B, Poirot JL, Tabouret M, et al. Combined detection of mannanaemia and antimannan antibodies as a strategy for the diagnosis of systemic infection caused by pathogenic *Candida* species. J Med Microbiol 2002; 51(5):433–42.

68. Philip A, Odabasi Z, Mattiuzzi G, Paetznick VL, Rex JH, Ostrosky-Zeichner L. SysCan3 for the detection of anti-Candida antibodies for the diagnosis of invasive candididiasis (IC). In: 43rd Interscience Conference on Antimicrobial Agents and Chemotherapy. Chicago, 2003 (Abstract M-2060).

69. Fung JC, Donta ST, Tilton RC. Candida detection system (CAND-TEC) to differentiate between *Candida albicans* colonization and disease. J Clin Microbiol 1986; 24(4):542–7.

70. Piens MA, Guyotat D, Archimbaud E, et al. Evaluation of a Candida antigen detection test (Cand-Tec) in the diagnosis of deep candidiasis in neutropenic patients. Eur J Cancer Clin Oncol 1988; 24(10):1655–9.

71. Pallavicini F, Izzi I, Pennisi MA, et al. Evaluation of the utility of serological tests in the diagnosis of candidemia. Minerva Anestesiol 1999; 65(9):637–9.

72. Bar W, Hecker H. Diagnosis of systemic Candida infections in patients of the intensive care unit. Significance of serum antigens and antibodies. Mycoses 2002; 45(1–2):22–8.

73. Misaki H, Iwasaki H, Ueda T. A comparison of the specificity and sensitivity of two Candida antigen assay systems for the diagnosis of deep candidiasis in patients with hematologic diseases. Med Sci Monit 2003; 9(2):MT1–T7.

74. Mitsutake K, Miyazaki T, Tashiro T, et al. Enolase antigen, mannan antigen, Cand-Tec antigen, and beta-glucan in patients with candidemia. J Clin Microbiol 1996; 34(8):1918–21.

75. Walsh TJ, Hathorn JW, Sobel JD, et al. Detection of circulating candida enolase by immunoassay in patients with cancer and invasive candidiasis. N Engl J Med 1991; 324(15):1026–31.

76. Kiehn TE, Bernard EM, Gold JW, Armstrong D. Candidiasis: detection by gas–liquid chromatography of D-arabinitol, a fungal metabolite, in human serum. Science 1979; 206(4418):577–80.

77. Pfaller MA. Laboratory aids in the diagnosis of invasive candidiasis. Mycopathologia 1992; 120(2):65–72.

78. Walsh TJ, Lee JW, Sien T, et al. Serum D-arabinitol measured by automated quantitative enzymatic assay for detection and therapeutic monitoring of experimental disseminated candidiasis: correlation with tissue concentrations of *Candida albicans*. J Med Vet Mycol 1994; 32(3):205–15.

79. Roboz J, Suzuki R, Holland JF. Quantification of arabinitol in serum by selected ion monitoring as a diagnostic technique in invasive candidiasis. J Clin Microbiol 1980; 12(4):594–601.

80. Holak EJ, Wu J, Spruance SL. Value of serum arabinitol for the management of Candida infections in clinical practice. Mycopathologia 1986; 93(2):99–104.

81. Lehtonen L, Anttila VJ, Ruutu T, et al. Diagnosis of disseminated candidiasis by measurement of urine D-arabinitol/L-arabinitol ratio. J Clin Microbiol 1996; 34(9):2175–9.

82. Chryssanthou E, Klingspor L, Tollemar J, et al. PCR and other non-culture methods for diagnosis of invasive Candida infections in allogeneic bone marrow and solid organ transplant recipients. Mycoses 1999; 42(4):239–47.

83. Sigmundsdottir G, Christensson B, Bjorklund LJ, Hakansson K, Pehrson C, Larsson L. Urine D-arabinitol/L-arabinitol ratio in diagnosis of invasive candidiasis in newborn infants. J Clin Microbiol 2000; 38(8):3039–42.

84. Tokunaga S, Ohkawa M, Takashima M, Seto C, Nakamura S. D-arabinitol versus mannan antigen and candidal protein antigen as a serum marker for *Candida pyelonephritis*. Eur J Clin Microbiol Infect Dis 1995; 14(2):118–21.

85. Hui M, Cheung SW, Chin ML, Chu KC, Chan RC, Cheng AF. Development and application of a rapid diagnostic method for invasive Candidiasis by the detection of D-/L-arabinitol using gas chromatography/mass spectrometry. Diagn Microbiol Infect Dis 2004; 49(2):117–23.

86. McSharry C, Lewis C, Cruickshank G, Richardson MD. Measurement of serum arabinitol by gas–liquid chromatography: limitations for detection of systemic candida infections. J Clin Pathol 1993; 46(5):475–6.

87. Obayashi T, Tamura H, Tanaka S, et al. A new chromogenic endotoxin-specific assay using recombined limulus coagulation enzymes and its clinical applications. Clin Chim Acta 1985; 149(1):55–65.

88. Miyazaki T, Kohno S, Mitsutake K, et al. Plasma (1-3)-beta-D-glucan and fungal antigenemia in patients with candidemia, aspergillosis, and cryptococcosis. J Clin Microbiol 1995; 33(12):3115–8.

89. Obayashi T, Yoshida M, Mori T, et al. Plasma (1-3)-beta-D-glucan measurement in diagnosis of invasive deep mycosis and fungal febrile episodes. Lancet 1995; 345(8941):17–20.

90. Ostrosky-Zeichner L, Alexander BD, Kett DH, et al. Multicenter clinical evaluation of the $(1\rightarrow3)$-β-D-glucan assay as an aid to diagnosis of fungal infections in humans. Clin Infect Dis 2005; 41:654–9.

91. Odabasi Z, Mattiuzzi G, Estey E, et al. Beta-D-glucan as a diagnostic adjunct for invasive fungal infections: validation, cutoff development, and performance in patients with acute myelogenous leukemia and myelodysplastic syndrome. Clin Infect Dis 2004; 39(2):199–205.

92. Kohno S, Mitsutake K, Maesaki S, et al. An evaluation of serodiagnostic tests in patients with candidemia: beta-glucan, mannan, candida antigen by Cand-Tec and D-arabinitol. Microbiol Immunol 1993; 37(3):207–12.

93. Takesue Y, Kakehashi M, Ohge H, et al. Combined assessment of beta-D-glucan and degree of candida colonization before starting empiric therapy for candidiasis in surgical patients. World J Surg 2004; 28(6):625–30.

94. Kitagawa T, Tsuboi I, Kimura S, Sasamoto Y. Rapid method for preparing a beta-glucan-specific sensitive fraction from Limulus (*Tachypleus tridentatus*) amebocyte lysate. J Chromatogr 1991; 567(1):267–73.

95. Iwanaga S. The limulus clotting reaction. Curr Opin Immunol 1993; 5(1):74–82.

96. Seki N, Muta T, Oda T, et al. Horseshoe crab (1,3)-beta-D-glucan-sensitive coagulation factor G. A serine protease zymogen heterodimer with similarities to beta-glucan-binding proteins. J Biol Chem 1994; 269(2):1370–4.

97. Zhang GH, Baek L, Buchardt O, Koch C. Differential blocking of coagulation-activating pathways of *Limulus* amebocyte lysate. J Clin Microbiol 1994; 32(6):1537–41.

98. Ohata A, Usami M, Horiuchi T, Nagasawa K, Kinoshita K. Release of (1-3)-beta-D-glucan from depth-type membrane filters and their in vitro effects on proinflammatory cytokine production. Artif Organs 2003; 27(8):728–35.

99. Kato A, Takita T, Furuhashi M, Takahashi T, Maruyama Y, Hishida A. Elevation of blood (1-3)-beta-D-glucan concentrations in hemodialysis patients. Nephron 2001; 89(1):15–9.

100. Nakao A, Yasui M, Kawagoe T, Tamura H, Tanaka S, Takagi H. False-positive endotoxemia derives from gauze glucan after hepatectomy for hepatocellular carcinoma with cirrhosis. Hepatogastroenterology 1997; 44(17):1413–8.

101. Kimura Y, Nakao A, Tamura H, Tanaka S, Takagi H. Clinical and experimental studies of the limulus test after digestive surgery. Surg Today 1995; 25(9):790–4.

102. Pfaller MA. Epidemiological typing methods for mycoses. Clin Infect Dis 1992; 14(Suppl. 1):S4–10.

103. Reiss E, Obayashi T, Orle K, Yoshida M, Zancope-Oliveira RM. Non-culture based diagnostic tests for mycotic infections. Med Mycol 2000; 38(Suppl. 1):147–59.

104. Wilson DA, Joyce MJ, Hall LS, et al. Multicenter evaluation of a *Candida albicans* peptide nucleic acid fluorescent in situ hybridization probe for characterization of yeast isolates from blood cultures. J Clin Microbiol 2005; 43(6):2909–12.

105. Alexander BD, Ashley ED, Reller LB, Reed SD. Cost savings with implementation of PNA FISH testing for identification of *Candida albicans* in blood cultures. Diagn Microbiol Infect Dis 2006; 54(4):277–82.

106. Forrest GN, Mankes K, Jabra-Rizk MA, et al. Peptide nucleic acid fluorescence in situ hybridization-based identification of *Candida albicans* and its impact on mortality and antifungal therapy costs. J Clin Microbiol 2006; 44(9):3381–3.

107. Iwen PC, Freifeld AG, Bruening TA, Hinrichs SH. Use of a panfungal PCR assay for detection of fungal pathogens in a commercial blood culture system. J Clin Microbiol 2004; 42(5):2292–3.

108. Maaroufi Y, Heymans C, De Bruyne JM, et al. Rapid detection of *Candida albicans* in clinical blood samples by using a TaqMan-based PCR assay. J Clin Microbiol 2003; 41(7):3293–8.

109. Tirodker UH, Nataro JP, Smith S, LasCasas L, Fairchild KD. Detection of fungemia by polymerase chain reaction in critically ill neonates and children. J Perinatol 2003; 23(2):117–22.

110. Dendis M, Horvath R, Michalek J, et al. PCR-RFLP detection and species identification of fungal pathogens in patients with febrile neutropenia. Clin Microbiol Infect 2003; 9(12):1191–202.

111. Posteraro B, Valentini P, Delogu A, et al. *Candida albicans* endocarditis diagnosed by PCR-based molecular assay in a critically ill pediatric patient. Scand J Infect Dis 2002; 34(2):145–7.

112. Lau JW. Rapid diagnosis of fungal infection in patients with acute necrotizing pancreatitis by polymerase chain reaction. Asian J Surg 2002; 25(3):214.

113. Fleming RV, Walsh TJ, Anaissie EJ. Emerging and less common fungal pathogens. Infect Dis Clin North Am 2002; 16(4):915–33 (see also vi–vii).

114. Peters RP, Agtmael MA, Danner SA, Savelkoul PH, Vandenbroucke-Grauls CM. New developments in the diagnosis of bloodstream infections. Lancet Infect Dis 2004; 4(12):751–60.

115. Hebart H, Loffler J, Reitze H, et al. Prospective screening by a panfungal polymerase chain reaction assay in patients at risk for fungal infections: implications for the management of febrile neutropenia. Br J Haematol 2000; 111(2):635–40.

116. Hendolin PH, Paulin L, Koukila-Kahkola P, et al. Panfungal PCR and multiplex liquid hybridization for detection of fungi in tissue specimens. J Clin Microbiol 2000; 38(11):4186–92.

117. Gueho E, Improvisi L, de Hoog GS, Dupont B. *Trichosporon* on humans: a practical account. Mycoses 1994; 37(1–2):3–10.

118. Segal BH, Bow EJ, Menichetti F. Fungal infections in nontransplant patients with hematologic malignancies. Infect Dis Clin North Am 2002; 16(4):935–64 (see also vii).

119. Krcmery V, Krupova I, Denning DW. Invasive yeast infections other than *Candida* spp. in acute leukaemia. J Hosp Infect 1999; 41(3):181–94.

120. Perfect JR, Schell WA. The new fungal opportunists are coming. Clin Infect Dis 1996; 22(Suppl. 2):S112–8.

121. Rowen JL, Atkins JT, Levy ML, Baer SC, Baker CJ. Invasive fungal dermatitis in the < or = 1000-gram neonate. Pediatrics 1995; 95(5):682–7.

122. Samonis G, Bafaloukos D. Fungal infections in cancer patients: an escalating problem. In Vivo 1992; 6(2):183–93.

123. Walsh TJ, Newman KR, Moody M, Wharton RC, Wade JC. Trichosporonosis in patients with neoplastic disease. Medicine (Baltimore) 1986; 65(4):268–79.

124. Morrison VA, Haake RJ, Weisdorf DJ. The spectrum of non-Candida fungal infections following bone marrow transplantation. Medicine (Baltimore) 1993; 72(2):78–89.

125. Lherm T, Monet C, Nougiere B, et al. Seven cases of fungemia with *Saccharomyces boulardii* in critically ill patients. Intensive Care Med 2002; 28(6):797–801.

126. Ponton J, Ruchel R, Clemons KV, et al. Emerging pathogens. Med Mycol 2000; 38(Suppl. 1):225–36.

127. Salonen JH, Richardson MD, Gallacher K, et al. Fungal colonization of haematological patients receiving cytotoxic chemotherapy: emergence of azole-resistant *Saccharomyces cerevisiae*. J Hosp Infect 2000; 45(4):293–301.

128. Powell DA, Hayes J, Durrell DE, Miller M, Marcon MJ. *Malassezia furfur* skin colonization of infants hospitalized in intensive care units. J Pediatr 1987; 111(2):217–20.

129. Marcon MJ, Powell DA. Epidemiology, diagnosis, and management of *Malassezia furfur* systemic infection. Diagn Microbiol Infect Dis 1987; 7(3):161–75.

130. Stenderup A. Ecology of yeast and epidemiology of yeast infections. Acta Derm Venereol Suppl (Stockh) 1986; 121:27–37.

131. Roberts SO. Pityriasis versicolor: a clinical and mycological investigation. Br J Dermatol 1969; 81(5):315–26.

132. Gupta AK, Madzia SE, Batra R. Etiology and management of seborrheic dermatitis. Dermatology 2004; 208(2):89–93.

133. Rolston K. Overview of systemic fungal infections. Oncology (Huntingt) 2001; 15(11 Suppl. 9):11–4.

134. Krcmery V, Laho L, Huttova M, et al. Aetiology, antifungal susceptibility, risk factors and outcome in 201 fungaemic children: data from a 12-year prospective national study from Slovakia. J Med Microbiol 2002; 51(2):110–6.

135. Costa SF, Marinho I, Araujo EA, Manrique AE, Medeiros EA, Levin AS. Nosocomial fungaemia: a 2-year prospective study. J Hosp Infect 2000; 45(1):69–72.

136. Nucci M, Pulcheri W, Spector N, et al. Fungal infections in neutropenic patients. A 8-year prospective study. Rev Inst Med Trop Sao Paulo 1995; 37(5):397–406.

137. Bodrossy L, Sessitsch A. Oligonucleotide microarrays in microbial diagnostics. Curr Opin Microbiol 2004; 7(3):245–54.

138. Quirk M. The genomics revolution has arrived in infectious diseases. Lancet Infect Dis 2003; 3(2):66.

139. Jones BL, McLintock LA. Impact of diagnostic markers on early antifungal therapy. Curr Opin Infect Dis 2003; 16(6):521–6.

140. Castagnola E, Bucci B, Montinaro E, Viscoli C. Fungal infections in patients undergoing bone marrow transplantation: an approach to a rational management protocol. Bone Marrow Transplant 1996; 18(Suppl. 2):97–106.

141. Imahara SD, Nathens AB. Antimicrobial strategies in surgical critical care. Curr Opin Crit Care 2003; 9(4):286–91.

142. Leather HL, Wingard JR. Prophylaxis, empirical therapy, or pre-emptive therapy of fungal infections in immunocompromised patients: which is better for whom? Curr Opin Infect Dis 2002; 15(4):369–75.

143. Martino P, Girmenia C. Diagnosis and treatment of invasive fungal infections in cancer patients. Support Care Cancer 1993; 1(5):240–4.

144. Penn RL, Lambert RS, George RB. Invasive fungal infections. The use of serologic tests in diagnosis and management. Arch Intern Med 1983; 143(6):1215–20.

10

Diagnosis of Cryptococcosis

Methee Chayakulkeeree

Division of Infectious Diseases, Department of Medicine, Duke University Medical Center, Durham, North Carolina, U.S.A., and Division of Infectious Diseases and Tropical Medicine, Department of Medicine, Siriraj Hospital, Mahidol University, Bangkok, Thailand

John R. Perfect

Division of Infectious Diseases, Department of Medicine and Department of Microbiology and Molecular Genetics, Duke University Medical Center, Durham, North Carolina, U.S.A.

INTRODUCTION

Cryptococcus neoformans is an encapsulated yeast that can cause life-threatening infectious diseases in both apparently immunocompetent and immunocompromised hosts in all areas of the world. This pathogenic yeast consists of four serotypes (A, B, C, and D) based on capsular agglutination reactions and three varieties or subspecies (1). Serotype A strains have been named *C. neoformans* var. *grubii*, serotype B and C strains were classified as *C. neoformans* var. *gattii* and recently considered to be a separate species, *Cryptococcus gattii*, and serotype D strains were named *C. neoformans* var. *neoformans* (2,3). About 95% of cryptococcal infections are caused by serotype A strains, whereas 4% to 5% of infections are caused by either serotype D or serotype B and C strains, depending on geographical location.

Early case reports of cryptococcal infections were primarily associated with cancer patients and those receiving corticosteroids (4,5). However, for more than two decades of the worldwide epidemic of Human Immunodeficiency Virus

(HIV) infection, cryptococcal infection has become an important opportunistic infection in HIV-infected patients, and in some populations without Highly Active Antiretroviral Therapy (HAART), about 5% to 10% of individuals with HIV/AIDS develop cryptococcosis (6). Therefore, it has become a major opportunistic pathogen, as it has been able to exploit immunosuppressive events of modern medicine such as AIDS, cancer, and immunosuppressive therapy (7,8). Even with the recent development of effective antiretroviral therapy (HAART), which decreases the rate of HIV-related cryptococcosis in developed countries (9,10), its prevalence is still high in developing countries and those without access to health care (11–13).

Although *C. neoformans* has a unique predisposition for establishing clinical infection in the central nervous system, this basidiomycetous fungus can cause not only meningoencephalitis but also infections involving other major organs such as lungs, skin, eyes, heart, and genitourinary tract (8,14–16). Furthermore, widely disseminated cryptococcal infection occurs in severely immunosuppressed patients and thus clinicians might observe cryptococcus at any site in the human body. Clinicians at all levels of care-providing may be faced with the challenge of identifying this encapsulated yeast. If left untreated, when the yeast reaches the central nervous system, patients with cryptococcal meningoencephalitis are uniformly fatal. Fortunately, many methods for making the diagnosis of cryptococcosis have been established and may be achieved by direct examination of the fungus in body fluids, cytology, or histopathology of infected tissues with several staining techniques, serological studies, and/ or culture.

DIRECT EXAMINATION OF SPECIMENS

Direct microscopic examination for the presence of encapsulated yeasts using India ink preparation of cerebrospinal fluid (CSF) is a basic and useful rapid diagnostic test for cryptococcal meningitis (8). This technique can be performed within a few minutes after a lumber puncture and provides a presumptive diagnosis as well as other important information for clinicians, including identification of patients at high risk for failure due to a heavy fungal burden. The globular encapsulated yeast cells range in size from 5 to 20 μm in diameter and are rapidly distinguished in a colloidal medium of India ink when mixed with CSF. Specimens for India ink examination should be sent in a sterile leak-proof container or tube and maintained at room temperature during transport. Routinely, 1 mL of CSF is acceptable to be used for this technique, although 5 mL of specimen is recommended to increase the sensitivity of the test. An India ink examination usually allows detection of yeasts in a CSF specimen when there are between 10^3 to 10^4 cfu of yeasts per milliliter of CSF or greater concentrations. This simple India ink preparation technique is 30% to 50% sensitive in cases of non-AIDS cryptococcal meningitis and up to 80% sensitive in AIDS-related cryptococcal meningitis. Centrifuging the CSF specimen at low speed (i.e., 500 rpm for 10 minutes) and using the pellet for India ink preparation can improve the sensitivity of the test. However, some authors suggest avoiding centrifugation before examination with the India ink technique because pseudo-cryptococcal artifacts produced from lysed lymphocytes might cause their misinterpretation as *C. neoformans* (17,18). This observation was proven by reproduction of such an artifact in cryptococcus-free CSF-leukocyte mixtures that had been subjected to high-speed centrifugation. Therefore, if centrifugation is to be used prior to India ink examination, caution is warranted in interpreting the result (18). Some authors also found that carbon particles in India ink may be repelled by leukocytes in the CSF, forming a halo around the cell that suggests presence of a capsule that might be misinterpreted as *C. neoformans*. This does not seem to occur with nigrosin, which is free from discernible particulate matter and therefore can avoid the pitfalls associated with the use of standard India ink (19,20). Myelin globules, fat droplets, and tissue cells can also cause a false-positive result and thus decrease specificity of this simple test. A modified India ink technique for the diagnosis of *C. neoformans* in CSF has been described. This technique employs 2% chromium mercury and India ink and allows a clear identification of some external and internal structures of the yeast (21).

Another simple, rapid positive stain technique for direct examination has been developed. This technique uses a fresh mixture of five part of Neisser stain I (0.1% methylene blue, 3.1% w/v ethanol, 5.0% glacial acetic acid) and one part of Gram stain I (2% crystal violet, 19.2% w/v ethanol, 0.8% ammonium oxalate) that help to clearly distinguish cryptococci from erythrocytes and leukocytes (22). The observation that dead yeast cells can remain in the CSF and be seen by India ink examination for varying periods of time during and after appropriate antifungal treatment and despite negative culture is a limitation for usefulness of direct microscopy of CSF during the management strategies of cryptococcal meningitis (23).

CYTOLOGY AND HISTOPATHOLOGY

C. neoformans, with its prominent capsule, can be prominently identified by histological stains of tissues from lungs, skin, bone marrow, brain, or other organs (24–29). Even though some authors have suggested that histopathology of bone marrow has a limited value in AIDS-related fungal infection (30), yeasts may be seen in bone marrow biopsies. Histopathological staining of centrifuged CSF sediment has proven to be more sensitive for rapid diagnosis of cryptococcal meningitis than the India ink method (31). Other body fluids as well as fine needle aspiration (FNA) specimens obtained from various body sites can also be properly used for cytological study (32). For instance, FNA cytology of peripheral lymph nodes (33), adrenal glands (34), or vitreous aspiration (35) has been used for obtaining tissues for cytology. Percutaneous transthoracic FNA under real-time ultrasound guidance for pulmonary nodules, masses, or infiltrative lesions can be performed safely and accurately for diagnosis of pulmonary cryptococcosis (36–38). Peritoneal fluid from chronic ambulatory peritoneal dialysis (CAPD) (39), seminal fluid (40), bronchial wash, or bronchoalveolar lavage fluid can also be used for cytology preparations in the diagnosis of cryptococcal infection (41,42).

However, with routine H&E stains, the yeast cell is almost colorless and difficult to see, and the organism is primarily identified when the yeast is surrounded by clear area within tissue that represents the non-staining capsule. A variety of positive staining methods have been described to demonstrate the yeast cells in tissue or fluids ranging from the nonspecific Papanicolaou, hematoxylin and eosin, Diff-Quick, May-Giemsa, Riu's, and acridine orange preparations to more specific fungal stains such as Calcifluor, which binds fungal chitin, or a Gomori-Grocott Chromic Acid Methenamine Silver Stain (GMS), which stains fungal cell wall (8,34,36,41,43). The fungus is seen as a yeast-like organism that reproduces in host tissue by the formation of narrow-based budding. Sensitivity of acridine orange staining followed by fluorescence microscopy is comparable to an India ink examination and detection of cryptococcal capsular polysaccharide antigen by latex agglutination (LA) (44). Riu's stain can be used in bronchoscopic brushing smears, or for needle aspiration and cytological studies (43). The silver staining technique, such as GMS and/or the Becker modification of the GMS Stain (BGMS), can be used to accentuate the wall of fungal organisms in the backscatter electron imaging (BEI) mode of the scanning electron microscopy. Therefore, BEI may be used in conjunction with a light microscopy stain for identification of these yeasts (45).

For *C. neoformans*, several specific stains that identify the polysaccharide capsular material surrounding the yeasts have been developed and are clinically useful. These staining techniques include Mayer's mucicarmine, periodic acid-Schiff (PAS), and alcian blue stains (8,46–48). In most cases of cryptococcosis, the yeast usually appears in tissue with enlarged capsular material surrounding the cell during infection, and the yeast is easily identified by these special staining techniques. However, there are cases in which *C. neoformans* in tissue is poorly encapsulated (49,50), and the yeast may be identified only by GMS or Fontana–Masson Silver (FMS) stain (51). Tissue sections stained with the FMS stain, which appears to identify melanin in the yeast cell wall, will show a dark brown to black color yeast for *C. neoformans* and also *Cryptococcus laurentii* but does not stain most other common pathogenic yeasts such as *Candida* species (52). Combinations of FMS stain and specific polysaccharide stains, such as alcian blue and mucicarmine will distinctively demonstrate both the cell wall and capsule of most cryptococci and not identify most other yeasts in one stain. In one study, more yeasts were recognized with the combined stains compared with either stain alone and no interference between the stains was noted (53). The alcian blue stain combined with the PAS reaction has also been shown to be helpful for identification of cryptococci (54). A reticulin stain of a bone marrow biopsy may give additional information compared to traditional hematoxylin and eosin stain in recognizing the characteristic budding yeast forms of cryptococci (55).

A simple Gram stain is not an optimal stain for identification of this yeast but it may show *C. neoformans* as a poorly stained gram-positive budding yeast (8,39). The recognition of *C. neoformans* in Gram-stained smears of purulent exudates may be hampered by the presence of the large gelatinous capsule, which apparently prevents definitive staining of the yeast-like cells. It also appears that the preparations of biopsies or other clinical specimens as well as modification of the staining technique for histopathology might alter the permeability properties of the yeast and, hence, the intensity of its staining. Therefore, in Gram-stained preparations, *C. neoformans* may appear either as round cells with gram-positive granular inclusions impressed upon a pale lavender cytoplasmic background or as gram-negative lipoid bodies and thus can be easily overlooked in such preparations (56).

The histological patterns of AIDS-related pulmonary cryptococcal lesions can be graded with respect to the degree and type of inflammatory reaction. The first pattern consists of small, scattered foci of intra-alveolar cryptococcal proliferation with a histiocytic response. The second pattern involves massive cryptococcal infection with few inflammatory cells but extensive numbers of yeasts with capillary involvement of the alveolar septa as a common finding (26). These histological findings were observed in patients with HIV infection who had not received antiretroviral treatment. The third pattern found in HIV-infected patients treated with antiretroviral drugs is characterized by the presence of CD4 + T cells, greater numbers of histiocytes and multinucleated giant cells, and lack of massive capillary involvement (57) and is typical of an apparent immune reconstitution reaction.

SEROLOGY

Diagnosis of cryptococcosis has been significantly improved over the last several decades by the development of serological tests for cryptococcal polysaccharide antigen and/or antibody. In seminal work, Kaufman and Blumer studied and compared five techniques, including an indirect fluorescent antibody (IFA) test, a tube agglutination (TA) test, a complement-fixation (CF) test, an immunodiffusion (ID) test, and a LA test, for detecting cryptococcal polysaccharide antigen and/or antibody in sera and/or CSF specimens of infected patients. They found that when the LA for cryptococcal antigen and IFA and TA tests for cryptococcal antibodies were used concurrently, 87% of the cryptococcosis case specimens were positive, permitting a presumptive diagnosis of *C. neoformans* infections in 61 of the 66 (92%) patients whose specimens were examined (58).

Using serum cryptococcal antibodies as the only diagnostic tool for cryptococcosis has had problems, although there has been some suggestion that its presence favors a good prognostic sign (23,59) and a better response to therapy (60). Bindschadler and Bennett found that IFA for serum cryptococcal antibodies can provide false positive results in patients receiving a cryptococcal skin test, and during infections with *Blastomyces dermatitidis*, and *Histoplasma capsulatum* (60). Widra et al. found that the sensitivity and specificity of the ID test for serum cryptococcal antibodies can vary widely depending upon the method of antigen preparation and a number of other factors (61). A bentonite flocculation technique to detect cryptococcal antibodies has been described by Kimball et al.; presumed false positives were found in only 2% of specimens from normal subjects and patients with non-fungal diseases. However, cross-reactions with sera from patients with other systemic fungal diseases were frequent (62). Other methods to detect serum cryptococcal antibodies have been described. These include a formalin-killed whole yeast cell agglutination test (59,63), enzyme immunoassay (EIA) (64), and monovalent charcoal particle agglutination test. The latter technique was developed by Gordon and Lapa and was claimed to be more sensitive and specific than the TA and IFA test (65). Use of cryptococcal antibodies for the diagnosis of cryptococcal infection is further complicated by the type of cryptococcal infection and the timing of antibody presence. Some evidence in non-HIV-infected patients has shown that antibody is positive mainly in the early stages of central nervous system (CNS) involvement and in infections with no CNS involvement. Furthermore, cryptococcal antibodies are often positive after institution of antifungal therapy and accompany a decline in antigen titers (59) . Walter and Jones found six cases of cryptococcosis that had antibody appear from 9 to 43 months after the sera had become culture-negative (63). This supports the theory that antibodies are neutralized by abundance of circulating antigen. Once it appears, the antibody can persist many years after the initial infection. Although IgA antibodies fall over one to two years in the recovery phase, IgG levels persist (64).

Thus, the antibody test was often positive in the absence of overt disease and thus devalued as a test for diagnosis of acute cryptococcal infections (65). On the other hand, the antibody test may be particularly useful for seroepidemiology studies of cryptococcosis. It was used to show the infection rate of children in New York City (66). Many investigators have attempted to determine the usefulness of cryptococcal antibodies in the diagnosis of infections caused by *C. neoformans* and have found that combined tests of both cryptococcal polysaccharide antigen and cryptococcal antibodies do provide sufficient specificity and sensitivity to be a useful aid in the rapid diagnosis of cryptococcosis (58–60). However, all of the studies of cryptococcal antibodies were performed before the HIV/AIDS epidemic; thus, the implementation of these antibody tests for use in diagnosis of cryptococcosis in immunologically paralyzed HIV-infected patients with high burden of yeasts is limited. Furthermore, the cryptococcal capsular polysaccharide antigen test performs at a sensitivity and specificity of over 90% by itself.

Although the tests of cryptococcal antibodies have not been adopted for early diagnosis of cryptococcosis, detection of cryptococcal capsular polysaccharide antigen in serum or body fluids has been robust in its performance and is the most currently useful diagnostic serological test in all fungal diseases. First developed in 1963 (67), Bloomfield et al. described the use of antibody-coated latex particles that detected soluble antigens of *C. neoformans* in sera or CSF of 7 of 9 patients with cryptococcosis. The technique is analogous to that employed by Singer et al. to detect C-reactive protein in serum (68). Although many methods for detection of cryptococcal polysaccharide antigen have been described (58,60,63), the LA technique has been studied to a great depth and it has been found to be a most useful method in the rapid diagnosis of cryptococcal infections.

A number of commercial kits using LA for detection of cryptococcal polysaccharide antigen have been made available. The accuracy and reproducibility of these commercial kits have been evaluated and compared with each other (69–74). There are at least seven commercial LA kits for detecting cryptococcal polysaccharide antigen: Crypto-LA® (International Biological Laboratories, Inc., Cranbury, New Jersey, U.S.A.), MYCO-Immune (American MicroScan, Inc., Mahwah, New Jersey, U.S.A.), IMMY (Immuno-Mycologics, Inc., Norman, Oklahoma, U.S.A.), CALAS (Meridian Bioscience, Inc., Cincinnati, Ohio, U.S.A.), Serodirect Cryptococcus (Eiken Chemical Co., Ltd., Tokyo, Japan), Pastorex Cryptococcus (Bio-Rad Laboratories, Inc., Marnes la Coquette, France), and Murex Cryptococcus Test (Murex Biotech, Ltd., Dartford, U.K.). Most tests use latex particles coated with polyclonal cryptococcal capsular antibodies. The latter two commercial kits use latex particles coated with anti-glucuronoxylomannan monoclonal antibodies. In general, all commercially available kits that rely on latex cryptococcal antigen agglutination can detect at least 10 ng of polysaccharide per milliliter of biologic fluids (75). The sensitivity and specificity of these LA kits for cryptococcal antigen depend on the commercial kits and type of specimens, but overall sensitivities and specificities have been found to be 93% to 100% and 93% to 98%, respectively, (70–74,76).

There have been some issues in LA tests for cryptococcal polysaccharide antigen that resulted in false-positive tests, and methods to eliminate these problems in clinical specimens have been developed and are implemented in most of the commercial kits. For example, Bennett and Bailey (77) reported false-positive results in 9.5% of 252 sera and CSF specimens and Dolan (78) reported false-positive reactions in 2.8% of sera and 1.4% of CSF specimens. However, after a couple decades of development, later reports revealed that the false-positive results of latex cryptococcal antigen agglutination tests have now decreased to 0% to 0.4% (72,73). Some misinterpretation may also cause incorrect positive results. These errors can be eliminated by interpretation of positive results when the reaction shows agglutination equivalent to or greater than 2 + or equivalent to a positive control (58,79). Some commercial latex cryptococcal antigen agglutination kits also provide a positive control with rheumatoid factor, which consistently produces a distinct positive agglutination reaction for comparison.

Rheumatoid factor is one of the most common causes of false-positive results in LA tests of cryptococcal polysaccharide antigen and has been found more frequently in serum specimens (67,77,80) than CSF specimens (81). Unlike the LA test, the old technique of complement fixation (CF) for cryptococcal polysaccharide antigen is not interfered by rheumatoid factors (77). Other unknown interference factors (67,70,82,83) have also been reported to produce the nonspecific agglutination of latex particles in both serum (67) and CSF (73), which is usually low grade. Stockman and Roberts reported a 1% interference incidence in their study of 9000 CSF specimens (83) whereas Wu and Koo found only one nonspecific agglutination out of 79 serum specimens (70). Normal globulin reagents have been used as a control to detect rheumatoid factor (67,77) and to validate the positive result in the presence of interference. The agglutination titers produced by anti-cryptococcal globulin reagents must be at least fourfold higher than that of normal globulin reagents to yield true-positive results (70).

There are many procedures used to eliminate rheumatoid factor or other unknown interfering substances in clinical specimens. By heating serum specimens to 56°C for 30 minutes (67) or CSF specimens to 100°C for 10 minutes (59), some of the low-grade non-specific agglutination can be eliminated. However, 9% false-positive results were still observed in CSF despite use of this boiling technique (73). Eng and Person reported a technique of ethylenediamine tetra-acetic acid (EDTA)-heat extraction by adding sera with EDTA and boiling it for five minutes before testing. They found that the technique possibly increases sensitivity as compared with the untreated sera, and the interfering rheumatoid factor activity was eliminated (84). Dithiothreitol (DTT) has been used to eliminate rheumatoid factor and interference factors in serum (80) and CSF specimens (81). Pretreatment with 2-β-mercaptoethanol can also be used to eliminate nonspecific reactivity in a LA test without affecting the true-positive results (85,86). An enzymatic method involving pronase, a protease enzyme, for elimination of interference factors in the LA test for cryptococcal polysaccharide antigen in sera and CSF has been developed. This technique requires no dilution of the specimens and uses less time for treatment than the DTT method (83). Pronase treatment produced positive results only in specimens from patients who were suspected of having cryptococcosis by virtue of increasing cryptococcal polysaccharide antigen titers in CSF and sera (82). Inactivation of the pronase vial in a commercial test kit has been reported to cause false-positive results (87).

Besides rheumatoid factor and certain interference factors, there are other situations that also cause false-positive results in LA tests for cryptococcal polysaccharide antigen. Infections with *Trichosporon beigelii*, a basidiomycetous fungus in the same family of Sporidiobolaceae as *C. neoformans*, has been reported to possess cross-reactivity, and subsequently cause false-positive results in the LA test (88,89). A study using immunoelectron microscopy in a rabbit model of experimental disseminated trichosporonosis revealed that the antigen that cross-reacts with the cryptococcal polysaccharide antigen is localized in the *T. beigelii* cell wall and in a fibrillar matrix extending from the cell wall (90). A glucuronoxylomannan-like antigen was found in *T. beigelii* that might cross-react with cryptococcal antibodies-coated latex particles (91). Infection caused by other microorganisms have also been reported to produce cross-reactivity with the latex cryptococcal polysaccharide antigen agglutination test. These include *Stomatococcus mucilaginosus* (92), *Capnocytophaga canimorsus* (93), and *Klebsiella pneumoniae* (94). There were also reports of false-positive results of latex cryptococcal polysaccharide antigen agglutination tests in CSF caused by contamination of syneresis fluid transferred from agar plates with pipetting. The cross reactive component was heat stable, was not eliminated by pronase treatment, and was not detected by the normal rabbit globulin controls (76,95).

Other reported causes of false-positive results in latex cryptococcal antigen tests include disinfectants and soaps (96), iron (Fe^{3+}) content in the tested sera (which can be eliminated by 2-β-mercaptoethanol) (97), hydroxyethyl starch (HES) for intravascular volume replacement (98), and malignancy (99,100). Except for patients with *T. beigelii* infections, in which the titers of cryptococcal polysaccharide antigen can be as high as 1000 and may help to substantiate the diagnosis of disseminated trichosporonosis (88,89), most of the false-positive results of LA tests for cryptococcal polysaccharide antigen had initial reciprocal titers of less than or equal to 8 (71). Results of such low titers must be carefully interpreted within the clinical context (59,101). However, a recent study by Kontoyiannis reported cancer patients with high titers of false-positive cryptococcal polysaccharide antigens in CSF despite use of a pronase-based cryptococcal polysaccharide antigen detection kit. The study showed that 7 patients had cryptococcal antigen titers less than or equal to 8, 2 patients had titers of 32, and 1 patient had a titer of 256 (100).

False-negative results of LA tests for cryptococcal polysaccharide antigen in the setting of cryptococcal meningitis are unusual (102–104). A prozone effect has been described as a cause of false-negative results in the latex cryptococcal polysaccharide antigen agglutination test of CSF (67,105). In this setting the excessive number of whole cryptococci in the patient's CSF can interfere with the test results. It has been suggested that a CSF specimen with positive findings on India ink examination and negative results for the latex cryptococcal polysaccharide antigen agglutination test should be diluted and retested in order to avoid the prozone effect (105). Low fungal burden as in chronic low-grade cryptococcal meningitis or in very early stages of cryptococcal infection can cause apparent false-negative results with latex cryptococcal polysaccharide antigen agglutination tests (67). One recent study has also shown that the immunoreactivity of cryptococcal capsular polysaccharide antigen is not stable with prolonged incubation in human serum and the loss of antigen reactivity depends upon pH and temperature (106). Therefore, improper storage of patients' sera before testing is probably a cause of false-negative results with the cryptococcal polysaccharide antigen agglutination test.

EIA for detection and quantification of cryptococcal polysaccharide antigen of all four serotypes of *C. neoformans* has been developed for sera and

CSF and is commercially available (PREMIER® Cryptococcal Antigen EIA; Meridian Bioscience, Inc., Cincinnati, Ohio, U.S.A.) (71,107–110). EIA for cryptococcal polysaccharide antigen detects the major component of the polysaccharide capsule, glucuronoxylomannan (GXM) (111). The EIA cryptococcal polysaccharide antigen test possesses sensitivities and specificities of 85.2% to 99% and 97%, respectively, (71,109). Previous studies compared EIA cryptococcal polysaccharide antigen tests and latex cryptococcal polysaccharide antigen agglutination tests and found that there was not significant differences between tests with 84.6% to 97.8% agreement (71,108,112). However other investigators reported that EIA cryptococcal polysaccharide antigen test possesses a 12-fold sensitivity advantage over latex cryptococcal polysaccharide antigen agglutination tests for serotype A and B strains (109). EIA for cryptococcal polysaccharide antigen do not give discrepant results with rheumatoid factor, syneresis fluid, or serum macroglobulins from systemic lupus erythematous patients and thus do not require pretreatment of specimens with pronase (107,109). EIA can potentially detect cryptococcal polysaccharide antigens at an earlier stage of cryptococcal infection by measuring a lower polysaccharide antigen concentration (8,109). EIA also provides spectrophotometrically determined objective results and is not affected by prozone reactions.

Although the presence of cryptococcal polysaccharide antigen in serum is undoubtedly suggestive for dissemination of cryptococcal infection outside the lung, the precise value of cryptococcal polysaccharide antigen for diagnosis of non-disseminated pulmonary cryptococcosis remains less certain. For instance, some clinicians have reported with a small number of subjects that immunocompromised patients who have cryptococcal pneumonia without apparent extrapulmonary cryptococcosis may have cryptococcal polysaccharide antigen in serum (113,114). On the other hand, other reports with larger numbers of patients revealed that the LA tests for cryptococcal polysaccharide antigen in CSF or sera were not useful for diagnosis of localized pulmonary or cutaneous cryptococcosis in the absence of dissemination (72,73,115). Prevost and Newell described 13 patients with culture-proven *C. neoformans* pulmonary infection and negative serum latex cryptococcal polysaccharide antigen tests who were later found not to have disseminated infections (73). Taelman et al. also reported a case series of 15 patients with primary pulmonary cryptococcosis and without extrapulmonary disease who were negative for latex cryptococcal antigen tests (115). Therefore, the serum cryptococcal polysaccharide antigen will not likely help to diagnose limited pulmonary disease, but its presence in serum should make clinicians consider that infection is now also located outside the lung.

LA tests for cryptococcal polysaccharide antigen have been used to identify polysaccharide antigen of all *C. neoformans* serotypes in sera, CSF, and various body fluids for diagnosis of invasive cryptococcosis. However, benefit of detection of cryptococcal polysaccharide antigen in other fluids such as bronchoalveolar lavage fluid is controversial. Early data from a prospective study by Baughman et al. found that all 8 patients who developed cryptococcal pneumonia had positive antigen titers of ≥ 8 in bronchoalveolar lavage fluid specimens, but they also detected four false-positive reactions with titers up to 8 (116). In a retrospective study by Kralovic and Rhodes, 42 bronchoalveolar lavage fluid specimens were positive but 17 were considered to be false-positive. The test gave a sensitivity of 71% for these specimens but a positive predictive value of only 59% (117). In contrast to bronchoalveolar lavage, detection of cryptococcal polysaccharide antigen from transthoracic needle aspiration biopsy tissue has reported yields as high as 97.5% accuracy. Liaw et al. reported 8 patients with pulmonary cryptococcosis and all of them had positive latex cryptococcal polysaccharide antigen agglutination tests from transthoracic needle aspiration of tissue. Only three of these patients had a positive serum cryptococcal polysaccharide antigen. The test had 100% sensitivity and 97% specificity with a positive and negative predictive value of 89% and 100%, respectively, (118). Determination of cryptococcal polysaccharide antigen in pleural fluid of 2 patients with pulmonary cryptococcosis has been reported (119). Detection of cryptococcal polysaccharide antigen in urine by the LA test can also be used for identifying patients with disseminated cryptococcosis but it is unlikely to replace the more standardized serum and CSF tests in most clinical situations (120).

In a high-risk patient, identification of cryptococcal antigen in CSF or serum is rapid, specific, noninvasive, and is virtually diagnostic of meningoencephalitic or disseminated cryptococcosis, even when the India ink examination or culture is negative (79,121,122). The LA test for serum cryptococcal polysaccharide antigen is widely used for detecting cryptococcal polysaccharide capsule in patients with AIDS as an initial screening test for patients with fever of unclear etiologies or neurological symptoms, and has become a part of routine clinical practice in the standard care of patients with or suspected of cryptococcal infections in geographical areas with a high density of disease (111,123–126). It may perform less well as a screening device in areas in which the incidence of cryptococcal disease is low (127,128). Some clinicians have found that the combined use of a cryptococcal polysaccharide antigen test and bacterial cultures of CSF might replace routine fungal cultures of CSF except in the setting in which fungal pathogens other than *C. neoformans* and *Candida* spp. remain important causes of meningitis (129). In some patients, it may represent the only means of achieving an etiologic diagnosis of invasive cryptococcosis (79).

Because the detection of cryptococcal polysaccharide antigen is highly sensitive and specific, it may precede a documented pulmonary or disseminated cryptococcal disease in severely immunosuppressed patients (130) and has created a series of cases identified as "isolated cryptococcal polysaccharidemia" (8,111,124). A study of HIV-infected patients in Uganda found that the frequency of asymptomatic isolated cryptococcal antigenemia among patients with positive serum cryptococcal polysaccharide antigen was 38.1% (8 of 21), and all of them were extremely immunosuppressed (124). The management of these laboratory findings, in which there is a positive serum antigen with no other signs or symptoms for *C. neoformans* infection in HIV-infected patients, is uncertain.

Feldmesser et al. identified 10 HIV-infected patients who had serum cryptococcal polysaccharide antigen ≥4 and met the criteria of asymptomatic cryptococcal antigenemia. Six patients were treated with fluconazole and did not develop cryptococcal meningitis within the follow-up period (3–22 months), 1 patient developed disseminated cryptococcosis later and died, and 3 patients were found to have disseminated cryptococcosis during initial evaluation. Yuen et al. reported 13 patients with isolated cryptococcal antigenemia who had serum cryptococcal polysaccharide antigen titers of ≥8. Ten patients received systemic antifungal therapy and did not develop disseminated diseases, whereas 2 of 3 patients who did not receive systemic antifungal therapy had cryptococcal meningitis later (131). Therefore, patients in a very high-risk group to have cryptococcal disease and have isolated cryptococcal antigenemia probably benefit from antifungal therapy to prevent or delay the development of overt cryptococcosis (111). There have also been reports of patients with isolated positive CSF cryptococcal antigens. Salom reported a patient without HIV infection who had a positive latex cryptococcal polysaccharide antigen agglutination test only in an undiluted CSF sample. All other laboratory results, including serum cryptococcal polysaccharide antigen, and cultures were initially negative but *C. neoformans* was identified by culture 17 days later in CSF from a cisternal tap (132). Manfredi et al. found that 5 of 27 HIV-infected patients who had positive CSF cryptococcal polysaccharide antigen titers and negative cultures and microscopic examinations eventually developed invasive crypto-coccosis clinically or at necropsy (123). Chakrabarti et al. also described isolated CSF antigen detection in 11 patients with immunosuppressive diseases other than HIV infection and in persons without apparent immunodeficiency (125,133). All of 11 patients had CSF cryptococcal polysaccharide antigen >8 and received systemic antifungal treatment. Eight of 11 patients responded well whereas 3 patients died. One of them was autopsied and encapsulated yeast cells were identified in meningeal tissue (125,133). Therefore, an isolated positive LA assay of ≥4 in serum or CSF should be regarded as an early sign of invasive cryptococcosis and will require prompt treatment if the patient is known to be at risk for disease. Generally, positive serum antigen tests at titers of ≥4 strongly suggest cryptococcal infections, and titers of ≥8 are probably indicative of active disease.

Baseline cryptococcal polysaccharide antigen titers in serum and CSF have been shown to be factors that may be used to predict outcome of patients with cryptococcal meningitis (60). Previous studies in patients without HIV infection suggested that high titers of cryptococcal polysaccharide antigen in serum and CSF at baseline are associated with a higher risk of death during treatment with amphotericin B (23,121,134,135). Diamond and Bennett found that initial CSF or serum cryptococcal polysaccharide antigen titers of ≥32 were associated with mortality during antifungal therapy and the post-treatment CSF or serum cryptococcal polysaccharide antigen titers of ≥8 predicted treatment failure (23). A retrospective study by Shih et al. found that only lymphoma and high initial CSF cryptococcal polysaccharide antigen titers of ≥ 512 were independent predictors of mortality in non-HIV-infected patients with cryptococcal meningitis in a multivariate analysis (121). Serum cryptococcal polysaccharide antigen titers may have less correlation with infection outcome in AIDS patients (136). However, an International Working Group on Cryptococcosis study on the discontinuation of maintenance therapy for cryptococcal meningitis in 100 HIV-infected patients with cryptococcal meningitis treated with antiretroviral treatment revealed that there were four relapse events for 262 person-years. Two of four patients with recurrent cases had negative serum cryptococcal polysaccharide antigen tests at the time of discontinuation of suppressive therapy, but serum antigen titers rose again when the patients relapsed (137). On the other hand, CSF cryptococcal polysaccharide antigen may be more precise in predicting outcome in HIV-infected patients with cryptococcal meningitis. A study in HIV-related acute cryptococcal meningitis indicated that a baseline titer of CSF cryptococcal polysaccharide antigen of ≥ 1024 was a predictor of death during systemic antifungal treatment (138). Therefore, initial CSF cryptococcal polysaccharide antigen titers may be used as a sign of poor prognosis in both AIDS or non-AIDS patients.

After initiation of systemic antifungal therapy and patients respond to treatment, titers of cryptococcal polysaccharide antigen usually fall (79). There is some correlation between unchanged or increased titers (titers rise by at least two dilutions or by fourfold) of CSF cryptococcal polysaccharide antigen and a higher risk for clinical and microbiological failure to response to treatment. The correlation is especially strong among patients whose baseline CSF cryptococcal polysaccharide antigen titers were ≥ 8. A rise in CSF cryptococcal polysaccharide antigen titers during suppressive therapy has been associated with relapse of cryptococcal meningitis (136). However, it is important to emphasize that the use of changing antigen titers to make therapeutic decisions during therapy is not precise and should probably be avoided. The kinetics of polysaccharide elimination remains unclear and despite the accuracy of commercial kits for diagnosis, the accuracy of titers can vary from kit to kit even with the same specimen.

CULTURE AND IDENTIFICATION

C. neoformans can be easily grown from biologic samples on routine standard fungal and bacterial culture media. Colonies can usually be observed on solid agar plates after 48 to 72 hours incubation at 30°C to 35°C in aerobic conditions. *C. neoformans* is generally the only *cryptococcal* species that can consistently grow at 37°C. The growth rates of *C. neoformans* strains are significantly reduced at temperatures between 39°C and 40°C and the more temperature-sensitive strains of *C. neoformans* var. *gattii* will die when temperature exceeds 40°C. In fact, in general *C. neoformans* var. *grubii* is more thermotolerant than *C. neoformans* var. *neoformans* and var. *gattii*. Some strains of *Cryptococcus albidus* and *C. laurentii*, which can rarely cause human diseases, can grow at 37°C but this characteristic is not common. Antibacterial agents, preferably chloramphenicol, can be added to the media when bacterial contamination is considered. The yeasts, however, do not grow in the presence of cycloheximide at the concentration used in selective isolation media (25 µg/ml). *C. neoformans* grows well in acidic media of pH 5 to 7 and does not tolerate alkaline pH above 7.6. Presence of some iron in the medium is essential for yeast growth (139). It should be noted that in patients who are receiving systemic antifungal therapy, *C. neoformans* may require longer time to produce visible colonies. Cultures should be held for three to four weeks before discarding, and is particularly important for patients already receiving antifungal treatment. Cultures may be negative despite positive microscopic examination (India ink) due to nonviable yeast cells that may have prolonged persistence at the site of infection. Aberrant strains of yeasts can be grown on hypertonic medium of salt and/or 0.3 M sucrose (140,141).

The radiometric methods such as the BACTEC system may not identify positive cultures when the numbers of yeasts in the blood are very low (142). Therefore, subculture of blood culture bottles from high-risk patients despite the low radiometric readings is occasionally recommended. Tinghitella and Lamagdeleine reported failure to detect *C. neoformans* in clinical specimens in the Difco ESP 384 blood culture system. The system failed to detect 1.4% (16 of 384) of the microorganisms, and 50% (8 of 16) of which were *C. neoformans*, indicating a deficiency in the detection mechanism of the system. Further studies demonstrated that while *C. neoformans* grew in the Difco media, the system did not detect its growth when the standard 5-day protocol was used (143). Continuous agitation of BACTEC blood culture bottles for the full incubation time can significantly improve the detection and recovery of *C. neoformans* (144). Furthermore, there has been a report that addition of hydrogen peroxide to blood in liquid culture can increase growth of *C. neoformans* (145). Positive blood cultures are frequently reported in AIDS patients, and this may actually represent the first sign of infection in a febrile high-risk patient.

Negative cultures of CSF in patients with cryptococcal meningitis may be due to a low burden of yeasts, which occurs in some cases of chronic cryptococcal meningitis. Because only a few *C. neoformans* cells may be present at the site of infection, there have been suggestions to culture pellets from centrifuged CSF, blood, and other body fluids. Other maneuvers to improve yield of positive cultures include large volume CSF lumbar taps (i.e., 15–20 mL) passed through sterile filter paper or withdrawal of CSF from the cisternal space in cases of chronic basilar meningitis.

C. neoformans colonies will appear on artificial media as opaque, white, creamy colonies that may turn orange-tan or brown after prolonged incubation. The mucoid appearance of the colony is related to the capsule size around the yeasts. Some textbooks described the colonial morphology as being "*Klebsiella*-like" because of a large amount of polysaccharide capsule material present (146).

On inhibitory mold agar, *C. neoformans* appears as a golden yellow, non-mucoid colony. Some colonies develop sectoring within the colonies after prolonged incubation on agar plates. There are three types of sectoring; mucoid, rough, and smooth (147). The sectoring is related to cells within the population that acquire thick capsules or tend to form pseudomycelium (148), and it is part of a well-described switching morphology system in *C. neoformans* (149).

Bronchial secretions and urine, especially from AIDS patients, are often contaminated by many microorganisms including *Candida* spp., which by their rapid growth may mask the growth of *C. neoformans*. The differential medium, niger seed (*Guizotia abyssinica*, birdseed) agar, as a primary culture medium can be used along with Sabouraud's dextrose agar to distinguish these two yeasts. *Candida* spp. will have white colonies, whereas *C. neoformans* colonies will turn brown because of their ability to break down caffeic acid to melanin (150,151). *Cryptococcus* spp. other than *C. neoformans* will appear on birdseed agar as white or greenish colonies. Birdseed agar can also be supplemented with several antibiotics and biphenyl to minimize the growth of bacterial contaminants and is frequently used in environmental sampling studies. A selective medium, inositol with chloramphenicol, has also been developed to inhibit *Candida* growth and enhance isolation of *Cryptococcus* species. On this medium, pellets from centrifuged bronchial secretions and urine can be inoculated. Inositol, as the unique carbon source, is assimilated by *Cryptococcus* species but not by *Candida* species that may be present in biologic fluids. After three to five days of incubation, *Cryptococcus* colonies can be recognized among the pinpoint *Candida* colonies, which develop as residual growth (75).

Characteristics of yeasts within genus *Cryptococcus* are that they do not produce hyphae or pseudohyphae or ballistospores and are not able to ferment sugars but assimilate inositol and hydrolyze urea. Among at least 38 species of *Cryptococcus*, *C. neoformans* is the only species which is apparently pathogenic, although there are a few reported cases of patients infected with *C. laurentii* (152–157), *C. albidus* (158,159), *Cryptococcus curvatus* (160), and *Cryptococcus adeliensis* (161). Because of ability to produce urease, a rapid test to identify *C. neoformans* urease activity has been developed (162). *C. neoformans* will become urease-positive within 15 minutes whereas other urease-positive species of yeasts from clinical specimens required more than three hours, and *Candida* spp., which do not produce urease, will be negative (162). Other formal biochemical profiles of *C. neoformans* show that it is not able to assimilate nitrate but has ability to use galactose, maltose, galactitol, and sucrose. It will not assimilate lactose and melibiose, and its growth is strain variable with erythritol. There have been many commercially available micromethod systems for identification of *C. neoformans* using carbohydrate assimilation, and these systems generally require 24-hour incubation (the API 20C System, the Flow Laboratories Uni-Yeast-Tek System, the BBL Minitek System, the Vitek Yeast Biochemical Card). There have also been commercial multi-test identification systems based on detection of pre-formed enzymes that can identify yeasts with chromogenic substrates within four hours of inoculation (API Yeast Identification System and Microscan Rapid Yeast Identification) (163). A DNA probe for ribosomal RNA (rRNA), AccuProbe® (GenProbe, Inc., San Diego, California, U.S.A.), can confirm or identify a yeast isolate as *C. neoformans* with 100% sensitivity and specificity and is also commercially available (164).

Recent advanced technology in fungal molecular biology has been developed and used for identification and diagnosis of cryptococcosis. Molecular probes for identification of *C. neoformans* from yeast colonies have been developed with high sensitivity and specificity (164,165). Amplification of a portion of cryptococcal ribosomal DNA (rDNA) directly from clinical specimens by polymerase chain reaction (PCR) techniques with or without restriction enzymes digestion has been used to identify the presence of *C. neoformans* in clinical specimens and thus can be used for diagnosis of cryptococcal infection (166–170). Although the more widely used methods of histological staining and serological tests for diagnosis of cryptococcal infection are more rapid, less time-consuming, and less expensive than the molecular techniques. These advanced molecular technologies can be incorporated as a part of diagnostic strategies for confirmation of cryptococcal infection in circumstances in which simple tests are inconclusive.

Furthermore, the molecular biological techniques are very useful for studies of molecular epidemiology and pathogenicity (171–182). Several molecular methods have been developed and used for genotyping of *C. neoformans* strains from both clinical and environmental isolates. These techniques include multilocus enzyme typing (183,184), electrophoretic karyotyping with pulse-field gel electrophoresis (PFGE) (172,185,186), restriction fragment length polymorphism (RFLP) analysis (179,180,187), DNA fingerprinting by hybridization of restricted DNA with various probes, random amplified polymorphic DNA (RAPD) analysis and PCR fingerprinting (172,173,175–182,188,189), and specific gene sequencing (multilocus sequence typing). The differences in chromosome sizes and numbers between varieties of *C. neoformans* by electrophoretic karyotyping with PFGE can separate strains (185). However, karyotype instability in vitro and microevolution in vivo for *C. neoformans* may be a limitation of this technique for confirming relatedness of strains (190). RFLP analysis using the repetitive multiple-copy rDNA genes of *C. neoformans* has been described (180,187) but these genes do not allow for much discrimination between strains. However, RFLP of the amplified *URA5* gene has been used for molecular typing of IberoAmerican *C. neoformans* isolates (179) and for rapid identification of varieties and serotypes in clinical samples (191). Furthermore, Chaturvedi et al. have also reported the use of mating-type locus (MAT)-α and MAT-β genes for PCR–RFLP that can be used to distinguish the three varieties of *C. neoformans* (192). Several probes have been used for hybridization of restricted DNA and help distinguish between strains of *C. neoformans*. These probes include CND1.4 and CND1.7 (193), *C. neoformans* repetitive element 1 (CNRE-1) (194–197), UT-4p

(198,199), mitochondrial DNA probes (200), and synthetic oligonucleotide probes to microsatellite sequences such as $5'$-(GACA)$_4$-$3'$, $5'$-(GATA)$_4$-$3'$, and $5'$-(GGAT)$_4$-$3'$ (201–203). DNA Hybridization with CNRE-1 and UT-4p, which contains the cryptococcal *URA5* gene, has been shown to be more stable in hybridization patterns during infection or with antifungal treatment and therefore may possess more reliable power for distinguishing between strains of *C. neoformans* (196,204). RAPD analysis and PCR fingerprinting with the oligonucleotide primers (GTG)$_5$, (GACA)$_4$, and the phage M13 core sequence has been successfully used to differentiate between strains of *C. neoformans* (173,176,180,189). Strains of serotype A, B/C, or D can be classified to serotype by their PCR fingerprint patterns. There have been reports of the use of RAPD to discriminate relapse from reinfection isolates of *C. neoformans* (201) and the use of Southern blot hybridization with two genomic DNA probes and pulsed-field electrophoresis of intact chromosomes to confirm the persistence of the original infecting strain in relapsed cryptococcal meningitis (196). Finally, with several cryptococcal genomes sequenced, multilocus sequencing tests can be performed to differentiate strains. Although use of these highly sensitive molecular techniques can probably identify specific *C. neoformans* strains and can be used for epidemiological studies, the techniques must be used carefully with proper controls since *C. neoformans* can microevolve during infection.

REFERENCES

1. Belay T, Cherniak R, O'Neill EB, Kozel TR. Serotyping of *Cryptococcus neoformans* by dot enzyme assay. J Clin Microbiol 1996; 34:466–70.
2. Franzot SP, Salkin IF, Casadevall A. *Cryptococcus neoformans* var. *grubii*: separate varietal status for *Cryptococcus neoformans* serotype A isolates. J Clin Microbiol 1999; 37:838–40.
3. Levitz SM. The ecology of *Cryptococcus neoformans* and the epidemiology of cryptococcosis. Rev Infect Dis 1991; 13:1163–9.
4. Mitchell TG, Perfect JR. Cryptococcosis in the era of AIDS—100 years after the discovery of *Cryptococcus neoformans*. Clin Microbiol Rev 1995; 8:515–48.
5. Kwon-Chung KJ. Cryptococcosis. In: Kwon-Chung KJ, Bennett JE, eds. Medical Mycology. Philadelphia, PA: Lea & Febiger, 1992:397–446.
6. Hajjeh RA, Conn LA, Stephens DS, et al. Cryptococcosis: population-based multistate active surveillance and risk factors in human immunodeficiency virus-infected persons. Cryptococcal Active Surveillance Group. J Infect Dis 1999; 179:449–54.
7. Perfect JR, Casadevall A. Cryptococcosis. Infect Dis Clin North Am 2002; 16:837–74 (see also v–vi).
8. Casadevall A, Perfect JR. *Cryptococcus neoformans*. 1st ed. Washington, DC: ASM Press, 1998.
9. Sorvillo F, Beall G, Turner PA, Beer VL, Kovacs AA, Kerndt PR. Incidence and factors associated with extrapulmonary cryptococcosis among persons with HIV infection in Los Angeles County. AIDS 1997; 11:673–9.

10. Haddad NE, Powderly WG. The changing face of mycoses in patients with HIV/AIDS. AIDS Read 2001; 11:365–8 (see also 375–368).

11. Senya C, Mehta A, Harwell JI, Pugatch D, Flanigan T, Mayer KH. Spectrum of opportunistic infections in hospitalized HIV-infected patients in Phnom Penh, Cambodia. Int J STD AIDS 2003; 14:411–6.

12. Inverarity D, Bradshaw Q, Wright P, Grant A. The spectrum of HIV-related disease in rural Central Thailand. Southeast Asian J Trop Med Public Health 2002; 33:822–31.

13. Bogaerts J, Rouvroy D, Taelman H, et al. AIDS-associated cryptococcal meningitis in Rwanda (1983–1992): epidemiologic and diagnostic features. J Infect 1999; 39:32–7.

14. Diamond R. *Cryptococcus neoformans*. In: Mandell GL, Bennett JE, Dolin R, eds. Mandell, Douglas, and Bennett's Principles and Practice of Infectious Diseases. Philadelphia, PA: Churchill Livingstone, 2000:2707–18.

15. Lewis JL, Rabinovich S. The wide spectrum of cryptococcal infections. Am J Med 1972; 53:315–22.

16. Perfect JR. Cryptococcosis. Infect Dis Clin North Am 1989; 3:77–102.

17. Merz W, Roberts GD. Detection and recovery of fungi from clinical specimens. In: Balows A, ed. Manual of Clinical Microbiology. Washington, DC: American Society for Microbiology, 1991:550.

18. Thiruchelvan N, Wuu KY, Arseculeratne SN, Ashraful-Haq J. A pseudo-cryptococcal artefact derived from leucocytes in wet India ink mounts of centrifuged cerebrospinal fluid. J Clin Pathol 1998; 51:246–8.

19. Portnoy D, Richards GK. Cryptococcal meningitis: misdiagnosis with India ink. Can Med Assoc J 1981; 124:891–2.

20. Dolan CT, Woodward MR. Identification of *Cryptococcus* species in the diagnostic laboratory. Am J Clin Pathol 1971; 55:591–5.

21. Zerpa R, Huicho L, Guillen A. Modified India ink preparation for *Cryptococcus neoformans* in cerebrospinal fluid specimens. J Clin Microbiol 1996; 34:2290–1.

22. Sobottka I, Freiesleben H, Laufs R. Simple, rapid stain technique for diagnosis of cryptococcosis. Eur J Clin Microbiol Infect Dis 1993; 12:479–81.

23. Diamond RD, Bennett JE. Prognostic factors in cryptococcal meningitis. A study in 111 cases. Ann Intern Med 1974; 80:176–81.

24. Davies SF. Diagnosis of pulmonary fungal infections. Semin Respir Infect 1988; 3:162–71.

25. Cunha BA. Central nervous system infections in the compromised host: a diagnostic approach. Infect Dis Clin North Am 2001; 15:567–90.

26. Shibuya K, Coulson WF, Wollman JS, et al. Histopathology of cryptococcosis and other fungal infections in patients with acquired immunodeficiency syndrome. Int J Infect Dis 2001; 5:78–85.

27. Picon L, Vaillant L, Duong T, et al. Cutaneous cryptococcosis resembling molluscum contagiosum: a first manifestation of AIDS. Acta Derm Venereol 1989; 69:365–7.

28. Pantanowitz L, Omar T, Sonnendecker H, Karstaedt AS. Bone marrow cryptococcal infection in the acquired immunodeficiency syndrome. J Infect 2000; 41:92–4.

29. Ferry JA, Pettit CK, Rosenberg AE, Harris NL. Fungi in megakaryocytes. An unusual manifestation of fungal infection of the bone marrow. Am J Clin Pathol 1991; 96:577–81.

30. Marques MB, Waites KB, Jaye DL, Kilby JM, Reddy VV. Histologic examination of bone marrow core biopsy specimens has limited value in the diagnosis of mycobacterial and fungal infections in patients with the acquired immunodeficiency syndrome. Ann Diagn Pathol 2000; 4:1–6.

31. Sato Y, Osabe S, Kuno H, Kaji M, Oizumi K. Rapid diagnosis of cryptococcal meningitis by microscopic examination of centrifuged cerebrospinal fluid sediment. J Neurol Sci 1999; 164:72–5.

32. Kumar S, Ferns S, Jatiya L. A rare case of cryptococcosis diagnosed by fine needle aspiration cytology. Acta Cytol 2003; 47:528–9.

33. Alfonso F, Gallo L, Winkler B, Suhrland MJ. Fine needle aspiration cytology of peripheral lymph node cryptococcosis. A report of three cases. Acta Cytol 1994; 38:459–62.

34. Powers CN, Rupp GM, Maygarden SJ, Frable WJ. Fine-needle aspiration cytology of adrenal cryptococcosis: a case report. Diagn Cytopathol 1991; 7:88–91.

35. O'Dowd GJ, Frable WJ. Cryptococcal endophthalmitis: diagnostic vitreous aspiration cytology. Am J Clin Pathol 1983; 79:382–5.

36. Hsu CY. Cytologic diagnosis of pulmonary cryptococcosis in immunocompetent hosts. Acta Cytol 1993; 37:667–72.

37. Kuo TH, Hsu WH, Chiang CD, Huang CM, Chen CY, Chang MC. Ultrasound-guided fine needle aspiration biopsy in the diagnosis of pulmonary cryptococcosis. J Formos Med Assoc 1998; 97:197–203.

38. Lee LN, Yang PC, Kuo SH, Luh KT, Chang DB, Yu CJ. Diagnosis of pulmonary cryptococcosis by ultrasound guided percutaneous aspiration. Thorax 1993; 48:75–8.

39. Morris B, Chan YF, Reddy J, Woodgyer A. Cryptococcal peritonitis in a CAPD patient. J Med Vet Mycol 1992; 30:309–15.

40. Staib F, Seibold M, L'Age M, et al. *Cryptococcus neoformans* in the seminal fluid of an AIDS patient. A contribution to the clinical course of cryptococcosis. Mycoses 1989; 32:171–80.

41. Kanjanavirojkul N, Sripa C, Puapairoj A. Cytologic diagnosis of *Cryptococcus neoformans* in HIV-positive patients. Acta Cytol 1997; 41:493–6.

42. Malabonga VM, Basti J, Kamholz SL. Utility of bronchoscopic sampling techniques for cryptococcal disease in AIDS. Chest 1991; 99:370–2.

43. Lee CH, Lan RS, Tsai YH, Chiang YC, Wang WJ. Riu's stain in the diagnosis of pulmonary cryptococcosis. Introduction of a new diagnostic method. Chest 1988; 93:467–70.

44. Cohen J. Comparison of the sensitivity of three methods for the rapid identification of *Cryptococcus neoformans*. J Clin Pathol 1984; 37:332–4.

45. Berman EL, Laudate A, Carter HW. Comparison of selective staining of fungi in paraffin sections by light microscopy, SEM and BEI. Scan Electron Microsc 1981; 2:115–22.

46. Vance AM. The use of the mucicarmine stain for a rapid presumptive identification of *Cryptococcus* from culture. Am J Med Technol 1961; 27:125–8.

47. Lopez JF, Lebron RF. *Cryptococcus neoformans*: their identification in body fluids and cultures by mucicarmine stain (Mayer). Bol Asoc Med P Rico 1972; 64:203–5.

48. Monteil RA, Hofman P, Michiels JF, Loubiere R. Oral cryptococcosis: case report of salivary gland involvement in an AIDS patient. J Oral Pathol Med 1997; 26:53–6.

49. Bottone EJ, Wormser GP. Poorly encapsulated *Cryptococcus neoformans* from patients with AIDS. II. Correlation of capsule size observed directly in cerebrospinal fluid with that after animal passage. AIDS Res 1986; 2:219–25.

50. Harding SA, Scheld WM, Feldman PS, Sande MA. Pulmonary infection with capsule-deficient *Cryptococcus neoformans*. Virchows Arch A Pathol Anat Histol 1979; 382:113–8.

51. Ro JY, Lee SS, Ayala AG. Advantage of Fontana–Masson stain in capsule-deficient cryptococcal infection. Arch Pathol Lab Med 1987; 111:53–7.

52. Kwon-Chung KJ, Hill WB, Bennett JE. New, special stain for histopathological diagnosis of cryptococcosis. J Clin Microbiol 1981; 13:383–7.

53. Lazcano O, Speights VO, Jr., Bilbao J, Becker J, Diaz J. Combined Fontana–Masson-mucin staining of *Cryptococcus neoformans*. Arch Pathol Lab Med 1991; 115:1145–9.

54. Lazcano O, Speights VO, Jr., Strickler JG, Bilbao JE, Becker J, Diaz J. Combined histochemical stains in the differential diagnosis of *Cryptococcus neoformans*. Mod Pathol 1993; 6:80–4.

55. Ahluwalia J, Garewal G, Das R, Vaiphei K. The reticulin stain in bone marrow biopsies—beyond marrow fibrosis. Br J Haematol 2003; 123:379.

56. Bottone EJ. *Cryptococcus neoformans*: pitfalls in diagnosis through evaluation of gram-stained smears of purulent exudates. J Clin Microbiol 1980; 12:790–1.

57. Shibuya K, Coulson WF, Naoe S. Histopathology of deep-seated fungal infections and detailed examination of granulomatous response against cryptococci in patients with acquired immunodeficiency syndrome. Nippon Ishinkin Gakkai Zasshi 2002; 43:143–51.

58. Kaufman L, Blumer S. Value and interpretation of serological tests for the diagnosis of cryptococcosis. Appl Microbiol 1968; 16:1907–12.

59. Gordon MA, Vedder DK. Serologic tests in diagnosis and prognosis of cryptococcosis. JAMA 1966; 197:961–7.

60. Bindschadler DD, Bennett JE. Serology of human cryptococcosis. Ann Intern Med 1968; 69:45–52.

61. Widra A, McMillen S, Rhodes HJ. Problems in serodiagnosis of cryptococcosis. Mycopathol Mycol Appl 1968; 36:353–8.

62. Kimball HR, Hasenclever HF, Wolff SM. Detection of circulating antibody in human cryptococcosis by means of a bentonite flocculation technique. Am Rev Respir Dis 1967; 95:631–7.

63. Walter JE, Jones RD. Serodiagnosis of clinical cryptococcosis. Am Rev Respir Dis 1968; 97:275–82.

64. Speed BR, Kaldor J, Cairns B, Pegorer M. Serum antibody response to active infection with *Cryptococcus neoformans* and its varieties in immunocompetent subjects. J Med Vet Mycol 1996; 34:187–93.

65. Gordon MA, Lapa E. Charcoal particle agglutination test for detection of antibody to *Cryptococcus neoformans*: a preliminary report. Am J Clin Pathol 1971; 56:354–9.

66. Goldman DL, Khine H, Abadi J, et al. Serologic evidence for *Cryptococcus neoformans* infection in early childhood. Pediatrics 2001; 107:E66.

67. Bloomfield N, Gordon MA, Elmendorf DF, Jr. Detection of *Cryptococcus neoformans* antigen in body fluids by latex particle agglutination. Proc Soc Exp Biol Med 1963; 114:64–7.

68. Singer JM, Plotz CM, Pader E, Elster SK. The latex-fixation test. III. Agglutination test for C-reactive protein and comparison with the capillary precipitin method. Am J Clin Pathol 1957; 28:611–7.

69. Kaufman L, Cowart G, Blumer S, Stine A, Wood R. Evaluation of a commercial latex agglutination test kit for cryptococcal antigen. Appl Microbiol 1974; 27:620–1.

70. Wu TC, Koo SY. Comparison of three commercial cryptococcal latex kits for detection of cryptococcal antigen. J Clin Microbiol 1983; 18:1127–30.

71. Tanner DC, Weinstein MP, Fedorciw B, Joho KL, Thorpe JJ, Reller L. Comparison of commercial kits for detection of cryptococcal antigen. J Clin Microbiol 1994; 32:1680–4.

72. Kauffman CA, Bergman AG, Severance PJ, McClatchey KD. Detection of cryptococcal antigen. Comparison of two latex agglutination tests. Am J Clin Pathol 1981; 75:106–9.

73. Prevost E, Newell R. Commercial cryptococcal latex kit: clinical evaluation in a medical center hospital. J Clin Microbiol 1978; 8:529–33.

74. Kiska DL, Orkiszewski DR, Howell D, Gilligan PH. Evaluation of new monoclonal antibody-based latex agglutination test for detection of cryptococcal polysaccharide antigen in serum and cerebrospinal fluid. J Clin Microbiol 1994; 32:2309–11.

75. Viviani MA, Tortorano AM, Ajello L. *Cryptococcus.* In: Anaissie EJ, McGinnis MR, Pfaller MA, eds. Clinical Mycology. Philadelphia, PA: Churchill Livingstone, 2003:240–59.

76. Boom WH, Piper DJ, Ruoff KL, Ferraro MJ. New cause for false-positive results with the cryptococcal antigen test by latex agglutination. J Clin Microbiol 1985; 22:856–7.

77. Bennett JE, Bailey JW. Control for rheumatoid factor in the latex test for cryptococcosis. Am J Clin Pathol 1971; 56:360–5.

78. Dolan CT. Specificity of the latex-cryptococcal antigen test. Am J Clin Pathol 1972; 58:358–64.

79. Goodman JS, Kaufman L, Koenig MG. Diagnosis of cryptococcal meningitis. Comparison of two latex agglutination tests. N Engl J Med 1971; 285:434–6.

80. Gordon MA, Lapa EW. Elimination of rheumatoid factor in the latex test for cryptococcosis. Am J Clin Pathol 1974; 61:488–94.

81. Hay RJ, Mackenzie DW. False positive latex tests for cryptococcal antigen in cerebrospinal fluid. J Clin Pathol 1982; 35:244–5.

82. Gray LD, Roberts GD. Experience with the use of pronase to eliminate interference factors in the latex agglutination test for cryptococcal antigen. J Clin Microbiol 1988; 26:2450–1.

83. Stockman L, Roberts GD. Specificity of the latex test for cryptococcal antigen: a rapid, simple method for eliminating interference factors. J Clin Microbiol 1982; 16:965–7.

84. Eng RH, Person A. Serum cryptococcal antigen determination in the presence of rheumatoid factor. J Clin Microbiol 1981; 14:700–2.

85. Whittier S, Hopfer RL, Gilligan P. Elimination of false-positive serum reactivity in latex agglutination test for cryptococcal antigen in human immunodeficiency virus-infected population. J Clin Microbiol 1994; 32:2158–61.

86. Sachs MK, Huang CM, Ost D, Jungkind DL. Failure of dithiothreitol and pronase to reveal a false-positive cryptococcal antigen determination in cerebrospinal fluid. Am J Clin Pathol 1991; 96:381–4.

87. Stoeckli TC, Burman WJ. Inactivated pronase as the cause of false-positive results of serum cryptococcal antigen tests. Clin Infect Dis 2001; 32:836–7.

88. Campbell CK, Payne AL, Teall AJ, Brownell A, Mackenzie DW. Cryptococcal latex antigen test positive in patient with *Trichosporon beigelii* infection. Lancet 1985; 2:43–4.

89. McManus EJ, Bozdech MJ, Jones JM. Role of the latex agglutination test for cryptococcal antigen in diagnosing disseminated infections with *Trichosporon beigelii*. J Infect Dis 1985; 151:1167–9.

90. Melcher GP, Reed KD, Rinaldi MG, Lee JW, Pizzo PA, Walsh TJ. Demonstration of a cell wall antigen cross-reacting with cryptococcal polysaccharide in experimental disseminated trichosporonosis. J Clin Microbiol 1991; 29:192–6.

91. Lyman CA, Devi SJ, Nathanson J, Frasch CE, Pizzo PA, Walsh TJ. Detection and quantitation of the glucuronoxylomannan-like polysaccharide antigen from clinical and nonclinical isolates of *Trichosporon beigelii* and implications for pathogenicity. J Clin Microbiol 1995; 33:126–30.

92. Chanock SJ, Toltzis P, Wilson C. Cross-reactivity between *Stomatococcus mucilaginosus* and latex agglutination for cryptococcal antigen. Lancet 1993; 342:1119–20.

93. Westerink MA, Amsterdam D, Petell RJ, Stram MN, Apicella MA. Septicemia due to DF-2. Cause of a false-positive cryptococcal latex agglutination result. Am J Med 1987; 83:155–8.

94. MacKinnon S, Kane JG, Parker RH. False-positive cryptococcal antigen test and cervical prevertebral abscess. JAMA 1978; 240:1982–3.

95. Heelan JS, Corpus L, Kessimian N. False-positive reactions in the latex agglutination test for *Cryptococcus neoformans* antigen. J Clin Microbiol 1991; 29:1260–1.

96. Blevins LB, Fenn J, Segal H, Newcomb-Gayman P, Carroll KC. False-positive cryptococcal antigen latex agglutination caused by disinfectants and soaps. J Clin Microbiol 1995; 33:1674–5.

97. Eberhard TH. False-positive reactions in cryptococcal antigen determination. Am J Clin Pathol 1993; 100:364.

98. Millon L, Barale T, Julliot MC, Martinez J, Mantion G. Interference by hydroxyethyl starch used for vascular filling in latex agglutination test for cryptococcal antigen. J Clin Microbiol 1995; 33:1917–9.

99. Hopper RL, Perry EV, Fainstein V. Diagnostic value of cryptococcal antigen in the cerebrospinal fluid of patients with malignant disease. J Infect Dis 1982; 145:915.

100. Kontoyiannis DP. What is the significance of an isolated positive cryptococcal antigen in the cerebrospinal fluid of cancer patients? Mycoses 2003; 46:161–3.

101. Snow RM, Dismukes WE. Cryptococcal meningitis: diagnostic value of cryptococcal antigen in cerebrospinal fluid. Arch Intern Med 1975; 135:1155–7.

102. Berlin L, Pincus JH. Cryptococcal meningitis. False-negative antigen test results and cultures in nonimmunosuppressed patients. Arch Neurol 1989; 46:1312–6.

103. Currie BP, Freundlich LF, Soto MA, Casadevall A. False-negative cerebrospinal fluid cryptococcal latex agglutination tests for patients with culture-positive cryptococcal meningitis. J Clin Microbiol 1993; 31:2519–22.

104. Haldane DJ, Bauman DS, Chow AW, et al. False negative latex agglutination test in cryptococcal meningitis. Ann Neurol 1986; 19:412–3.
105. Stamm AM, Polt SS. False-negative cryptococcal antigen test. JAMA 1980; 244:1359.
106. McFadden DC, Zaragoza O, Casadevall A. Immunoreactivity of cryptococcal antigen is not stable under prolonged incubations in human serum. J Clin Microbiol 2004; 42:2786–8.
107. Engler HD, Shea YR. Effect of potential interference factors on performance of enzyme immunoassay and latex agglutination assay for cryptococcal antigen. J Clin Microbiol 1994; 32:2307–8.
108. Frank UK, Nishimura SL, Li NC, et al. Evaluation of an enzyme immunoassay for detection of cryptococcal capsular polysaccharide antigen in serum and cerebrospinal fluid. J Clin Microbiol 1993; 31:97–101.
109. Gade W, Hinnefeld SW, Babcock LS, et al. Comparison of the PREMIER cryptococcal antigen enzyme immunoassay and the latex agglutination assay for detection of cryptococcal antigens. J Clin Microbiol 1991; 29:1616–9.
110. Knight FR. New enzyme immunoassay for detecting cryptococcal antigen. J Clin Pathol 1992; 45:836–7.
111. Feldmesser M, Harris C, Reichberg S, Khan S, Casadevall A. Serum cryptococcal antigen in patients with AIDS. Clin Infect Dis 1996; 23:827–30.
112. Sekhon AS, Garg AK, Kaufman L, et al. Evaluation of a commercial enzyme immunoassay for the detection of cryptococcal antigen. Mycoses 1993; 36:31–4.
113. Fisher BD, Armstrong D. Cryptococcal interstitial pneumonia: value of antigen determination. N Engl J Med 1977; 297:1440–1.
114. Mueller NJ, Fishman JA. Asymptomatic pulmonary cryptococcosis in solid organ transplantation: report of four cases and review of the literature. Transpl Infect Dis 2003; 5:140–3.
115. Taelman H, Bogaerts J, Batungwanayo J, Van de Perre P, Lucas S, Allen S. Failure of the cryptococcal serum antigen test to detect primary pulmonary cryptococcosis in patients infected with human immunodeficiency virus. Clin Infect Dis 1994; 18:119–20.
116. Baughman RP, Rhodes JC, Dohn MN, Henderson H, Frame PT. Detection of cryptococcal antigen in bronchoalveolar lavage fluid: a prospective study of diagnostic utility. Am Rev Respir Dis 1992; 145:1226–9.
117. Kralovic SM, Rhodes JC. Utility of routine testing of bronchoalveolar lavage fluid for cryptococcal antigen. J Clin Microbiol 1998; 36:3088–9.
118. Liaw YS, Yang PC, Yu CJ, et al. Direct determination of cryptococcal antigen in transthoracic needle aspirate for diagnosis of pulmonary cryptococcosis. J Clin Microbiol 1995; 33:1588–91.
119. Young EJ, Hirsh DD, Fainstein V, Williams TW. Pleural effusions due to *Cryptococcus neoformans*: a review of the literature and report of two cases with cryptococcal antigen determinations. Am Rev Respir Dis 1980; 121:743–7.
120. Chapin-Robertson K, Bechtel C, Waycott S, Kontnick C, Edberg SC. Cryptococcal antigen detection from the urine of AIDS patients. Diagn Microbiol Infect Dis 1993; 17:197–201.
121. Shih CC, Chen YC, Chang SC, Luh KT, Hsieh WC. Cryptococcal meningitis in non-HIV-infected patients. QJM 2000; 93:245–51.

122. Chuck SL, Sande MA. Infections with *Cryptococcus neoformans* in the acquired immunodeficiency syndrome. N Engl J Med 1989; 321:794–9.

123. Manfredi R, Moroni A, Mazzoni A, et al. Isolated detection of cryptococcal polysaccharide antigen in cerebrospinal fluid samples from patients with AIDS. Clin Infect Dis 1996; 23:849–50.

124. Tassie JM, Pepper L, Fogg C, et al. Systematic screening of cryptococcal antigenemia in HIV-positive adults in Uganda. J Acquir Immune Defic Syndr 2003; 33:411–2.

125. Chakrabarti A, Gupta V. Isolated detection of cryptococcal polysaccharide antigen in patients with cryptococcosis. Clin Infect Dis 1997; 25:1494–5.

126. Desmet P, Kayembe KD, De Vroey C. The value of cryptococcal serum antigen screening among HIV-positive/AIDS patients in Kinshasa, Zaire. AIDS 1989; 3:77–8.

127. Hoffmann S, Stenderup J, Mathiesen LR. Low yield of screening for cryptococcal antigen by latex agglutination assay on serum and cerebrospinal fluid from Danish patients with AIDS or ARC. Scand J Infect Dis 1991; 23:697–702.

128. Nelson MR, Bower M, Smith D, Reed C, Shanson D, Gazzard B. The value of serum cryptococcal antigen in the diagnosis of cryptococcal infection in patients infected with the human immunodeficiency virus. J Infect 1990; 21:175–81.

129. Barenfanger J, Lawhorn J, Drake C. Nonvalue of culturing cerebrospinal fluid for fungi. J Clin Microbiol 2004; 42:236–8.

130. French N, Gray K, Watera C, et al. Cryptococcal infection in a cohort of HIV-1-infected Ugandan adults. AIDS 2002; 16:1031–8.

131. Yuan C, Graziani A, Pietroski N, Macgregor R, Schuster M. Cryptococcal antigenemia in HIV-infected patients. Clin Infect Dis 1994; 19:579.

132. Salom IL. Cryptococcal meningitis; significance of positive antigen test on undiluted spinal fluid. N Y State J Med 1981; 81:1369–70.

133. Chakrabarti A, Vama S, Roy P. Cryptococcosis in and around Chandigarh: an analysis of 65 cases. Indian J Med Microbiol 1995; 13:65–9.

134. Bennett JE, Dismukes WE, Duma RJ, et al. A comparison of amphotericin B alone and combined with flucytosine in the treatment of cryptoccal meningitis. N Engl J Med 1979; 301:126–31.

135. Dismukes WE, Cloud G, Gallis HA, et al. Treatment of cryptococcal meningitis with combination amphotericin B and flucytosine for four as compared with six weeks. N Engl J Med 1987; 317:334–41.

136. Powderly WG, Cloud GA, Dismukes WE, Saag MS. Measurement of cryptococcal antigen in serum and cerebrospinal fluid: value in the management of AIDS-associated cryptococcal meningitis. Clin Infect Dis 1994; 18:789–92.

137. Mussini C, Pezzotti P, Miro JM, et al. Discontinuation of maintenance therapy for cryptococcal meningitis in patients with AIDS treated with highly active antiretroviral therapy: an international observational study. Clin Infect Dis 2004; 38:565–71.

138. Saag MS, Powderly WG, Cloud GA, et al. Comparison of amphotericin B with fluconazole in the treatment of acute AIDS-associated cryptococcal meningitis. The NIAID Mycoses Study Group and the AIDS Clinical Trials Group. N Engl J Med 1992; 326:83–9.

139. Vartivarian SE, Cowart RE, Anaissie EJ, Tashiro T, Sprigg HA. Iron acquisition by *Cryptococcus neoformans*. J Med Vet Mycol 1995; 33:151–6.

140. Dunne WM, Jr., Bhandarkar G, Nafziger D. Isolation of a nutritionally aberrant strain of *Cryptococcus neoformans* from a patient with AIDS. Clin Infect Dis 1995; 21:1512–3.

141. Louria DB, Kaminski T, Grieco M, Singer J. Aberrant forms of bacteria and fungi found in blood or cerebrospinal fluid. Arch Intern Med 1969; 124:39–48.

142. Robinson PG, Sulita MJ, Matthews EK, Warren JR. Failure of the BACTEC 460 radiometer to detect *Cryptococcus neoformans* fungemia in an AIDS patient. Am J Clin Pathol 1987; 87:783–6.

143. Tinghitella TJ, Lamagdeleine MD. Assessment of Difco ESP 384 blood culture system by terminal subcultures: failure to detect *Cryptococcus neoformans* in clinical specimens. J Clin Microbiol 1995; 33:3031–3.

144. Prevost-Smith E, Hutton N. Improved detection of *Cryptococcus neoformans* in the BACTEC NR 660 blood culture system. Am J Clin Pathol 1994; 102:741–5.

145. Huahua T, Rudy J, Kunin CM. Effect of hydrogen peroxide on growth of Candida, *Cryptococcus*, and other yeasts in simulated blood culture bottles. J Clin Microbiol 1991; 29:328–32.

146. Forbes BA, Sahm DF, Weissfeld AS. Bailey & Scott's Diagnostic Microbiology. 11th ed. St. Louis, MO: Andrew Allen, 2002.

147. Drouhet E, Couteau M. Sectorial variations of colonies of *Torulopsis neoformans*. Ann Inst Pasteur 1951; 80:456–7.

148. Littman ML. Cryptococcosis (torulosis). Current concepts and therapy. Am J Med 1959; 27:976–98.

149. Fries BC, Goldman DL, Casadevall A. Phenotypic switching in *Cryptococcus neoformans*. Microbes Infect 2002; 4:1345–52.

150. Staib F, Seibold M, Antweiler E, Frohlich B, Weber S, Blisse A. The brown colour effect (BCE) of *Cryptococcus neoformans* in the diagnosis, control and epidemiology of *C. neoformans* infections in AIDS patients. Zentralbl Bakteriol Mikrobiol Hyg A 1987; 266:167–77.

151. Staib F, Seibold M, Antweiler E, Frohlich B. Staib agar supplemented with a triple antibiotic combination for the detection of *Cryptococcus neoformans* in clinical specimens. Mycoses 1989; 32:448–54.

152. Lynch JP, III, Schaberg DR, Kissner DG, Kauffman CA. *Cryptococcus laurentii* lung abscess. Am Rev Respir Dis 1981; 123:135–8.

153. Johnson LB, Bradley SF, Kauffman CA. Fungaemia due to *Cryptococcus laurentii* and a review of non-neoformans cryptococcaemia. Mycoses 1998; 41:277–80.

154. Kordossis T, Avlami A, Velegraki A, et al. First report of *Cryptococcus laurentii* meningitis and a fatal case of *Cryptococcus albidus* cryptococcaemia in AIDS patients. Med Mycol 1998; 36:335–9.

155. Kunova A, Krcmery V. Fungaemia due to thermophilic cryptococci: 3 cases of *Cryptococcus laurentii* bloodstream infections in cancer patients receiving antifungals. Scand J Infect Dis 1999; 31:328.

156. Cheng MF, Chiou CC, Liu YC, Wang HZ, Hsieh KS. *Cryptococcus laurentii* fungemia in a premature neonate. J Clin Microbiol 2001; 39:1608–11.

157. Sinnott JT, IV, Rodnite J, Emmanuel PJ, Campos A. *Cryptococcus laurentii* infection complicating peritoneal dialysis. Pediatr Infect Dis J 1989; 8:803–5.

158. Lee YA, Kim HJ, Lee TW, et al. First report of *Cryptococcus albidus*—induced disseminated cryptococcosis in a renal transplant recipient. Korean J Intern Med 2004; 19:53–7.

159. Ramchandren R, Gladstone DE. *Cryptococcus albidus* infection in a patient undergoing autologous progenitor cell transplant. Transplantation 2004; 77:956.

160. Dromer F, Moulignier A, Dupont B, et al. Myeloradiculitis due to *Cryptococcus curvatus* in AIDS. AIDS 1995; 9:395–6.

161. Rimek D, Haase G, Luck A, Casper J, Podbielski A. First report of a case of meningitis caused by *Cryptococcus adeliensis* in a patient with acute myeloid leukemia. J Clin Microbiol 2004; 42:481–3.

162. Zimmer BL, Roberts GD. Rapid selective urease test for presumptive identification of *Cryptococcus neoformans*. J Clin Microbiol 1979; 10:380–1.

163. Buesching WJ, Kurek K, Roberts GD. Evaluation of the modified API 20C system for identification of clinically important yeasts. J Clin Microbiol 1979; 9:565–9.

164. Huffnagle KE, Gander RM. Evaluation of Gen-Probe's *Histoplasma capsulatum* and *Cryptococcus neoformans* AccuProbes. J Clin Microbiol 1993; 31:419–21.

165. Stockman L, Clark KA, Hunt JM, Roberts GD. Evaluation of commercially available acridinium ester-labeled chemiluminescent DNA probes for culture identification of *Blastomyces dermatitidis*, *Coccidioides immitis*, *Cryptococcus neoformans*, and *Histoplasma capsulatum*. J Clin Microbiol 1993; 31:845–50.

166. Fell JW. rDNA targeted oligonucleotide primers for the identification of pathogenic yeasts in a polymerase chain reaction. J Ind Microbiol 1995; 14:475–7.

167. Hopfer RL, Walden P, Setterquist S, Highsmith WE. Detection and differentiation of fungi in clinical specimens using polymerase chain reaction (PCR) amplification and restriction enzyme analysis. J Med Vet Mycol 1993; 31:65–75.

168. Mitchell TG, Freedman EZ, White TJ, Taylor JW. Unique oligonucleotide primers in PCR for identification of *Cryptococcus neoformans*. J Clin Microbiol 1994; 32:253–5.

169. Mitchell TG, Sandin RL, Bowman BH, Meyer W, Merz WG. Molecular mycology: DNA probes and applications of PCR technology. J Med Vet Mycol 1994; 32(Suppl. 1):351–66.

170. Prariyachatigul C, Chaiprasert A, Meevootisom V, Pattanakitsakul S. Assessment of a PCR technique for the detection and identification of *Cryptococcus neoformans*. J Med Vet Mycol 1996; 34:251–8.

171. Reiss E, Tanaka K, Bruker G, et al. Molecular diagnosis and epidemiology of fungal infections. Med Mycol 1998; 36(Suppl. 1):249–57.

172. Boekhout T, van Belkum A, Leenders AC, et al. Molecular typing of *Cryptococcus neoformans*: taxonomic and epidemiological aspects. Int J Syst Bacteriol 1997; 47:432–42.

173. Casali AK, Goulart L, Rosa e Silva LK, et al. Molecular typing of clinical and environmental *Cryptococcus neoformans* isolates in the Brazilian state Rio Grande do Sul. FEMS Yeast Res 2003; 3:405–15.

174. Ellis D, Marriott D, Hajjeh RA, Warnock D, Meyer W, Barton R. Epidemiology: surveillance of fungal infections. Med Mycol 2000; 38(Suppl. 1):173–82.

175. Horta JA, Staats CC, Casali AK, et al. Epidemiological aspects of clinical and environmental *Cryptococcus neoformans* isolates in the Brazilian state Rio Grande do Sul. Med Mycol 2002; 40:565–71.

176. Igreja RP, Lazera Mdos S, Wanke B, Galhardo MC, Kidd SE, Meyer W. Molecular epidemiology of *Cryptococcus neoformans* isolates from AIDS patients of the Brazilian city, Rio de Janeiro. Med Mycol 2004; 42:229–38.

177. Lo Passo C, Pernice I, Gallo M, et al. Genetic relatedness and diversity of *Cryptococcus neoform*ans strains in the Maltese Islands. J Clin Microbiol 1997; 35:751–5.

178. Meyer W, Marszewska K, Amirmostofian M, et al. Molecular typing of global isolates of *Cryptococcus neoformans* var. *neoformans* by polymerase chain reaction fingerprinting and randomly amplified polymorphic DNA—a pilot study to standardize techniques on which to base a detailed epidemiological survey. Electrophoresis 1999; 20:1790–9.

179. Meyer W, Castaneda A, Jackson S, Huynh M, Castaneda E. Molecular typing of IberoAmerican *Cryptococcus neoformans* isolates. Emerg Infect Dis 2003; 9:189–95.

180. Pernice I, Lo Passo C, Criseo G, Pernice A, Todaro-Luck F. Molecular subtyping of clinical and environmental strains of *Cryptococcus neoformans* variety *neoformans* serotype A isolated from southern Italy. Mycoses 1998; 41:117–24.

181. Yamamoto Y, Kohno S, Koga H, et al. Random amplified polymorphic DNA analysis of clinically and environmentally isolated *Cryptococcus neoformans* in Nagasaki. J Clin Microbiol 1995; 33:3328–32.

182. Poonwan N, Mikami Y, Poosuwan S, et al. Serotyping of *Cryptococcus neoformans* strains isolated from clinical specimens in Thailand and their susceptibility to various antifungal agents. Eur J Epidemiol 1997; 13:335–40.

183. Brandt ME, Hutwagner LC, Klug LA, et al. Molecular subtype distribution of *Cryptococcus neoformans* in four areas of the United States. Cryptococcal Disease Active Surveillance Group. J Clin Microbiol 1996; 34:912–7.

184. Brandt ME, Hutwagner LC, Kuykendall RJ, Pinner RW. Comparison of multilocus enzyme electrophoresis and random amplified polymorphic DNA analysis for molecular subtyping of *Cryptococcus neoformans*. The Cryplococcal Disease Active Surveillance Group. J Clin Microbiol 1995; 33:1890–5.

185. Perfect JR, Ketabchi N, Cox GM, Ingram CW, Beiser CL. Karyotyping of *Cryptococcus neoformans* as an epidemiological tool. J Clin Microbiol 1993; 31:3305–9.

186. Pfaller M, Zhang J, Messer S, et al. Molecular epidemiology and antifungal susceptibility of *Cryptococcus neoformans* isolates from Ugandan AIDS patients. Diagn Microbiol Infect Dis 1998; 32:191–9.

187. Fan M, Currie BP, Gutell RR, Ragan MA, Casadevall A. The 16S-like, 5.8S and 23S-like rRNAs of the two varieties of *Cryptococcus neoformans*: sequence, secondary structure, phylogenetic analysis and restriction fragment polymorphisms. J Med Vet Mycol 1994; 32:163–80.

188. Aoki FH, Imai T, Tanaka R, et al. New PCR primer pairs specific for *Cryptococcus neoformans* serotype A or B prepared on the basis of random amplified polymorphic DNA fingerprint pattern analyses. J Clin Microbiol 1999; 37:315–20.

189. Sorrell TC, Chen SC, Ruma P, et al. Concordance of clinical and environmental isolates of *Cryptococcus neoformans* var. *gattii* by random amplification of polymorphic DNA analysis and PCR fingerprinting. J Clin Microbiol 1996; 34:1253–60.

190. Fries BC, Chen F, Currie BP, Casadevall A. Karyotype instability in *Cryptococcus neoformans* infection. J Clin Microbiol 1996; 34:1531–4.

191. Velegraki A, Kiosses VG, Kansouzidou A, Smilakou S, Mitroussia-Ziouva A, Legakis NJ. Prospective use of RFLP analysis on amplified *Cryptococcus neoformans* URA5 gene sequences for rapid identification of varieties and serotypes in clinical samples. Med Mycol 2001; 39:409–17.

192. Chaturvedi S, Rodeghier B, Fan J, McClelland CM, Wickes BL, Chaturvedi V. Direct PCR of *Cryptococcus neoformans MAT*alpha and *MAT*a pheromones to determine mating type, ploidy, and variety: a tool for epidemiological and molecular pathogenesis studies. J Clin Microbiol 2000; 38:2007–9.

193. Polacheck I, Lebens G, Hicks JB. Development of DNA probes for early diagnosis and epidemiological study of cryptococcosis in AIDS patients. J Clin Microbiol 1992; 30:925–30.

194. Franzot SP, Fries BC, Cleare W, Casadevall A. Genetic relationship between *Cryptococcus neoformans* var. *neoformans* strains of serotypes A and D. J Clin Microbiol 1998; 36:2200–4.

195. Franzot SP, Hamdan JS, Currie BP, Casadevall A. Molecular epidemiology of *Cryptococcus neoformans* in Brazil and the United States: evidence for both local genetic differences and a global clonal population structure. J Clin Microbiol 1997; 35:2243–51.

196. Spitzer ED, Spitzer SG, Freundlich LF, Casadevall A. Persistence of initial infection in recurrent *Cryptococcus neoformans* meningitis. Lancet 1993; 341:595–6.

197. Spitzer SG, Spitzer ED. Characterization of the CNRE-1 family of repetitive DNA elements in *Cryptococcus neoformans*. Gene 1994; 144:103–6.

198. Varma A, Kwon-Chung KJ. DNA probe for strain typing of *Cryptococcus neoformans*. J Clin Microbiol 1992; 30:2960–7.

199. Garcia-Hermoso D, Mathoulin-Pelissier S, Couprie B, Ronin O, Dupont B, Dromer F. DNA typing suggests pigeon droppings as a source of pathogenic *Cryptococcus neoformans* serotype D. J Clin Microbiol 1997; 35:2683–5.

200. Varma A, Kwon-Chung KJ. Restriction fragment polymorphism in mitochondrial DNA of *Cryptococcus neoformans*. J Gen Microbiol 1989; 135:3353–62.

201. Haynes KA, Sullivan DJ, Coleman DC, et al. Involvement of multiple *Cryptococcus neoformans* strains in a single episode of cryptococcosis and reinfection with novel strains in recurrent infection demonstrated by random amplification of polymorphic DNA and DNA fingerprinting. J Clin Microbiol 1995; 33:99–102.

202. Meyer W, Mitchell TG, Freedman EZ, Vilgalys R. Hybridization probes for conventional DNA fingerprinting used as single primers in the polymerase chain reaction to distinguish strains of *Cryptococcus neoformans*. J Clin Microbiol 1993; 31:2274–80.

203. Meyer W, Mitchell TG. Polymerase chain reaction fingerprinting in fungi using single primers specific to minisatellites and simple repetitive DNA sequences: strain variation in *Cryptococcus neoformans*. Electrophoresis 1995; 16:1648–56.

204. Currie BP, Freundlich LF, Casadevall A. Restriction fragment length polymorphism analysis of *Cryptococcus neoformans* isolates from environmental (pigeon excreta) and clinical sources in New York City. J Clin Microbiol 1994; 32:1188–92.

11

A Diagnostic Approach to
Pneumocystis jiroveci Pneumonia

Abigail Orenstein

*Division of Pulmonary and Critical Care Medicine,
Department of Medicine, University of Maryland School of
Medicine, Baltimore, Maryland, U.S.A.*

Henry Masur

*Critical Care Medicine Department, National Institutes of Health,
Clinical Center, Bethesda, Maryland, U.S.A.*

INTRODUCTION

Pneumocystis jiroveci, the etiologic agent of pneumocystis infection in humans, was first described in 1909 by Carlos Chagas, who, in his study of guinea pigs, mistook the cysts for the sexual state of *Trypanosoma cruzi* (1). Several years later, the Delanoës, a husband-and-wife team of scientists, realized that the cysts were a separate entity when they found them in the lungs of Parisian sewer rats that did not have trypanosomiasis (2). They named the organism *Pneumocystis carinii* in honor of Antonio Carini, a contemporary of Chagas, even though he, too, had thought it was a trypanosome (3). Since then, pneumocystis organisms have been identified in a wide range of other host species, including humans. Not until the 1960s, however, was pneumocystis deemed a significant opportunistic pathogen in humans. With the aid of bronchoscopy in the 1970s, the organism was identified with increasing frequency in patients with malignant neoplasms and in patients with congenital or drug-induced immunosuppression. Then, in the 1980s, pneumocystis pneumonia (PCP) became widely recognized as one of the most common presenting manifestations of the Acquired Immunodeficiency Syndrome (AIDS) in North America and Europe.

With the development of more sophisticated laboratory techniques, the diagnosis of PCP can be definitively established by rapid, noninvasive methods. Focused and directed treatment can be implemented promptly, avoiding, or at least limiting, the use of unnecessary therapies that may cause adverse drug reactions (4). Overall outcome may also be improved by establishing a specific diagnosis, as was found in a retrospective analysis of 1021 AIDS patients who had been treated for PCP. Cytologic confirmation, which required bronchoscopy in the majority of cases, was associated with significantly reduced in-hospital mortality from 22% to 14% ($p < 0.01$), even after adjusting for severity of illness (5). Furthermore, in a study of 171 HIV-infected patients with 227 episodes of PCP, the case fatality rate for the 47 empirically treated episodes was significantly higher than that of the 180 cytologically proven episodes (55% vs. 18%, $p < 0.0001$) (6).

INFECTION

The inability to successfully culture human pneumocystis has limited knowledge and understanding of its biology. Unique among fungi, pneumocysts have only a single copy of the nuclear ribosomal RNA locus (7) (most fungi contain hundreds) and plasma membranes that do not contain ergosterol (8). Thus, until fairly recently, pneumocystis was classified as a protozoon. Detailed genetic analysis has since proven it to be a fungus (9). Subsequent sequencing and antigenic analysis have shown that the organisms that infect various mammalian species are distinct (10) and specific (11). Those strains that infect humans have been designated *P. jiroveci* (12), whereas *P. carinii* and *P. muris* now refer to those that infect rats and mice, respectively (13).

Numerous studies have shown that at least 85% of healthy children throughout the world develop antibodies to pneumocystis by age three years (14–16). Yet, despite this worldwide prevalence, PCP has been documented less often in developing countries than in the United States or Western Europe. Why this is the case is not entirely clear, although lack of access to diagnostic testing and deaths due to other causes (primarily tuberculosis) before a sufficient drop in CD4+ count is reached seem to be contributing factors. Another possibility is that there are less pathogenic strains of *P. jiroveci*. Nonetheless, post-mortem studies have detected pneumocystis in as many as 52% of HIV-positive infants who died from pneumonia in South Africa (17) and 67% in Zimbabwe (18).

Pneumocystis appears to be a ubiquitous organism, but how it is transmitted to humans is unknown. Without any convincing evidence that different pneumocystis species can infect more than one host species (11), *P. jiroveci* pneumonia is no longer considered a zoonosis; yet, whether the source of infection is environmental or person-to-person spread has not been resolved. In rodents, pneumocystis is transmitted via a respiratory route. Susceptible mice and rats can be infected by exposure to air directed into their holding facility from areas where infected mice or rats are housed. Intriguing case clusters suggest this route for humans, but there has been no definitive proof (19–21).

Human disease has been attributed to reactivation of latent disease acquired in childhood. There is a growing body of evidence to suggest that re-infection also takes place. Multiple reports in the literature describe patients with recurrent episodes of PCP who were found to have strains that were genotypically different from prior episodes (22–26). Genotype frequency distribution patterns have been shown to vary with place of diagnosis, not birth (27). Individuals with newly diagnosed HIV have been found to have mutant strains associated with prior use of PCP prophylaxis, despite never having received prophylaxis (28–30). Studies are ongoing to determine the relative importance of latency versus re-infection in human pneumocystis infection.

SUSCEPTIBLE PATIENT POPULATIONS

Overview

Patients with PCP have a wide variety of underlying diseases, both congenital and acquired. While most of these involve disorders in T-cell function, pure B-cell defects can also predispose to infection. In HIV-infected patients, the risk of developing PCP closely correlates with the CD4+ lymphocyte count. In the Pulmonary Complications of HIV Infection Study, 95% of 145 episodes of PCP occurred in patients with CD4+ counts less than 200 cells/μL and 79% occurred in those with counts less than 100 cells/μL (31). In other immunocompromised patients, the relationship between CD4+ counts and susceptibility to PCP is less well defined. Findings from one small study of HIV-negative individuals suggest that there may be an association. Of the 22 immunosuppressed patients diagnosed with PCP (reasons for immunosuppression: recent solid organ transplantation, chemotherapy for malignancy, systemic corticosteroids), 55% had CD4+ counts less than 100, 73% had counts less than 200, and 91% had counts less than 300 CD4+ cells/μL (32).

Although cell-mediated immunity is thought to play the predominant role in host defense against pneumocystis, individuals with antibody deficiencies do develop PCP. There is no known quantitative immunoglobulin level that marks susceptibility, but children with primary agammaglobulinemia present more often than their adult counterparts, which may be due to their concomitant immature T-cell function. Animal models suggest that the humoral arm of the immune system is necessary, but not sufficient, for the host to resist and recover from PCP. In adoptive transfer experiments using mice with severe combined immuno-deficiency (SCID) and PCP, investigators found that those who were given infusions of B-cell depleted thymus or spleen cells did not resolve their infection (33). The precise role B cells play in host defense against pneumocystis is uncertain.

Patients with disorders of neutrophils are not considered to be at increased risk and, yet, there are a few case reports in the literature of PCP in patients with chronic granulomatous disease (34,35), underscoring the fact that our under-standing of the immunology of pneumocystis is far from complete.

HIV

Eighty to 90% of cases of PCP in HIV-infected patients occur in those with CD4+ lymphocyte counts less than 200 cells/μL (36). Patients with counts less than 200 cells/μL have an approximately five times higher risk of developing PCP than those with counts greater than 200 cells/μL (37). Other risk factors, independent of CD4+ count, include a history of non-PCP AIDS-related illness, a previous episode of pneumonia of any type, oral thrush, and high viral load (38,39).

Malignancy, Organ Transplantation, and Immunosuppressive Therapy

PCP in patients with cancer or post-transplantation is almost always a result of immunosuppressive therapy. Hence, the principal determinants of risk are the intensity and duration of immunosuppression. Corticosteroids and cyclosporine, both of which have inhibitory effects on T lymphocytes, are among the agents most closely associated with pneumocystis infection. Other agents that specifically target T cells are tacrolimus (FK506) and monoclonal anti-T cell antibodies, e.g., OKT3 and alefuzamab (CAMPATH). Cytotoxic drugs, e.g., methotrexate, cyclophosphamide, fluorouracil, and cytarabine, have been implicated as well, but their mechanism of suppression is not well understood (Table 1).

CLINICAL PRESENTATION

Pulmonary

There is no clinical presentation pathognomonic for PCP. The diagnosis should be considered in any immunocompromised patient with a nonproductive cough and dyspnea. Although pleuritic chest pain is unusual (except in association with a pneumothorax), substernal chest tightness is a frequent complaint. The absence of any of these signs or symptoms, however, does not rule out the possibility of PCP. Even the chest exam may be remarkably normal without adventitious breath sounds.

PCP presents more subtly in AIDS patients as opposed to other immunocompromised hosts. Whereas other immunocompromised hosts tend to present with acute illness, several days after symptom onset, AIDS patients' symptoms may be so mild as to be ignored for weeks to months. This is especially problematic in those unaware of their HIV status, as this may significantly delay their pursuit of medical attention (Table 2).

Extrapulmonary

Pneumocystis can disseminate to virtually any anatomic site, yet it is unusual to have extrapulmonary disease that is clinically important. The most frequent reports of extrapulmonary pneumocystosis involve the liver, lymph

Table 1 Patients at Risk for Pneumocystis Pneumonia

Risk factor	Associated with highest risk	Estimated rates without prophylaxis
HIV	CD4 + count < 200 cells/μL	> 75%
Immune deficiencies	SCID	> 20%
Hematologic Malignancies	ALL in children HD	10–25%
Allogeneic SCT	1st 30–100 days Severe GVHD	5–15%
Autologous SCT	Intense conditioning CAMPATH	Rare
Solid tumors	Rhabdomyosarcoma Brain tumor[a]	> 20%
Solid transplants	1st 6 months Lung Heart	5–15%
Immunosuppressive therapy	Taper or discontinuation Long-term systemic corticosteroids[b] and cytotoxic agent(s) Underlying immunologic disorder Wegener's granulomatosis	Unknown
Protein—calorie malnutrition	Premature infants	Unknown

[a] Brain tumor may be primary or metastatic. Risk related to use of high-dose dexamethasone.
[b] Long-term usually defined as greater than 1-month duration.
Abbreviations: ALL, acute lymphocytic leukemia; CAMPATH, alefuzamab; HD, Hodgkin's disease; SCID, severe combined immunodeficiency; SCT, stem-cell transplant.

nodes, spleen, and bone marrow. Less common sites are the eye, gastrointestinal tract, ear canal, skin, nasopharynx, trachea, adrenals, genitourinary system, pituitary, meninges, cerebral cortex, thyroid, pancreas, heart, omentum, thymus, and muscle. Extrapulmonary pneumocystosis can be clinically silent or present

Table 2 Differences in Clinical Presentation

Signs and symptoms at presentation	Patients with AIDS ($n=49$)	Patients with other immunosuppressive diseases ($n=39$)
Duration of symptoms prior to presentation: median number of days (range)	28 (1–270)	5 (1–42)
Fever (%)	81	87
Temperature $\geq 38.0°C$ (%)	76	92
Median respiratory rate per minute (range)	24 (14–40)	26 (16–60)
PaO$_2$ on room air (mmHg)	69	52

Source: Adapted from Ref. 4.

as a nonspecific debilitating illness, which may be overlooked in the absence of pulmonary symptoms. Aerosolized pentamidine has been theorized as a possible risk factor for dissemination, but, to date, studies have been inconclusive (40).

DIAGNOSIS

Overview

Since *P. jiroveci* cannot be propagated in vitro, alternative strategies must be used to definitively establish the organism as the cause of disease. Until recently, this required visualization of the organism in the host, stained by any one of a number of methods. Evolving molecular techniques have begun to provide another option.

Although the spectrum of histopathology due to PCP is similar among immunocompromised hosts, in HIV-infected patients there is often a surprising discordance between severity of illness and number of organisms. That is, despite their subtle and often subacute presentation, patients with AIDS and PCP tend to have a higher organism burden, although this does not necessarily predict a worse outcome (4). In fact, in examining bronchoalveolar lavage (BAL) fluid from a series of 75 patients with PCP, Limper and colleagues found greater numbers of neutrophils in the lungs of those without AIDS, which correlated with poorer oxygenation and poorer survival, despite a lower organism burden than was seen in the lungs of patients with AIDS (41). In this study, the patients with HIV-related PCP had fewer BAL neutrophils, which was thought to explain their higher arterial oxygen tensions. The investigators concluded that inflammation contributes substantially to respiratory impairment in PCP. Other studies have confirmed the predictive value of BAL neutrophilia. One retrospective analysis of 144 patients with AIDS determined that the presence of an increased proportion of BAL neutrophils (greater than 10%) was an independent risk factor for 90-day mortality and significantly correlated with the occurrence of pneumothorax and the need for mechanical ventilation (42).

Blood Tests and Exercise Pulse Oximetry

Lactate Dehydrogenase

At present, there is no blood test specific for pneumocystis. While lactate dehydrogenase (LDH) is frequently elevated in patients with PCP and may reflect the severity of pulmonary dysfunction, many other pathologic entities increase LDH levels, including multiple other etiologies of lung damage in immunocompromised patients. Moreover, a normal LDH does not exclude the diagnosis of PCP. A retrospective analysis of LDH values in a cohort of 54 HIV-infected patients treated for PCP found that 93% had elevated LDH levels, 7% had normal values, and gradual decreases in serial measurements predicted survival, while rising values predicted death (43).

Arterial Blood Gas

As dyspnea is a common clinical feature of PCP, abnormalities are frequently detected on arterial blood gas (ABG) analysis. In Kovacs and colleagues' study comparing the presentation of PCP in patients with and without HIV, normal room air arterial oxygen tension (i.e., PaO_2 of 80 mmHg or greater) was found in a minority of both groups of patients (20% in those with AIDS and 10% of those with other immunosuppressive diseases) (4). However, hypoxemia on ABG, similar to an elevated LDH, cannot reliably be used to rule in or rule out PCP. Rather, ABG abnormalities serve as markers of the severity of lung inflammation and injury. In a retrospective analysis of HIV-infected patients with PCP ($n = 94$), early fatal outcome was 17 times more likely with an alveolar to arterial oxygen (A–a) gradient greater than 35 mmHg (44). With such severe impairment in gas exchange, the fact that the addition of steroids improves outcome should come as little surprise.

Exercise Pulse Oximetry

In lieu of obtaining an ABG, exercise pulse oximetry may provide similarly useful, but non-specific data. A retrospective review of HIV-infected patients with pneumonia found that exertional dyspnea plus interstitial infiltrate were the most useful variables for differentiating PCP from bacterial pneumonia and pulmonary tuberculosis (45). In a study of HIV-infected patients who presented to the hospital with cough, fever, or exertional dyspnea, 85% of those with biopsy proven PCP desaturated with exercise as compared to only 10% of those with other chest disorders, e.g., bacterial pneumonia (46). Perhaps even more interesting is the fact that more than half of the patients with PCP who desaturated had normal resting arterial oxygen pressures, as well as normal chest radiographs. In another study, a decrease in oxygen saturation of only three points was 100% sensitive for PCP and 77% specific (47). Thus, exercise pulse oximetry may help identify patients in need of further work-up for possible PCP, but cannot be used alone to make the diagnosis.

Serum Enzyme-Linked Immunosorbent Assay

Although a high quality quantitative serum enzyme-linked immunosorbent assay (ELISA) has been developed using a recombinant *P. jiroveci* antigen, reactivity is unlikely to have any diagnostic utility since most adults are seropositive. In the small number of HIV-positive patients with PCP who have been studied, no consistent pattern of antibody response was seen. Patterns of persistent increase were observed in a few healthy persons, which may have reflected recent exposure (48). At present, it is unclear whether the absence of anti-pneumocystis IgG antibodies would be evidence against the diagnosis of PCP.

Polymerase Chain Reaction

The diagnostic value of polymerase chain reaction (PCR) for serum is not yet well delineated. One small study of 15 HIV-infected patients with clinically active PCP was unable to detect any DNA in blood by PCR prior to therapy (49), while another ($n = 14$) found positive results in 71%, which was reduced to 0% after they received a mean of 8.8 days of treatment (50). The discrepancy between these two studies may be explained by the effect of transient dissemination of pneumocystis organisms into the blood, given that the diagnostic yield in an additional study increased from 10% to 67% when only cases of disseminated pneumocystosis were sought (51).

Pulmonary Function Tests

Pulmonary function tests (PFTs) provide data regarding the presence of pulmonary dysfunction, but there is no abnormality specific for PCP. The diffusing capacity of the lung for carbon monoxide (DLCO) is the most common abnormality associated with PCP. An abnormal DLCO, when defined as less than 75% of the predicted value, has a reported sensitivity of 89% to 100% for PCP (52–54). Since reduced levels are also seen in other respiratory diseases, as well as intravenous drug users, this test is non-specific.

Radiology

Chest Radiography

The most typical chest radiograph associated with PCP shows symmetric, bilateral increased interstitial markings, but a substantial number of patients will have atypical findings. Normal chest radiographs have been reported in as many as 39% of cases, although they are more commonly seen in HIV-infected patients than in non-HIV patients (55). Consolidation, lymphadenopathy, cavitation, nodular lesions, and pleural effusions are uncommon, but have been attributed to PCP. A spontaneous pneumothorax in a patient with HIV should be presumed to be due to PCP until proven otherwise (56,57). Pneumatoceles (air-filled cysts), which are being seen with increased frequency, are often the precursor. Pneumothoraces and upper-lobe disease are probably more common in patients on aerosolized pentamidine.

High-Resolution Chest Computerized Tomography

"Patchy ground-glass" is the most characteristic appearance of PCP seen on high-resolution chest computerized tomography (HRCT). One small study ($n = 53$) found that the presence of ground-glass opacities was 90% accurate in diagnosing BAL-proven PCP with a sensitivity of 100% and a specificity of 89% (58). Many clinicians use HRCT to determine the need for bronchoscopy in patients with equivocal clinical findings.

Gallium Scintigraphy

Gallium scans are based on the principle that gallium-67 (^{67}Ga) citrate concentrates in areas of inflammation, infection, and tumor, which may not be visible on radiograph. The most common pattern seen in PCP is of diffuse radionuclide uptake in the lungs with a sparing of the heart. In patients who have received aerosolized pentamidine, uptake tends to be more localized to the apices, where the drug often fails to reach.

A useful, though somewhat expensive, screening tool (sensitivity up to 100%), a positive gallium scan can suggest pulmonary pathology well before radiographic abnormalities appear, but provides little in the way of distinguishing among potential etiologies (specificity 20%). Use of a graded score (1–4), instead of simply "normal" or "abnormal," can improve specificity markedly ($\geq 80\%$), as can a radiolabeled monoclonal antibody (immunoscintigraphy) directed against *P. jiroveci* (59). The latter technique has the added advantage of being more rapid (less than 24 hours) to complete, whereas standard gallium scans require a delay of at least 48 hours, but may require as long as 72 hours (60).

Diethylenetriamine Pentaacetate Scanning

Measuring the lung clearance of aerosolized diethylenetriamine pentaacetate (DTPA) labeled with radioactive technetium-99m (^{99m}Tc) is a sensitive way of identifying alveolar damage, permitting the detection of subtle abnormalities before they become apparent on chest radiograph. ^{99m}Tc-DTPA clearance is increased in patients with PCP due to increased alveolar-capillary membrane permeability. Although DTPA clearance is increased in a number of conditions, including smoking, with PCP the pattern is characteristically biphasic. The sensitivity and specificity of this test can be as high as 100% (61,62). The disadvantages with this technique, as with gallium scanning, are time and cost. In addition, to perform DTPA scanning, the nuclear medicine department must have a gamma camera, as well as experienced personnel to interpret the results, neither of which may be readily available.

Respiratory Samples

Specimen Acquisition

Tissue biopsy: *Open or Percutaneous (Closed).* Prior to the AIDS epidemic, diagnosis of PCP typically involved open lung biopsy (OLB). Now, OLB is performed when bronchoscopy cannot be safely performed or when a preceding bronchoscopic procedure is nondiagnostic, which is more likely to be the case in non–HIV-immunocompromised patients due to their lower organism burden. Due to the significant morbidity associated with OLB, the procedure is reserved for the evaluation of unusual manifestations or when other diagnoses are strongly considered (e.g., Kaposi's sarcoma). If there is a peripheral lesion, video-assisted thoracoscopic surgery (VATS) may be employed instead of conventional thoracotomy. Percutaneous biopsy with or without CT-guidance, e.g., fine needle aspiration, may obviate the need for an open procedure, but obtains a smaller sample of tissue.

Transbronchial.   With transbronchial biopsy (TBB), multiple specimens can be obtained using a fiberoptic bronchoscope. Under fluoroscopic guidance, the diagnostic yield approaches 100% with a 5% to 10% incidence of pneumothorax (63–65). Nonetheless, in diagnosing PCP, TBB, which samples only a few alveoli, provides marginal advantage over bronchoalveolar lavage, which samples over a million alveoli. TBB does, however, increase the overall yield for other diagnoses such as CMV and should be considered if the BAL is non-diagnostic or if the patient fails to improve following a BAL-based diagnosis (65,66).

TBB is generally performed under the guidance of fluoroscopy. Diagnostic yield is thereby increased, particularly if the radiologic abnormality is focal (67), while also decreasing the risk of pneumothorax and hemorrhage. Contraindications to TBB are mechanical ventilation, pulmonary hypertension, and bleeding diatheses.

Bronchial washings and brushings: The bronchoscope may also be used to obtain bronchial washings (BWs) or brushings (BBs). The diagnostic yield of both BWs and BBs is highly variable, ranging from 30% to 70% (64,68,69). In a retrospective review of 35 AIDS patients with PCP, the sensitivity of BWs was 55% and BBs 39% (70). Consequently, these techniques are rarely used anymore to establish a diagnosis of PCP.

BWs are the pooled samples from the airways collected during the entire bronchoscopy. When compared with lavage fluid (obtained immediately after instilling saline), BWs have a lower diagnostic yield for pneumocystis even if they include post-BAL material. In contrast, BBs may improve the diagnostic yield of BAL, but at the added risk of bleeding and pneumothorax (71).

Bronchoalveolar lavage: Bronchoscopy with bronchoalveolar lavage samples approximately one million alveoli. Remembering that PCP is an alveolar process (the organism attaches to the surface of pneumocytes), the similarity in cellular composition of lavage fluid to that found in OLB specimens is to be expected. BAL has become the diagnostic procedure with which all others are compared. When performed properly, this technique rarely misses cases of PCP, particularly if both lungs are sampled (bilateral BAL) or if sampling is directed towards the sites of greatest involvement (site-directed BAL) (72,73). Sensitivities range from 85% to more than 98% (65,69,70,74–76). In patients who have received aerosolized pentamidine prophylaxis, regardless of radiographic findings, BAL should include at least one upper lobe (77–79).

Like TBB, BAL is usually obtained using a flexible fiberoptic bronchoscope and requires the expertise of a bronchoscopist. BAL is an invasive, time-consuming, and expensive procedure, but generally well tolerated without complications. BAL can be performed in patients with thrombocytopenia (i.e., less than 50,000 platelets/μL) or other bleeding problems. Rarely, individuals will develop fever, transient hypoxemia, or over-sedation afterwards.

Other devices have been designed to be reasonably priced, readily available alternatives. The Ballard BAL catheter, unlike the fiberoptic bronchoscope, is inexpensive, disposable, and easy to use. The Ballard catheter is introduced through the selected naris and advanced blindly past the vocal cords. However, without direct visualization, non-bronchoscopic BAL is only appropriate if there is a diffuse disease process in at least one lung. In such situations, the Ballard BAL catheter has been shown to perform as well as bronchoscopic BAL in the quality of the sample and diagnostic utility for PCP (80,81). In practice, however, the Ballard catheter is seldom used to establish a diagnosis of PCP. Pulmonologists and intensivists generally prefer a bronchoscope, and those less experienced in bronchoscopy should probably avoid the Ballard catheter unless they are competent to manage acute laryngospasm.

For both the fiberoptic bronchoscope and the Ballard BAL catheter, the technique is the same; the device is wedged into a subsegmental bronchus (usually in the right middle lobe) and varying amounts of sterile normal saline (100–280 mL in 10–60 mL aliquots) are instilled and immediately suctioned back into a sterile trap. Approximately 50%, or at least 30 to 40 mL, of the instilled volume is recovered. The specimen is then centrifuged and the resulting pellet is smeared, air dried, and prepared for staining.

Expectorated sputum: Expectorated sputum has a low sensitivity (10–30%) in the diagnosis of PCP (82). This should not be surprising given that there are very few pneumocystis organisms in the upper respiratory tract and that the majority of patients with PCP have a non-productive cough. The sensitivity may be improved with the use of a direct fluorescent antibody, but has not been shown to exceed 55% in HIV-positive patients (83,84).

Induced sputum: To induce sputum, the patient inhales hypertonic (3%) saline solution from a high-flow nebulizer for 15 to 30 minutes and is then asked to cough. Sputum induction is a noninvasive, safe, inexpensive, and quick procedure that does not require specialized personnel, specifically engineered rooms, or expensive equipment to obtain. In some health care settings, sputum induction is rarely diagnostic. Poor quality specimens are often to blame. Contamination with food or cellular debris and insufficient volume may be contributing factors. Acquiring an adequate induced sputum (IS) specimen relies not only on the respiratory therapist, but also on the active participation of the patient, which depending on his or her condition may not be possible. The procedure is poorly tolerated in a patient with altered mental status, severe dyspnea, or bronchospasm. (Adequate specimens usually require at least one alveolar macrophage and less than 25 epithelial cells/LPF.) Also, a technologist accustomed to reading BAL specimens may have difficulty with an IS specimen, which has relatively few pneumocystis organisms and an abundance of upper-airway flora (85,86). For these reasons, the diagnostic yield from specimens of IS is largely institution dependent.

Initially, centers reported diagnostic yields of approximately 55% with sputum induction (87–89). Enhancements, such as concentrating the sputum by mucolysis or liquefaction, have improved them to as high as 74% to 78% (90,91) with conventional stains, 95% with fluorescent antibody stains (92), and 98% to 100% with PCR (93,94). The yield remains lower in patients who have received aerosolized pentamidine prophylaxis, but sputum induction should still be attempted (95,96).

Oral wash: Though PCP is characteristically an alveolar disease, sufficient organisms reach the oropharynx to be detected by highly sensitive PCR methods. Accordingly, oral wash offers an alternative to sputum induction, while requiring much less commitment and coordination to obtain an adequate specimen. The patient gargles approximately 10 mL of sterile saline for one minute and then rinses.

Utilizing PCR, oral washes have been shown to achieve a sensitivity as high as 91% and a specificity of 100% (50,97–100). However, most of these studies looked only at patients with HIV and those that included other populations did not stratify their results. The one small study that did look at patients with hematologic malignancies ($n = 26$), though, found PCR on oral washes to perform just as well with a sensitivity and specificity of 100% (101).

Studies are ongoing to define factors that may diminish the diagnostic utility of oral washes, such as quality and quantity of specimens, cough, and severity of PCP. Larsen and colleagues have already found that prior treatment for only one day can lead to a statistically significant ($p < 0.0001$) decrease in sensitivity (99).

Organism Identification

Tinctorial stains: In spite of extensive efforts, a reliable in vitro system for cultivation of *P. jiroveci* does not exist. As a result, tinctorial staining has been the method most relied on to identify organisms in respiratory specimens. Although each technique has its own sensitivity, specificity, speed, and cost, the tinctorial stains can be divided into two broad categories for the sake of comparison: (*i*) cyst wall selective stains and (*ii*) "indirect" or non-cyst wall selective stains. Persistence of organisms detected by tinctorial stains in a treated host does not necessarily indicate treatment failure since both viable and nonviable organisms are stained.

Cyst Wall Stains.   With the cyst wall stains, cysts in different stages of development can be visualized. When the organism burden is low, these stains appear to be more sensitive than indirect ones. The stains include Gomori's methenamine silver (GMS), toluidine blue O, cresyl echt violet, Gram–Weigert, periodic acid-Schiff (PAS), and calcifluor white. In general, these stains can be performed in less than two hours and analyzed rapidly with minimal expertise. The GMS stain, with its high background staining, requires more expertise in interpreting, as yeast and fungal elements can be confused with pneumocysts.

The same can be said for the toluidine blue O and calcofluor white (viewed under a fluorescent microscope) stains, although at least with the latter the pneumocysts' highly characteristic staining pattern aids in their rapid recognition.

Indirect Stains. Although trophozoite forms can occasionally be stained with the Gram–Weigert and PAS techniques, true "indirect" stains are primarily taken up by non-cyst forms, i.e., intracystic bodies (sporozoites) and (extracystic) trophozoites. Cysts can be visualized by their inability to take up stain and therefore appear "negatively" stained. Indirect stains can be performed more rapidly than the direct stains, but require more time and experience to interpret more information, although adequate skill can be achieved without extensive training. Care must be taken so as to not confuse organisms with host cells and debris; neutrophils entrapped in mucus can appear to be clusters of organisms. However, if correctly identified, the presence of neutrophils can be helpful in assessing prognosis. Wright–Giemsa, the prototypical indirect stain, can be completed within 30 minutes. A modified version, Diff-Quik, is inexpensive and takes only several minutes to prepare. Polychrome methylene blue is another indirect stain, although not commonly used.

Other Stains. Smears stained by the routine Papanicolaou method can be used with or without a fluorescent microscope to identify pneumocystis. Using this method, an experienced cytopathologist may be able to distinguish organisms from smoker's pigment, red blood cells, and mucus, while also identifying associated infections and cellular changes.

Direct and indirect fluorescent antibody stains: The development of antibody-directed fluorescent stains has resulted in a rapid (1–2 hours), sensitive, and relatively simple way to diagnose PCP. Direct and Indirect Fluorescent Antibody (DFA and IFA) stains have the added advantage of being able to reliably stain extrapulmonary tissue (102). Whereas the IFA stain usually relies on the use of polyclonal antibodies, the DFA technique employs a monoclonal antibody, the specificity of which determines what will be stained. Potentially, all developmental stages, i.e., both cysts and trophozoites, can be seen, rendering fluorescent stains more sensitive than conventional cytochemical stains for both BAL fluid and IS specimens. In practice, this difference is only significant for the latter (77,85).

PCR: With the application of PCR assays, the sensitivity of IS (51,94, 103) and even oral washes (97–100,104) may reach that of BAL, permitting the routine use of less invasive means for diagnosis. However, a bronchoscopy with BAL may still be necessary to diagnose other respiratory diseases that may present concomitantly.

While differences in patient population, PCR technique, and study design make comparing the data from varied clinical studies difficult, protocols targeting the major surface glycoprotein (MSG) gene (105), a gene which belongs to a multi-copy gene family, have been the most sensitive. (More so than those that use the mitochondrial ribosomal RNA gene, another multi-copy target.) Furthermore, at least for diagnostic purposes, single-round touchdown

PCR (TD-PCR) seems to be superior to nested PCR (106). Although they have not been compared head-to-head, given that nested PCR requires at least two rounds of amplification, an inherently greater risk of contamination and false positive results is to be expected.

Studies have begun to specifically examine the diagnostic yield of PCR when used on symptomatic immunosuppressed patients without HIV infection. One such study looked at nested PCR on BAL specimens from 63 HIV-positive patients and 128 non–HIV-immunosuppressed patients and found no difference in sensitivity (100% in both groups), but a significant decline in the positive predictive value (PPV) of the assay in the non-HIV patients. Whereas the PPV was 96% in the HIV-positive patients, it was less than 40% in the other patients (107). These results may, in part, reflect the loss of specificity that can be seen when using PCR on BAL (108) and, also, the lower prevalence of PCP in the non–HIV-immunosuppressed population.

While a negative PCR result has reasonable power to rule out PCP, a positive PCR result must be carefully interpreted in the context of clinical findings (97). A positive result may reflect the recent administration of therapy or subclinical infection, some of which may become clinically significant. Alternatively, a positive result may represent colonization (105,109–111). Modifications employing a cut-off value, as well as assays which can distinguish viable from non-viable organisms, show promise in improving specificity (112,113). With further validation, a quantitative PCR assay will likely come into widespread clinical use for making the diagnosis of pneumocystis infection.

A CLINICAL APPROACH

Diagnostic Work-Up

PCP should be included in the differential diagnosis of any high-risk patient with new or worsening respiratory symptoms, or simply unexplained fever. Among HIV-infected patients, greatest attention should be focused on those with CD4 + lymphocyte counts less than or equal to 200 cells/μL. Among patients with other types of immunocompromise, those who have received prolonged courses of high-dose corticosteroid therapy should be considered especially (Fig. 1).

When to Repeat Bronchoscopy

Regardless of the etiology of immunosuppression, if a patient with confirmed PCP fails to improve or worsens after 4 to 8 days of therapy, a repeat bronchos-copy can be useful. Although repeat bronchoscopy will allow a histologic assessment of response to therapy, the main purpose should be to look for other, previously undiagnosed, pathogens. In a review of 420 HIV-infected patients diagnosed with PCP by BAL, 18% were found to have at least one other organism (114). In another study, 67 AIDS patients with pulmonary disease (37 of whom had PCP) underwent repeat bronchoscopy due to persistent or recurrent infiltrates

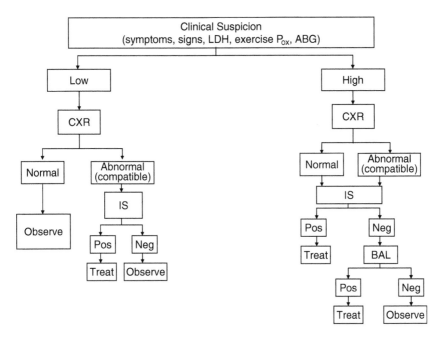

Figure 1 Algorithm for the approach to the diagnosis of pneumocystis pneumonia. *Abbreviations*: ABG, arterial blood gas; BAL, bronchoalveolar lavage; pos, positive; neg, negative; CXR, chest radiograph; IS, induced sputum; LDH, lactate dehydrogenase; P_{ox}, oxygen saturation.

despite therapy. A new treatable diagnosis was found in 28 (42%) (115). If a repeat bronchoscopy is done, if possible, a TBB should be performed as well.

Concomitant Pathogens

Cytomegalovirus

In bone marrow and lung transplant patients in whom cytomegalovirus (CMV) pneumonia is a major cause of morbidity and mortality, viral isolation from BAL fluid has been shown to correlate with active or soon-to-be active clinical disease. In HIV-infected patients, however, the role CMV plays is unclear. Frequently grown from BAL fluid, even when asymptomatic, the clinical significance of a positive CMV culture, particularly in the context of a confirmed diagnosis of pneumocystis, is doubted (116). In fact, a retrospective study of 112 AIDS patients found no survival difference between patients with PCP alone and dual (PCP and CMV) pulmonary infection (117). If a patient with PCP is not responding appropriately to therapy, obtaining transbronchial biopsies for the evaluation of viral cytopathic effect may assist in making a decision whether to treat CMV.

Mycobacterium avium Complex

Especially in the United States, *M. avium* complex (MAC) is frequently cultured from respiratory samples of AIDS patients with CD4+ lymphocyte counts less than 100 cells/μL. Yet, without evidence of disseminated disease, MAC virtually never causes isolated pulmonary disease and may be considered a respiratory colonizer.

CONCLUSION

Among susceptible patients, pneumocystis continues to be a significant opportunistic pathogen. Experience gained over the last 20 years of the AIDS epidemic has led to improved outcomes, in part, because of the ability to make a definitive diagnosis by more rapid and less invasive means. Molecular techniques have made diagnosis from even non-invasive, upper respiratory samples possible. Given the ease of specimen acquisition and high diagnostic yield, the degree to which this technology is utilized will, undoubtedly, increase. Moreover, with further research and refinements, perhaps PCR detection of pneumocystis in serum or blood samples will achieve diagnostic utility, eliminating the need for respiratory specimens of any kind to confirm a clinical suspicion of *P. jiroveci* pneumonia.

REFERENCES

1. Chagas C. Nova tripanomiaza humana. Estudos sobre a morfolojia e o ciclo evolutivo do Schiztrypanum cruzi n. gen., n. sp. ajente etiolojico de nova entidade morbida do homen. Mem Inst Oswaldo Cruz 1909; 1:159–218.
2. Delanoe P, Delanoe M. Sur les rapports des kystes *Pneumocystis carinii* du poumon des rats avec Trypanosoma lewisi. C R Acad Sci (Paris) 1912; 155:658–60.
3. Carini A. Formas de eschizogonia do *Typanosoma lewisi*. Soc Med Ci Sao Paulo 1910; 38:8.
4. Kovacs JA, Hiemenz JW, Macher AM, et al. *Pneumocystis carinii* pneumonia— a comparison between patients with the acquired immunodeficiency syndrome and patients with other immunodeficiencies. Ann Intern Med 1984; 100:663–71.
5. Bennett CL, Horner RD, Weinstein RA, et al. Empirically treated *Pneumocystis carinii* pneumonia in Los Angeles, Chicago, and Miami: 1987–1990. J Infect Dis 1995; 172:312–5.
6. Beck EJ, French PD, Helbert MH, et al. Empirically treated *Pneumocystis carinii* pneumonia in London, 1983–1989. Int J STD AIDS 1992; 3:285–7.
7. Tang X, Bartlett MS, Smith JW, Lu J, Lee C. Determination of copy number of rRNA genes in *Pneumocystis carinii* f. sp. hominis. J Clin Microbiol 1998; 36:2492–3.
8. Kaneshiro ES, Ellis JE, Jayasimhulu K, Beach DH. Evidence for the presence of "metabolic sterols" in Pneumocystis: identification and initial characterization of *Pneumocystis carinii* sterols. J Eukaryot Microbiol 1994; 41:78–85.

9. Edman JC, Kovacs JA, Masur H, Santi SV, Elwood HJ, Sogin ML. Ribosomal RNA sequence shows *Pneumocystis carinii* to be a member of the fungi. Nature 1988; 334:519–22.

10. Sinclair K, Wakefield AE, Banerji S, Hopkin JM. *Pneumocystis carinii* organisms derived from rat and human hosts are distinct. Mol Biochem Parasitol 1991; 45:183–4.

11. Gigliotti F, Harmsen AG, Haidaris CG, Haidaris PJ. *Pneumocystis carinii* is not universally transmissible between mammalian species. Infect Immun 1993; 51:2886–90.

12. Stringer JR, Beard CB, Miller RF, Wakefield AE. A new name (*Pneumocystis jiroveci*) for pneumocystis from humans. Emerg Infect Dis 2002; 8:891–6.

13. Stringer JR, Cushion MT, Wakefield AE. New nomenclature for the genus Pneumocystis. J Eukaryot Microbiol 2001; 49(Suppl.):184S–9.

14. Peglow SL, Smulian AG, Linke MJ, et al. Serologic responses to *Pneumocystis carinii* antigens in health and disease. J Infect Dis 1990; 161:296–306.

15. Vargas SL, Hughes WT, Santolaya ME, et al. Search for a primary infection by *Pneumocystis carinii* in a cohort of normal, healthy infants. CID 2001; 32:855–61.

16. Meuwisswen JHET, Tauber I, Leeuwenberg ADEM, Beckers PJA, Sieben M. Parasitologic and serologic observations of infection with Pneumocystis in humans. J Infect Dis 1977; 136:43–9.

17. Jeena PM, Coovadia HM, Chrystal V. *Pneumocystis carinii* and cytomegalovirus infections in severely ill, HIV-infected African infants. Ann Trop Paediatr 1996; 16:361–8.

18. Nathoo KJ, Gondo M, Gwanzura L, Mhlanga BR, Mavetera T, Mason PR. Fatal *Pneumocystis carinii* pneumonia in HIV-seropositive infants in Harare, Zimbabwe. Trans R Soc Trop Med Hyg 2001; 95:37–9.

19. Chave JP, David S, Wauters JP, Van Melle G, Rancioli P. Transmission of *Pneumocystis carinii* from AIDS patients to other immunosuppressed patients: a cluster of *Pneumocystis carinii* pneumonia in renal transplant recipients. AIDS 1991; 5:927–32.

20. Goesch TR, Gotz G, Stellbrinck KH, Albrecht H, Weh HJ, Hossfeld DK. Possible transfer of *Pneumocystis carinii* between immunodeficient patients. Lancet 1990; 336:627.

21. Bensousan T, Garo B, Islam S, Bourbigot B, Cledes J, Garre M. Possible transfer of *Pneumocystis carinii* between kidney transplant recipients. Lancet 1990; 336:1066–7.

22. Latouche S, Poirot JL, Bernard C, Roux P. Study of internal transcribed spacer and mitochondrial large-subunit genes of *Pneumocystis carinii* hominis isolated by repeated bronchoalveolar lavage from human immunodeficiency virus-infected patients during one or several episodes of pneumonia. J Clin Microbiol 1997; 35:1687–90.

23. Keely SP, Baughman RP, Smulian AG, Dohn MN, Stringer JR. Source of *Pneumocystis carinii* in recurrent episodes of pneumonia in AIDS patients. AIDS 1996; 10:881–8.

24. Keely SP, Stringer JR, Baughman RP, Linke MJ, Walzer PD, Smulian AG. Genetic variation among *Pneumocystis carinii* hominis isolated in recurrent pneumocystosis. J Infect Dis 1995; 172:595–8.

25. Tsolaki AG, Miller F, Underwood AP, Banerji S, Wakefield AE. Genetic diversity at the internal transcribed spacer regions of the rRNA operon among isolates of *Pneumocystis carinii* from AIDS patients with recurrent pneumonia. J Infect Dis 1996; 174:14–156.

26. Keely SP, Stringer JR. Sequences of *Pneumocystis carinii* f. sp. hominis strains associated with recurrent pneumonia vary at multiple loci. J Clin Microbiol 1997; 35:2745–7.

27. Beard CB, Carter JL, Keely SP, et al. Genetic variation in *Pneumocystis carinii* isolates from different geographic regions: implications for transmission. Emerg Infect Dis 2000; 6:265–72.

28. Kazanjian P, Armstrong W, Hossler PA, et al. *Pneumocystis carinii* mutations are associated with duration of sulfa or sulfone prophylaxis exposure in AIDS patients. J Infect Dis 2000; 182:551–7.

29. Huang L, Beard CB, Creasman J, et al. Sulfa or sulfone prophylaxis and geographic region predict mutations in the *Pneumocystis carinii* dihydropteroate synthase gene. J Infect Dis 2000; 182:1192–8.

30. Crothers K, Huang L, Morris A, et al. Pneumocystis dihydropteroate synthase mutations in patients with Pneumocystis pneumonia who are newly diagnosed with HIV infection. J Eukaryot Microbiol 2003; 50(Suppl.):609–10.

31. Stansell JD, Osmond DH, Charlebois E, et al. Pulmonary complications of HIV infection study group. Predictors of Pneumocystis carinii pneumonia in HIV-infected persons. Am J Respir Crit Care Med 1997; 155:60–6.

32. Mansharamani NG, Balachandran D, Vernovsky I, Garland R, Koziel H. Peripheral CD4+ counts during *Pneumocystis carinii* pneumonia in immunocompromised patients without HIV infection. Chest 2000; 118:712–20.

33. Harmsen AG, Stankiewicz M. T cells are not sufficient for resistance to Pneumocystis carinii pneumonia in mice. J Protozool 1991; 38:44–5S.

34. Pedersen FK, Johansen KS, Rosenkvist J, Tygstrup I, Valerius NH. Refractory Pneumocystis carinii infection in chronic granulomatous disease: successful treatment with granulocytes. Pediatrics 1979; 64:935–8.

35. Adinoff AD, Johnston RB, Dolen J, South MA. Chronic granulomatous disease and *Pneumocystis carinii* pneumonia. Pediatrics 1982; 69:133–4.

36. Masur H, Ognibene FP, Yarchoan R, et al. CD4 counts as predictors of opportunistic pneumonias in human immunodeficiency virus (HIV) infection. Ann Intern Med 1989; 111:223–31.

37. Phair J, Munoz A, Detels R, Kaslow R, Rinaldo C, Saah A. The risk of *Pneumocystis carinii* pneumonia among men infected with human immunodeficiency virus type 1. Multicenter AIDS Cohort Study Group. N Engl J Med 1990; 322:161–5.

38. Kaplan JE, Hanson DL, Navin TR, Jones JL. Risk factors for primary *Pneumocystis carinii* pneumonia in human immunodeficiency virus-infected adolescents and adults in the United States: reassessment of indications for chemoprophylaxis. J Infect Dis 1998; 178:1126–32.

39. Kaplan JE, Hanson DL, Jones JL, Dworkin MS. Viral load as an independent risk factor for opportunistic infections in HIV-infected adults and adolescents. AIDS 2001; 15:1831–6.

40. Cohen OJ, Stoeckle MY. Extrapulmonary *Pneumocystis carinii* infections in the acquired immunodeficiency syndrome. Arch Intern Med 1991; 151:1205–14.

41. Limper AH, Offord KP, Smith TF, Martin WJ, II. Pneumocystis carinii pneumonia: differences in lung parasite number and inflammation in patients with and without AIDS. Am Rev Respir Dis 1989; 140:1204–9.
42. Azoulay E, Parrot A, Flahault A, et al. AIDS-related *Pneumocystis carinii* pneumonia in the era of adjunctive steroids: implication of BAL neutrophilia. Am J Respir Crit Care Med 1999; 160:493–9.
43. Zaman MK, White DA. Serum lactate dehydrogenase levels and *Pneumocystis carinii* pneumonia: diagnostic and prognostic significance. Am Rev Respir Dis 1988; 137:796–800.
44. Speich R, Opravil M, Weber R, Hess T, Luethy R, Russi EW. Prospective evaluation of a prognostic score for *Pneumocystis carinii* pneumonia in HIV-infected patients. Chest 1992; 102:1045–8.
45. Selwyn PA, Pumerantz AS, Durante A, et al. Clinical predictors of *Pneumocystis carinii* pneumonia, bacterial pneumonia and tuberculosis in HIV-infected patients. AIDS 1998; 12:885–93.
46. Smith DE, McLuckie A, Wyatt J, Gazzard B. Severe exercise hypoxaemia with normal or near normal X-rays: a feature of *Pneumocystis carinii* infection. Lancet 1988; 2:1049–51.
47. Chouaid C, Maillard C, Housser B, Febvre M, Zaoui D, Lebeau B. Cost effectiveness of noninvasive oxygen saturation measurement during exercise for the diagnosis of *Pneumocystis carinii* pneumonia. Am Rev Respir Dis 1993; 147:1360–3.
48. Bishop LR, Kovacs JA. Quantitation of anti-*Pneumocystis jiroveci* antibodies in healthy persons and immunocompromised patients. J Infect Dis 2003; 187:1844–8.
49. Tamburrini E, Mencarini P, Visconti E, et al. Detection of *Pneumocystis carinii* DNA in blood by PCR is not of value for diagnosis of P. carinii pneumonia. J Clin Microbiol 1996; 34:1586–8.
50. Atzori C, Agostoni F, Angeli E, Mainini A, Orlando G, Cargnel A. Combined use of blood and oropharyngeal samples for noninvasive diagnosis of *Pneumocystis carinii* pneumonia using the polymerase chain reaction. Eur J Clin Microbiol Infect Dis 1998; 17:241–6.
51. Lipschick GY, Gill VJ, Lundgren JD, et al. Improved diagnosis of *Pneumocystis carinii* infection by polymerase chain reaction on induced sputum and blood. Lancet 1992; 340:203–6.
52. Huang L, Stansell J, Osmond D, et al. Performance of an algorithm to detect *Pneumocystis carinii* pneumonia in symptomatic HIV-infected persons. Chest 1999; 115:1025–32.
53. Coleman DL, Dodek PM, Golden JA, et al. Correlation between serial pulmonary function tests and fiberoptic bronchoscopy in patients with *Pneumocystis carinii* pneumonia and the acquired immune deficiency syndrome. Am Rev Respir Dis 1984; 129:491–3.
54. Hopewell PC, Luce JM. Pulmonary involvement in the acquired immunodeficiency syndrome. Chest 1985; 87:104–12.
55. Opravil M, Marincek B, Fuchs WA, et al. Shortcomings of chest radiography in detecting *Pneumocystis carinii* pneumonia. J Acquir Immune Defic Syndr 1994; 7:39–45.
56. Sepkowitz KA, Telzak EE, Gold JWM, et al. Pneumothorax in AIDS. Ann Intern Med 1991; 114:455–9.

57. Metersky ML, Colt HG, Olson LK, Shanks MS. AIDS-related spontaneous pneumothorax, risk factors and treatment. Chest 1995; 108:946–51.
58. Gruden JF, Huang L, Turner J, et al. High-resolution CT in the evaluation of clinically suspected *Pneumocystis carinii* pneumonia in AIDS patients with normal, equivocal, or nonspecific radiographic findings. Am J Roentgenol 1997; 169:967–75.
59. Goldenberg DM, Sharkey RM, Udem S, et al. Immunoscintigraphy of *Pneumocystis carinii* pneumonia in AIDS patients. J Nucl Med 1994; 35:1028–34.
60. Coleman DL, Hattner RS, Luce JM, Dodek PM, Golden JA, Murray JF. Correlation between gallium lung scans and fiberoptic bronchoscopy in patients with suspected *Pneumocystis carinii* pneumonia and the acquired immune deficiency syndrome. Am Rev Respir Dis 1984; 130:1166–9.
61. Robinson DS, Cunningham DA, Dave S, Fleming J, Mitchell DM. Diagnostic value of lung clearance of ^{99m}Tc DTPA compared with other non-invasive investigations in *Pneumocystis carinii* pneumonia in AIDS. Thorax 1991; 46:722–6.
62. Picard C, Meignan M, Rosso J, Cinotti L, Mayaud C, Revuz J. Technetium-99m DTPA aerosol and gallium scanning in acquired immune deficiency syndrome. Clin Nucl Med 1987; 12:501–6.
63. Stover DE, White DA, Romano PA, Gellene RA. Diagnosis of pulmonary disease in acquired immune deficiency syndrome (AIDS): role of bronchoscopy and bronchoalveolar lavage. Am Rev Respir Dis 1980;659–62.
64. Mones JM, Saldana MJ, Oldham SA. Diagnosis of Pneumocystis pneumonia: Roentgenographic-pathologic correlates based on fiberoptic bronchoscopy specimens from patients with the acquired immunodeficiency syndrome. Chest 1986; 89:522–6.
65. Broaddus C, Dake MD, Stulbarg MS, et al. Bronchoalveolar lavage and transbronchial biopsy for the diagnosis of pulmonary infections in the acquired immunodeficiency syndrome. Ann Intern Med 1985; 102:747–52.
66. Tuan IZ, Dennison D, Weisdorf DJ. *Pneumocystis carinii* pneumonitis following bone marrow transplantation. Bone Marrow Transplant 1992; 10:267–72.
67. Milligan SA, Luce JM, Golden J, Stulbarg M, Hopewell PC. Transbronchial biopsy without fluoroscopy in patients with diffuse roentgenographic infiltrates and the acquired immunodeficiency syndrome. Am Rev Respir Dis 1988; 137:486–8.
68. Stover DE, Zaman MB, Hajdu SI, Lange M, Gold J, Armstrong D. Bronchoalveolar lavage in the diagnosis of diffuse pulmonary infiltrates in the immunosuppressed host. Ann Intern Med 1984; 101:1–7.
69. Ognibene FP, Shelhamer J, Gill V, et al. The diagnosis of *Pneumocystis carinii* pneumonia in patients with the acquired immunodeficiency syndrome using subsegmental bronchoalveolar lavage. Am Rev Respir Dis 1984; 129:929–32.
70. Coleman DL, Dodek PM, Luce JM, Golden JA, Gold WM, Murray JF. Diagnostic utility of fiberoptic bronchoscopy in patients with *Pneumocystis carinii* pneumonia and the acquired immune deficiency syndrome. Am Rev Respir Dis 1983; 128:795–9.
71. Djamin RS, Drent M, Schreurs AJM, Groen EAH, Wagenaar SS. Diagnosis of *Pneumocystis carinii* pneumonia in HIV-positive patients. Acta Cytologica 1998; 42:933–8.

72. Meduri GU, Stover DE, Greeno RA, Nash T, Zaman MB. Bilateral bronchoalveolar lavage in the diagnosis of opportunistic pulmonary infections. Chest 1991; 100:1272–6.
73. Cadranel J, Gillet-Juvin K, Antoine M, et al. Site-directed bronchoalveolar lavage and transbronchial biopsy in HIV-infected patients with pneumonia. Am J Respir Crit Care Med 1995; 152:1103–6.
74. Golden JA, Hollander H, Stulbarg MS, Gamsu G. Bronchoalveolar lavage as the exclusive diagnostic modality for *Pneumocystis carinii* pneumonia: a prospective study among patients with the acquired immunodeficiency syndrome. Chest 1986; 90:18–22.
75. Huang L, Hecht FM, Stansell JD, Montanti R, Hadley WK, Hopewell PC. Suspected *Pneumocystis carinii* pneumonia with a negative sputum examination. Am J Respir Crit Care Med 1995; 151:1866–71.
76. Orenstein M, Webber CA, Cash M, Heurich AE. Value of bronchoalveolar lavage in the diagnosis of pulmonary infection in acquired immune deficiency syndrome. Thorax 1986; 41:345–9.
77. Levine SJ, Kennedy D, Shelhamer JH, et al. Diagnosis of *Pneumocystis carinii* pneumonia by multiple lobe, site-directed bronchoalveolar lavage with immuno-fluorescent monoclonal antibody staining in human immunodeficiency virus-infected patients receiving aerosolized pentamidine prophylaxis. Am Rev Respir Dis 1992; 146:838–43.
78. Yung RC, Weinacker AB, Steiger DJ, et al. Upper and middle lobe bronchoalveolar lavage to diagnose *Pneumocystis carinii* pneumonia. Am Rev Respir Dis 1993; 148:1563–6.
79. Jules-Elysee KM, Stover DE, Zaman MB, Bernard EM, White DA. Aerosolized pentamidine: effect on diagnosis and presentation in *Pneumocystis carinii* pneumonia. Ann Intern Med 1990; 112:750–7.
80. Levy H. Comparison of Ballard catheter bronchoalveolar lavage with broncho-scopic bronchoalveolar lavage. Chest 1994; 106:1753–6.
81. Levy H. Comparison of Ballard BAL catheter with bronchoscopic bronchoalveolar lavage. Chest 1992; 102:143S (Abstract).
82. del Rio C, Guarner J, Honig EG, Slade B. Sputum examination in the diagnosis of *Pneumocystis carinii* pneumonia in the acquired immunodeficiency syndrome. Arch Pathol Lab Med 1988; 112:1229–32.
83. Metersky ML, Aslenzadeh J, Stelmach P. A comparison of induced and expectorated sputum for the diagnosis of *Pneumocystis carinii* pneumonia. Chest 1998; 113:1555–9.
84. Rafanan AL, Klevjer-Anderson P, Metersky ML. *Pneumocystis carinii* pneumonia diagnosed by non-induced sputum stained with a direct fluorescent antibody. Ann Clin Lab Sci 1998; 28:99–103.
85. Kovacs JA, Ng VL, Masur H, et al. Diagnosis of *Pneumocystis carinii* pneumonia—improved detection in sputum with use of monoclonal antibodies. N Engl J Med 1988; 318:589–93.
86. Miller RF, Semple SJG, Kocjan G. Difficulties with sputum induction for diagnosis of *Pneumocystis carinii* pneumonia. Lancet 1990; 335:112.
87. Pitchenik AE, Ganjei P, Torres A, Evans DA, Rubin E, Baier H. Sputum examination for the diagnosis of *Pneumocystis carinii* pneumonia in the Acquired Immunodeficiency Syndrome. Am Rev Respir Dis 1986; 133:226–9.

88. Bigby TD, Margolskii D, Curtis JL, et al. The usefulness of induced sputum in the diagnosis of *Pneumocystis carinii* pneumonia in patients with the acquired immunodeficiency syndrome. Am Rev Respir Dis 1986; 133:515–8.

89. Cruciani M, Marcati P, Malena M, Bosco O, Serpelloni G, Mengoli C. Meta-analysis of diagnostic procedures for *Pneumocystis carinii* pneumonia in HIV-1 infected patients. Eur Respir J 2002; 20:982–9.

90. Ng VL, Garner I, Weymouth LA, Goodman CD, Hopewell PC, Hadley WK. The use of mucolysed induced sputum for the identification of pulmonary pathogens associated with human immunodeficiency virus infection. Arch Pathol Lab Med 1989; 113:488–93.

91. Zaman MK, Wooten OJ, Suprahmanya B, Ankobiah W, Finch PJP, Kamholz SL. Rapid noninvasive diagnosis of *Pneumocystis carinii* from the induced liquefied sputum. Ann Intern Med 1988; 107:7.

92. Willocks L, Burns S, Cossar R, Brettle R. Diagnosis of *Pneumocystis carinii* in a population of HIV-positive drug users, with particular reference to sputum induction and fluorescent antibody techniques. J Infect 1993; 26:257–64.

93. Cartwright CP, Nelson NA, Gill VJ. Development and evaluation of a rapid and simple procedure for detection of *Pneumocystis carinii* by PCR. J Clin Microbiol 1994; 32:1634–8.

94. Chouaid C, Roux P, Lavard I, Poirot JL, Housset B. Use of the polymerase chain reaction technique on induced sputum samples for the diagnosis of *Pneumocystis carinii* pneumonia in HIV-infected patients. A clinical and cost-analysis study. Am J Clin Pathol 1995; 104:72–5.

95. Levine SJ, Masur H, Gill VJ, et al. Effect of aerosolized pentamidine prophylaxis on the diagnosis of *Pneumocystis carinii* pneumonia by induced sputum examination in patients infected with the human immunodeficiency virus. Am Rev Respir Dis 1991; 144:760–4.

96. Metersky ML, Catanzaro A. Diagnostic approach to *Pneumocystis carinii* pneumonia in the setting of prophylactic aerosolized pentamidine. Chest 1991; 100:1345–9.

97. Helweg-Larsen J, Jensen JS, Benfield T, Svendsen UG, Lundgren JD, Lundgren B. Diagnostic use of PCR for detection of *Pneumocystis carinii* in oral wash samples. J Clin Microbiol 1998; 36:2068–72.

98. Fischer S, Gill VJ, Kovacs J, et al. The use of oral washes to diagnose *Pneumocystis carinii* pneumonia: a blinded retrospective study using a polymerase chain reaction-based detection system. J Infect Dis 2001; 184:1485–8.

99. Larsen HH, Huang L, Kovacs JA, et al. A prospective, blinded study of quantitative touch-down polymerase chain reaction using oral-wash samples for diagnosis of Pneumocystis pneumonia in HIV-infected patients. J Infect Dis 2004; 189:1679–83.

100. Wakefield AE, Miller RF, Guiver LA, Hopkin JM. Oropharyngeal samples for detection of *Pneumocystis carinii* by DNA amplification. Q J Med 1993; 86:401–6.

101. Helweg-Larsen J, Jensen JS, Lundgren B. Non-invasive diagnosis of *Pneumocystis carinii* pneumonia by PCR on oral washes. Lancet 1997; 350:1363.

102. Radio SJ, Hansen S, Goldsmith J, Linder J. Immunohistochemistry of *Pneumocystis carinii* infection. Mod Pathol 1990; 3:462–9.

103. Wakefield AE, Guiver L, Miller RF, Hopkin JM. DNA amplification of induced sputum samples for diagnosis of *Pneumocystis carinii* pneumonia. Lancer 1991; 337:1378–9.

104. Tsolaki AG, Miller RF, Wakefield AE. Oropharyngeal samples for genotyping and monitoring response to treatment in AIDS patients with *Pneumocystis carinii* pneumonia. J Med Microbiol 1999; 48:897–905.
105. Huang SN, Fischer SH, O'Shaughnessy E, Gill VJ, Masur H, Kovacs JA. Development of a PCR assay for diagnosis of Pneumocystis carinii pneumonia based on amplification of the multicopy major surface glycoprotein gene family. Diagn Microbiol Infect Dis 1999; 35:27–32.
106. Lu JJ, Chen CH, Bartlett MS, Smith JW, Lee CH. Comparison of six different PCR methods for detection of Pneumocystis carinii. J Clin Microbiol 1995; 33:2785–8.
107. Sing A, Trebesius K, Roggenkamp A, et al. Evaluation of diagnostic value and epidemiological implications of PCR for *Pneumocystis carinii* in different immunosuppressed and immunocompetent patient groups. J Clin Microbiol 2000; 38:1461–7.
108. Olsson M, Stralin K, Holmberg H. Clinical significance of nested polymerase chain reaction and immunofluorescence for detection of Pneumocystis carinii pneumonia. Clin Microbiol Infect 2001; 9:492–7.
109. Tuncer S, Erguven S, Kocagoz S, Unal S. Comparison of cytochemical staining, immunofluorescence and PCR for diagnosis of *Pneumocystis carinii* on sputum samples. Scand J Infect Dis 1998; 30:125–8.
110. Torres J, Goldman M, Wheat LJ, et al. Diagnosis of *Pneumocystis carinii* pneumonia in human immunodeficiency virus-infected patients with polymerase chain reaction: a blinded comparison to standard methods. Clin Infect Dis 2000; 30:141–5.
111. Olsson M, Elvin K, Lofdahl S, Linder E. Detection of *Pneumocystis carinii* DNA in sputum and bronchoalveolar lavage samples by polymerase chain reaction. J Clin Microbiol 1993; 31:221–6.
112. Larsen HH, Masur H, Kovacs JA, et al. Development of and evaluation of a quantitative, touch-down, real-time PCR assay for diagnosing *Pneumocystis carinii* pneumonia. J Clin Microbiol 2002; 40:490–4.
113. Huang L, Crothers K, DeOliveira A, et al. Application of an mRNA-based molecular viability assay to oropharyngeal washes for the diagnosis of Pneumocystis pneumonia in HIV-infected patients, a pilot study. J Eukaryot Microbiol 2003; 50:618–20.
114. Baughman RP, Dohn MN, Frame PT. The continuing utility of bronchoalveolar lavage to diagnose opportunistic infections in AIDS patients. Am J Med 1994; 97:515–22.
115. Barrio JL, Harcup C, Baier HJ, Pitchenik AE. Value of repeated bronchoscopies and significance of nondiagnostic bronchoscopic results in patients with the acquired immunodeficiency syndrome. Am Rev Respir Dis 1987; 135:422–5.
116. Mann M, Shelhamer JH, Masur H, et al. Lack of clinical utility of bronchoalveolar cultures for cytomegalovirus in HIV infection. Am J Respir Crit Care Med 1997; 155:1723–8.
117. Bower M, Barton SE, Nelson MR, et al. The significance of the detection of cytomegalovirus in the bronchoalveolar lavage fluid in AIDS patients with pneumonia. AIDS 1990; 4:317–20.

12

The Diagnosis of Endemic Mycoses

John R. Graybill
Division of Infectious Diseases, Department of Medicine, University of Texas Health Science Center, San Antonio, Texas, U.S.A.

Gregory M. Anstead
Division of Infectious Diseases, Department of Medicine, University of Texas Health Science Center, and Medical Service, South Texas Veterans Healthcare System, San Antonio, Texas, U.S.A.

Flavio Queiroz-Telles
Department of Communitarian Health, Hospital de Clínicas, Universidade Federal do Paraná, Curitiba, Paraná, Brazil

INTRODUCTION

The major endemic mycoses are defined by their heightened prevalence in specific geographic regions. In the Americas, *Histoplasma capsulatum* is concentrated in the Midwestern United States, most densely within the Ohio and Mississippi River basins, and south through Mexico, Central America, into South America, particularly Colombia, Venezuela, Brazil, and Argentina (1). African histoplasmosis, due to *H. capsulatum* var. *duboisii* is a much less common disease and is found in Central and Western Africa (2). There have also been cases of *H. capsulatum* var. *capsulatum* reported in South Africa.

"North American" blastomycosis, caused by *Blastomyces dermatitidis*, has some overlap with *H. capsulatum* in North America, ranging up into Canada as far as Manitoba, and is scattered uncommonly in Africa and other parts of the world (3–7). South American blastomycosis, or paracoccidioidomycosis, is caused by *Paracoccidioides braziliensis*, and is restricted to the

Latin Americas, with the endemic zone extending south from Tampico, Mexico, to Buenos Aires, Argentina (8–10). For coccidioidomycosis, the principle endemic area is the American Southwest and Northern Mexico. It is also found in scattered areas of Latin America; it is caused by *Coccidioides immitis* [more recently subdivided on the basis of genomics into *C. immitis* (California isolates) and *Coccidioides posadasii* (isolates outside of California)] (11–18). With no clear clinical differences, both *C. immitis* and *C. posadasii* are referred to as *C. immitis* in this chapter. *C. immitis* is not found naturally outside of the Americas. Penicilliosis marneffei, caused by *Penicillium marneffei*, is found predominantly in parts of Indochina, Southern China, and the Malay Peninsula (19–21).

All of these fungal pathogens are dimorphic, that is, they have a mycelial free-living form, which is the infectious propagule, and a parasitic form, which is responsible for disease. Because all of these pathogens were seen with unique parasitic forms and first observed in people with advanced and often disseminated diseases, they were thought to be exceedingly rare. When the free-living mycelial forms were discovered, and antigens were prepared for skin testing and for measurement of antibody titers, the truly wide range and often frequent evidence of prior infection was appreciated.

The endemic mycoses all commence following inhalation of fungal conidia from free-living mycelial forms. They are small enough to reach the alveoli, are ingested by alveolar macrophages, and, over the course of a few days, convert to the parasitic forms and begin to replicate. During the course of the next weeks to months there is often progression of pulmonary nodular or infiltrative lesions, and dissemination of daughter cells via the regional lymphatics and bloodstream to other organs. In this early period, the patient may be asymptomatic, or may develop a non-specific syndrome of cough, malaise, fever, and myalgias. As tissue antigens are processed and a specific immune response is developed, the patient may experience immunologic reactions including eosinophilia, erythema nodosum or multiforme, arthralgias, and arthritis. These are associated with resolution of infection. Normally, in the weeks following acute infection, the host develops delayed-type skin test reactivity to antigens of the offending pathogen, and usually develops antibody titers as well. Resolution may be accompanied by complete disappearance of all clinical and radiographic criteria of infection. Alternatively, the patient may develop gradual regression, and, in some cases, calcification of the infiltrates. These may persist, in the case of histoplasmosis, as "shotgun" calcifications, or as onion-skin rings of calcification around a pulmonary or mediastinal lymph node histoplasmoma. Calcifications may also occur in the liver and spleen at the sites of *Histoplasma* granulomas. The latter may vary in size over months and years. These may resolve completely, though the larger ones tend to persist. Thus, the normal presentation of primary infection varies from an acute flu-like syndrome or rheumatic manifestations of immune response to no symptoms at all.

However, the host response so characteristic of most of these mycoses may not quite completely ensnare all of the fungi, and slowly replicating organisms may stimulate ongoing fibrosing and necrotizing responses (22). Episodes of pulmonary infiltration, cavitation, and resolution characterize chronic pulmonary histoplasmosis. Unchecked, eventually large cavities may replace lung parenchyma and the patient dies of respiratory insufficiency, but not disseminated disease (23). Coccidioidomycosis, blastomycosis, and especially paracoccidioidomycosis also have chronic pulmonary fibrotic forms, which cause progressive lung destruction. In these patients one tends to have a positive skin test and variable titers of antibodies to the fungus.

By contrast, the absence of a competent host immune response is associated with chronic or rapidly progressing disseminated disease, typically involving the reticuloendothelial system. Splenomegaly, hepatomegaly, lymphadenopathy, and bone marrow involvement are common. Nodular skin lesions may reflect hematogenous dissemination. Lymphocytic meningitis may also occur. In these forms of disease the skin test tends to be negative and the antibody titers are variable. Fever may be present. Weight loss, cachexia, and death follow. Rapidly progressing disease has been seen in children with dissemination, and in patients with AIDS. Slowly progressing disease, often over years, is sometimes associated with chronic adrenal involvement and adrenal insufficiency, most prominent in histoplasmosis and paracoccidioidomycosis (24).

Although the above general pattern of pathogenesis is common to these fungi, each tends to cause unique clinical and immunologic responses to infection. In the following discussion we highlight epidemiologic and clinical cues for diagnosis of specific mycoses, direct demonstration of the pathogen, and various serologic techniques used to make the diagnosis. These differ with the varied presentations of the mycoses.

HISTOPLASMOSIS

Epidemiologic Clues to Diagnosis

The classic endemic range of *H. capsulatum* is indicated in Figure 1. This figure reflects the well-known traditional zones in which the pathogen has been cultured, and in which skin test surveys with Histoplasmin antigen testing have revealed heightened reactivity (25). Histoplasmin is a culture filtrate containing multiple antigens, including the M and H antigens used for serology. Cross-reactivity with coccidioidal antigens is reflected in the skin test positivity in non-endemic zones for histoplasmosis, including West Texas, Phoenix, Arizona, and the San Joaquin Valley in California (25). Cross-reactivity of Histoplasmin in patients with blastomycosis has also been recognized, so the tests are not totally disease-specific. After conversion, the skin test may remain positive indefinitely. A positive test does not distinguish a person with recent infection from prior exposure years ago. Therefore, the skin test is not useful to determine whether

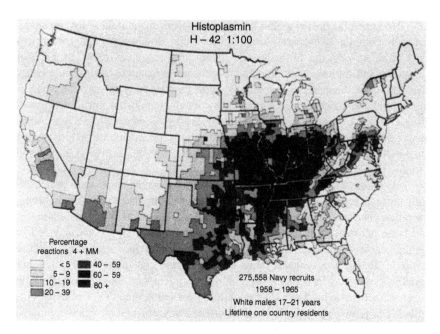

Figure 1 Distribution of positive histoplasmin skin sensitivity testing in naval recruits. *Source*: From Ref. 25.

a patient has active histoplasmosis. Conversely, it has long been known that Histoplasmin skin tests may be negative in persons with active histoplasmosis and depressed immune response (26). Indeed, anergic skin test responses in patients with advanced HIV infection increase as the CD4 count declines, from 49% of patients with CD4 > 400 to 76% of those with CD4 < 200. Of seven patients in one series who had serial skin testing, and developed histoplasmosis, six were anergic (27).

Finally, a positive Histoplasmin skin test may stimulate the increase of anti-*Histoplasma* antibodies to titers > 1:8, level suggesting active histoplasmosis (28). Given the interaction of the skin test and serologic titers of antibody, cross-reactivity with other endemic mycoses, and insensitivity among the immune suppressed, the use of the Histoplasmin skin test has been primarily to define areas of endemicity, and to explore populations exposed in epidemics. If the skin test is used to study outbreaks, sera for antibodies should be drawn before the test is applied.

There has been a major change since the above map was published. This is the "expansion" of the zone of endemicity, which was revealed by the HIV outbreak in the 1980s. Hospitals in cities such as San Antonio and Austin, Texas, long thought to be to the west of the major Mississippi River Valley endemic region, had a sharp upsurge in patients with histoplasmosis in the setting of advanced AIDS. This reached as many as 20 cases per year in some Texas hospitals (29). Various Caribbean islands and Latin American countries such as Guatemala, Honduras, Colombia, Brazil, Argentina, and Peru experienced similar problems. We now appreciate that *H. capsulatum* is endemic at least to south central Texas, and focally in many areas as far south as Buenos Aires.

While transmission of *H. capsulatum* in the southeastern United States has been associated with exposure to blackbirds and chickens, bat roosts appear to be a major *Source* in Texas and much of Latin America (30). However, most HIV patients cannot give a definite history of exposure, in part because some disease is primary and some is reactivation from previously infected foci. Thus patients may develop active histoplasmosis thousands of miles where they were infected. Histoplasmin for skin testing at present is not commercially available (25). Prior travel to or residence in an area of endemicity is useful in the medical history of patients suspected to have histoplasmosis.

Clinical Clues to Diagnosis

Primary Infection

With a low intensity inoculum, histoplasmosis is often clinically silent in the immunocompetent patient. In the patient exposed to a very heavy inoculum, or with severe immunosuppression, the disease may progress directly to dissemination with diffuse pulmonary, lymphatic, splenic, hepatic, and bone marrow involvement. Fever and wasting accompany this most severe form of disease. In about 1% of immunocompetent patients, during the first weeks after infection, histoplasmosis manifests as a non-specific pneumonia, with dry cough, fever, and occasionally pleuritic chest pain. A large outbreak in Indianapolis revealed that some patients have immunologic manifestations similar to those of acute coccidioidomycosis, including rashes (such as erythema nodosum), pericarditis, and arthralgias (31–33). Mediastinal lymphadenopathy may occur. In connection with a bird or bat exposure, these rheumatologic findings may suggest a diagnosis of histoplasmosis rather than bacterial or viral pneumonia. Primary histoplasmosis commonly resolves without sequelae, but multiple alternative courses can be followed. These depend essentially on the immunocompetence and pulmonary anatomy (typically related to the smoking habits) of the patient.

Resolution with Chronic Residua

Uncommonly, the cell-mediated immune responses of the host react excessively to fungal antigens, producing foci of caseating necrosis and calcification.

"Buckshot" calcification: This is asymptomatic, and appears as small calcifications, which superficially resemble shotgun pellets on the chest radiograph. They can be seen not only in the lungs but also in the liver and spleen, where the organism has disseminated during primary infection. Severe varicella pneumonia may leave a similar pattern, but the "buckshot" appearance on chest radiographs is generally quite suggestive of prior histoplasmosis that is presently inactive.

Mediastinal granuloma/histoplasmoma: Mediastinal granulomas may follow primary disease, and be seen as large, sometimes caseous or liquefied, mediastinal lymph nodes. They may obstruct the esophagus or airways, and may progress to calcification. Such granulomas, or histoplasmomas, may appear elsewhere in the lungs, and in these sites the contraction of infiltrates into nodular granulomas occurs. These lesions are generally asymptomatic, and are discovered on routine chest radiography. The lesions may have a characteristic onion-skin series of calcified layers about a central core. They may enlarge or shrink over long periods of time (34). They are often incidentally diagnosed at surgery to remove a potential carcinoma. Small numbers of organisms may be seen but are rarely cultured. Particularly for a resident of an endemic area who is non-smoker, the radiographic pattern may prompt the physician to wait and observe over some months to determine whether the lesion remains stable in size rather than immediately undertake surgical resection.

Fibrosing mediastinitis: This very rare manifestation also represents an excessively robust host response, and the targets are again the mediastinal lymph nodes. These may scar and constrict the esophagus, the primary or secondary bronchi, and/or major mediastinal blood vessels (Fig. 2). Radiographs may not confirm this and tissue diagnosis may be required. Peripheral fibrosis and sometimes calcification surround a central caseous necrotic core, in which scattered yeast cells may occasionally be seen, particularly with Gomori's

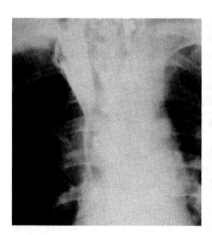
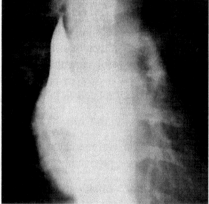

Figure 2   Chronic pulmonary histoplasmosis with fibrosing mediastinitis compressing great vessels. Note the abrupt narrowing of the superior vena cava as it enters the mediastinum. *Source*: From Ref. 35.

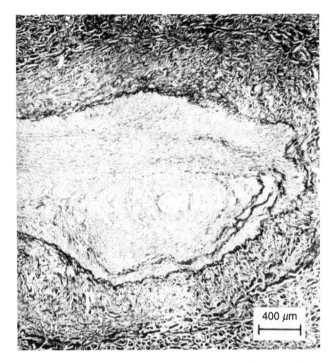

Figure 3 Chronic pulmonary histoplasmosis. Section of a mediastinal lymph node showing fibrosis surrounding central necrotic core. *Source*: From Ref. 35.

methenamine silver (GMS) or the periodic acid Schiff (PAS) tissue stains (Fig. 3). Cultures are rarely positive (35,36).

High-Inoculum Infection/Reinfection Immune Response

Intense exposure is often associated with extensive pulmonary infiltrates and respiratory insufficiency (37). Occasionally, in the setting of a very intense exposure, a subject with previously documented histoplasmosis will have an acute flare of cough and a flu-like illness. This appears somewhat more abruptly than primary histoplasmosis, and may cause acute hypoxemia due to the host immune response. Generally, epidemiologic history of exposure with acute pneumonia, should suggest this re-infection pattern, which in essence is pulmonary hypersensitivity disease.

Syndrome of Presumed Ocular Histoplasmosis

This asymptomatic retinal lesion is a favorite diagnosis of some ophthalmologists, but with no microbiologic confirmation that it is actually caused by *H. capsulatum* (38). It is not considered further here.

Chronic Pulmonary Histoplasmosis

This used to be one of the more commonly recognized forms of histoplasmosis in the central United States. Patients in general are white male smokers who have some degree of underlying lung damage, usually chronic obstructive pulmonary disease (23). The illness manifests as irregularly recurrent episodes of dyspnea, and occasionally productive cough. Chest radiographs commonly reveal upper lobe infiltrates, with heightened lymphangitic tracking down to the hilum. The infiltrative lesions may resolve or may progress to cavitation, or may gradually constrict the involved lobes of the lung from progressive fibrosis (Fig. 4). The illness may be caused by the repeated exposure of fungal antigens released from sequestered endogenous sites, associated with a strong and ultimately destructive immune response. If episodes continue to recur, they may progress into necrotic cavities. As fungal antigen spreads through the lungs, an increased reaction occurs, with enlarging "marching" cavities. Although death may occur from progressive lung destruction, dissemination in chronic pulmonary histoplasmosis is uncommon (Fig. 5) (23,32). This illness may be mistaken for tuberculosis.

Disseminated Histoplasmosis

At one end of the spectrum is chronic disseminated histoplasmosis. This may present solely as adrenal insufficiency, caused by slowly progressing (over years)

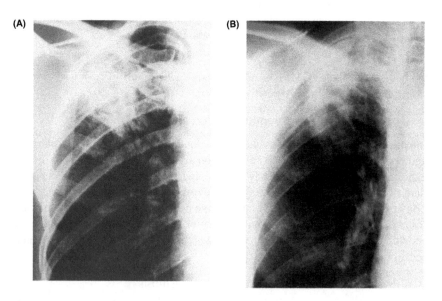

(A)   (B)

Figure 4 (A) Acute infiltrate in a patient with chronic pulmonary histoplasmosis. (B) Same patient six weeks later, showing contraction of lung and fibrosis, with resolution of the infiltrate. *Source*: From Ref. 23.

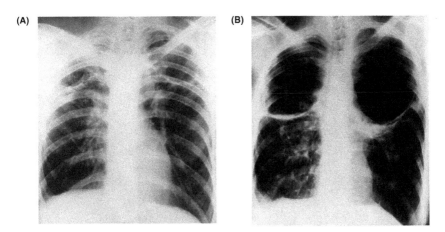

Figure 5 (**A**) Chronic pulmonary histoplasmosis with large cavities, bullae, and fibrosis. (**B**) Same patients as (**A**), showing progressively enlarging "marching" cavities thought to be due to dribbling of *H. capsulatum* antigens into dependent areas of lungs, with fibrosing and necrotizing host response. This radiograph was obtained shortly before the patient died of progressive pulmonary insufficiency. *Source*: From Ref. 23.

destruction of the adrenal glands. Dehydration due to sodium loss, hyperpigmentation of the palms and soles, orthostatic hypotension, and other manifestations may be present. Computerized tomography may show calcification of the adrenals with central necrosis. In subacute disease there may be adrenal involvement but, in addition, the patient has generalized wasting and may have skin or mucous membrane ulcers containing *H. capsulatum*. There may or may not be evidence of reticuloendothelial tissue involvement, such as hepatosplenomegaly. This disease may wax and wane spontaneously. The third form, infantile or juvenile disease, was named because of the immature immune responsiveness found in most patients. This previously rare form is what we most commonly see today, in AIDS patients. In patients with late stages of AIDS, the presentation with fever, wasting, markedly elevated serum lactate dehydrogenase (LDH), and anemia or pancytopenia, especially in African-Americans, should prompt the clinician to consider histoplasmosis (39). Chest radiographs may show reticulonodular or military infiltrates, but may be normal in as many as 40% of patients. These patients have cachexia, and may also have hematochezia or diarrhea from involvement of the ileum or colon. Bone marrow involvement is often associated with pancytopenia. Mucosal ulcers are commonly seen, and can be found anywhere from the mouth to the rectum. Skin rashes and ulcers may also appear, and are infiltrated with intracellular yeast cells (Figs. 6 and 7). Histoplasmosis may progress to death within a month if undiagnosed. Lymphocytic meningitis may occur, especially in AIDS patients, but commonly is asymptomatic.

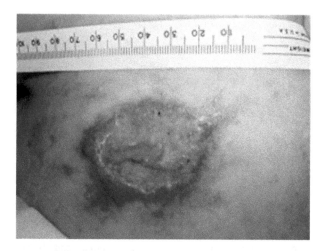

Figure 6 Shoulder ulcer in patients with disseminated histoplasmosis and AIDS. The lesion is filled with macrophages containing abundant *Histoplasma capsulatum* yeast. *Source*: Courtesy of G. Crawford, University of Texas Health Science Center at San Antonio, San Antonio, Texas, U.S.A.

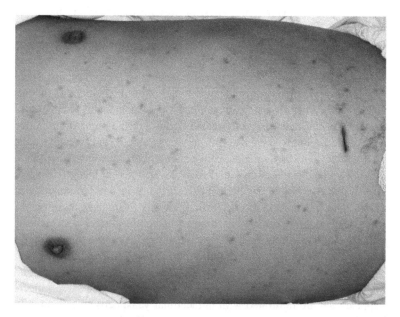

Figure 7 Cutaneous rash in a patient with disseminated histoplasmosis and AIDS. *Source*: Courtesy of G. Crawford, University of Texas Health Science Center at San Antonio, San Antonio, Texas, U.S.A.

Microbiologic Clues to Diagnosis

H. capsulatum is relatively easy to identify provided one thinks of looking for it. In general, the more intense the host inflammatory response, the lesser the burden of fungal cells. Microbiologic and serologic methods of diagnosis have been reviewed extensively by Wheat, and serodiagnostic methods are discussed in detail by Warnock and Morrison elsewhere in this book (40–42).

Culture

Although culture is the most specific diagnostic method, the organism may require up to four weeks to grow. Yeast cells growing in culture may be rapidly identified by DNA homology (GenProbe) with *H. capsulatum*. Initial cultures, if done on Sabouraud's agar, grow mycelial colonies that often (but not always) contain characteristic tuberculate macroconidia (Fig. 8). These resemble World War II naval mines. *H. capsulatum* is the only human pathogen with such conidia. Mycelia can be converted to the yeast phase, which is somewhat tedious. Prior to the appearance of AIDS, *H. capsulatum* was only occasionally cultured from patients with primary disease (Table 1). If the patients had only rheumatologic syndromes or pericarditis as manifestations of primary infection, cultures were commonly negative. Patients with disseminated histoplasmosis and cavitary pulmonary histoplasmosis were frequently culture positive, although they could be negative in up to 35% of cases (43). Late syndromes of aberrant healing, such as mediastinal fibrosis and histoplasmoma are often culture-negative (22,34).

Blood and tissue cultures are often positive for yeast in patients with AIDS and disseminated histoplasmosis. The MYCO/F Lytic method using the BACTEC 9240 blood culture system was compared to the Isolator system of Wampole Laboratories (44). There were no significant differences for detection of *H. capsulatum*, though of 14 samples positive for *Histoplasma*, seven grew

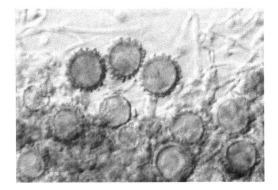

Figure 8 Mycelium of *Histoplasma capsulatum*, showing tuberculate macroconidia. Nomarski optics. *Source*: Courtesy of D. Sutton, Fungal Testing Laboratory, University of Texas Health Science Center at San Antonio, San Antonio, Texas, U.S.A.

Table 1 Fungal Cultures in Histoplasmosis

	Acute self-limited positive/total N	% Positive	Disseminated positive/total N	% Positive	Cavitary positive/total N	% Positive
Sputum	7/72	9.7	7/10	70	22/36	61.1
Lung	3/14	21.4	9/13	69.2	4/6	66.6
Lymph nodes	1/9	11.1	5/6	71.4	ND	0
Bone marrow	0/16	0	33/43	76.7	1/11	9
Liver	0/2	0	8/24	33.3	ND	0
Cerebrospinal fluid	0/13	0	2/14	14.3	0/1	0
Blood	0/15	0	11/21	52.3	0/1	0
Any	11/28	8.6	58/66	87.8	23/40	57.5

Source: From Ref. 1.
Abbreviation: ND, no data available.

using both methods, and only from the BACTEC in seven cases. The yeast cells are not of unique appearance. However, for a patient in which there is a high clinical suspicion for histoplasmosis (AIDS, wasting syndrome, lymphadenopathy, etc.) cultures of yeast cells can be rapidly identified using GenProbe for DNA homology.

Histopathology

The yeast form can be identified by its size of 3 to 5 μm diameter, narrow-based budding, lack of a capsule, and localization within host phagocytic cells, particularly monocytes and macrophages (Fig. 9). *H. capsulatum* can be readily identified by its strong affinity for GMS stain; it also stains well with PAS reagent. Patients with AIDS may have such intense infection that the organisms can be seen in Giemsa or silver stains of circulating leukocytes. The small size

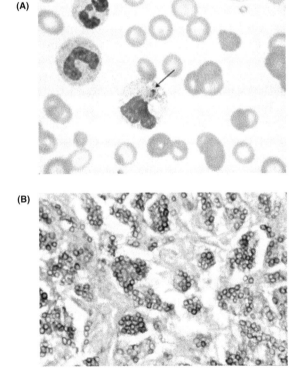

Figure 9 (**A**) *Histoplasma capsulatum* yeast in peripheral blood smear. Wright-Giemsa stain. Note relatively small size of yeast cell (*arrow*) in relation to nucleus of monocytes/macrophages. (**B**) *Histoplasma* yeast cells in dense masses in a patient with AIDS and disseminated histoplasmosis. Gomori's methenamine silver stain. *Source:* (**A**) Courtesy of J. R. Graybill; (**B**) Courtesy of D. Sutton.

of the yeast, narrow neck of buds for daughter cells, absence of capsule on mucicarmine stain, and lack of pseudomycelia help distinguish *H. capsulatum* from other fungi. *H. capsulatum* can also be stained with immunochemical techniques, although this has not found widespread application (45–47).

Serologic Clues to Diagnosis

Antibody Detection Methods

In the United States, antibody detection methods have largely been replaced by antigen detection for the diagnosis of histoplasmosis (discussed below). However, in Latin America and other parts of the world they are still used (48). Methods and general applications are discussed elsewhere in this text (40). Serodiagnostic methods have included immunoprecipitin, complement fixation, radioimmunoassay (RIA), and enzyme-linked immunosorbent assays (ELISA). Histoplasmin is a crude extract of *H. capsulatum* cells. Antigens used in serodiagnosis have been extracted from Histoplasmin, purified by gel chromatography, and designated the H and M antigens. A positive precipitin test to H antigen usually indicates active histoplasmosis (49). There is some cross-reactivity of the complement fixation test in patients with blastomycosis, particularly at lower titers (50).

As one example of non-specificity for diagnosing acute disease, using the RIA technique, sera for IgM and IgG anti-*Histoplasma* antibodies were tested from 92 patients in a large outbreak. Patients were compared with, residents living near and far from the outbreak as controls (51). Elevated IgM antibodies were found in 59% of outbreak subjects (within three months of illness), 10% of controls with pulmonary disease, and 6.7% of residents of South Dakota (a non-endemic area). Conversely, elevated IgG antibodies were found in 80% of subjects with recent histoplasmosis, 27% of controls with other lung diseases, 4.7% of normal controls attending sexually transmitted disease (STD) clinics, and fully 34% of "controls" attending STD clinics in Indianapolis, the site of the outbreak. This means that controls from a hyperendemic site are of no help in determining who was exposed during an acute outbreak. Of the 92 patients with histoplasmosis, the RIA and complement fixation titers were positive in 81.5%, while the RIA alone was positive in 9.8%, the complement fixation titer was positive alone in 4.3%, and both were negative in 4.3% (51). In the year following infection (and resolution) the IgM antibodies tend to clear in about half of patients, while the IgG antibodies tend to persist. Wheat et al. considered the RIA to be superior to the prior complement fixation and z tests for diagnosis of histoplasmosis (51).

In the most severe forms of disease, the acute disseminated type, host response may be so feeble that no antibodies are generated (52). Unfortunately, antibody detection systems may detect as few as 30% of the patients with severe disseminated histoplasmosis. Cross-reactivity with other fungal antigens is also a significant problem, and is mediated in part by carbohydrate epitopes present in Histoplasmin (53). Deglycosylation using periodate may reduce this cross-reactivity (54,55). Deglycosylated Histoplasmin, when used as the antigen for measuring antibodies in an ELISA test, also was more sensitive than native Histoplasmin, with relatively few cross reactions (54). The test was reproducible, with an r^2 of >0.98 for both glycosylated and deglycosylated antigens. Both H and M antigens were readily measured in deglycosylated antigens.

Antigen Test

In recent years, in the United States, serologic methods of diagnosis have been replaced with an assay that quantifies *Histoplasma* antigens, now performed solely at Miravista Diagnostics (Indianapolis, Indiana, U.S.A.). The test is highly sensitive and *Histoplasma* antigens can be detected in urine, blood, and cerebrospinal fluid (in the case of meningitis). The test as presently done was initially developed as a RIA using polyclonal rabbit antibody to *H. capsulatum* antigen (56). This was recently changed to a solid phase enzyme immunoassay (57). Antigen levels that are 50% higher than the mean value for normal sera are considered positive. The RIA test is reproducible in 92% of sera and 93% of urines (58). There are rare false positives in sera with negative urine tests, and sera are recommended to be tested only when accompanied by urine testing. The assay is very sensitive for *H. capsulatum*, but also detects antigens involved in other endemic mycoses, such as blastomycosis (cross-reactivity 63%), para-coccidioidomycosis (cross-reactivity 89%), and penicilliosis marneffei (cross-reactivity 94%). There is little cross-reactivity in patients with disseminated coccidioidomycosis (Fig. 10) (59). The specificity of the test is reported as 98% for histoplasmosis. In patients with AIDS and histoplasmosis, the urine assay sensitivity is 94% and that of the serum assay is 86% (Table 2). In patients

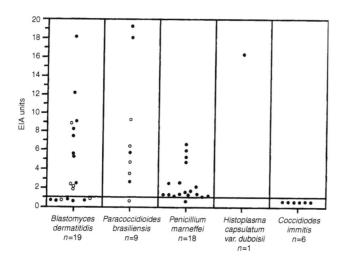

Figure 10   Cross Reaction of *Histoplasma* urine antigen in patients with other mycoses. *Abbreviation*: EIA, enzyme immunoassay. *Source*: From Ref. 59.

Table 2   Antigen Detection in Patients with Histoplasmosis

Percent positive antigen tests in patients with AIDS	
Urine only	7%
Serum only	0%
Urine and serum	86%
Neither urine nor serum	7%

Source: From Ref. 58.

with no underlying immunosuppression, the sensitivity is 82% for the urine assay and 62% for the serum assay (52). Patients with acute pulmonary histoplasmosis have a positive urine antigen test of 75% to 83% of the time. In chronic pulmonary histoplasmosis, the sensitivity of the urine antigen test is 6% to 14%, consistent with the lower amount of antigen present in this disease. For patients with only rheumatologic manifestations of histoplasmosis, antigen testing also has low sensitivity. Cerebrospinal fluid is antigen-positive in 25% to 75% of patients with *Histoplasma* meningitis, and may cross-react in specimens from patients with coccidioidal meningitis (60). In rare cases, with negative serology and absent clinical findings elsewhere, a brain or meningeal biopsy may be required to determine the diagnosis.

The *Histoplasma* antigen test has also been used to follow the course of histoplasmosis. Successful treatment is associated with declining antigen titers (Fig. 11) (61). In patients with AIDS and histoplasmosis, antigen is cleared more rapidly from serum than from the urine during induction treatment. Urine antigen tests reverted to negative in 17% of patients during induction treatment. A more rapid decline was seen in patients receiving amphotericin B as compared with itraconazole (62). By two weeks into treatment, antigen was negative in 6 of 31 patients receiving liposomal amphotericin B versus only 1 in 29 patients in the itraconazole group. By 12 weeks of therapy, antigens were negative in urine of 21% of the liposomal amphotericin B group, versus 19% of itraconazole recipients. Conversely, clinical relapse is associated with a rise in titer of ≥ 2 optical density units (Fig. 12) (63). A larger rise of ≥ 4 units is an even more clear indication of relapse. In patients with relapsed histoplasmosis, the rise in antigen levels (seroreversion) may precede clinical findings.

The *Histoplasma* antigen detection test of Wheat et al. has become very widely used in the United States. It is positive in patients with severe and non-severe manifestations of histoplasmosis (Table 3) (39). Many patients with HIV infection who present with fever or wasting will have *Histoplasma* urine antigen determinations performed to screen for the presence of this organism. Because of increasing concerns about shipments of infected sera and tissues, it has become very difficult to send specimens across national borders for testing *Histoplasma* antigens. An antigen test has been developed in Columbia, by Gomez et al. (64). However, this test is not widely available. Thus, the countries in Latin America at present are at a major disadvantage regarding the use of antigen testing for the

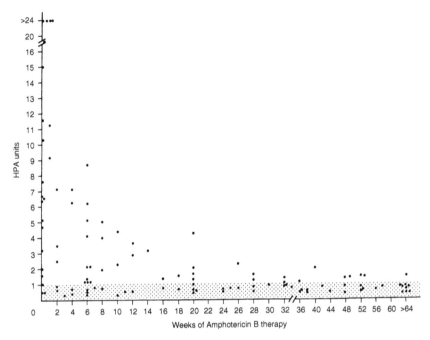

Figure 11 *Histoplasma* serum antigen in patients with histoplasmosis in the setting of AIDS, during induction and maintenance antifungal therapy with amphotericin B. *Abbreviation*: HPA, *Histoplasma* polysaccharide antigen. *Source*: From Ref. 61.

diagnosis of histoplasmosis. In these countries the older antibody testing systems are still being used for diagnosis, although antibody techniques have largely fallen out of favor in the United States. The Mycology Branch of Centers for Disease Control and Prevention is developing alternative methods for antigen detection to be established in Latin American and other Countries.

Polymerase Chain Reaction

The goal of the polymerase chain reaction (PCR) is to detect low levels of fungal DNA in serum or tissues. The PCR technique has been developed to a high levels of sensitivity and specificity in a mouse model, with a 50% quantile result at three yeast form colony-forming units per milligram of tissue (65). DNA hybridization can also be done on tissue specimens. It is far more sensitive than the hematoxylin and eosin stain. The PCR technique has also been applied to human paraffinized tissues. In a follow-up study, the test was positive in 50% of 11 skin biopsies, 6 of 20 oropharyngeal specimens, and 3 of 16 lymph node specimens (66). Tissue samples of 50 patients without histoplasmosis were negative. The inability to detect *H. capsulatum* in all infected tissues was likely to due to formalin fixation, which adversely affects these procedures. In the GenBank database, 18S rDNA PCR detects a target identical in *H. capsulatum*

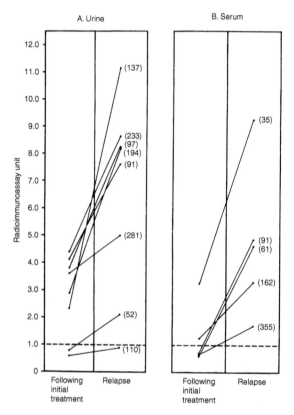

Figure 12   Rise in antigen titer associated with relapse of histoplasmosis. *Source*: From Ref. 63.

var. *capsulatum* and var. *duboisii*, so the test should be useful in patients with African histoplasmosis. It is not clear whether PCR-based methods will have any clinical advantage over direct testing for fungal antigens.

Less Specific Laboratory Findings

Disseminated histoplasmosis is associated with marked elevations of serum LDH, sometimes above 1000 units/L (67). While infection with *Pneumocystis jiroveci* may also be associated with high LDH, this is uncommonly to the high levels seen with disseminated histoplasmosis. Disseminated disease is also associated with the pattern of elevated levels of serum alkaline phosphatase, sometimes with modest elevation of the aspartate or alanine aminotransferase levels. Bilirubin is elevated only with the most severe liver involvement, and generally only mildly. Bone marrow involvement is associated with pancytopenia in overwhelming disseminated disease. Rarely, the leukemoid reaction or

Table 3 Comparison of Laboratory Diagnostic Methods in Histoplasmosis in Patients with AIDS

Diagnosis	Severe ($N=28$)	Non-severe ($N=127$)	Total ($N=155$)
Classification			
Pulmonary	2(7)	8(6)	10(6)
Disseminated	12(43)	70(55)	82(53)
Both	14(50)	49(39)	63(41)
Method			
Culture	22(85)	83(80)	105(81)
Histopathology	11(73)	38(64)	49(66)
Complement fixation antibody	10(67)	32(57)	42(59)
Immunodiffusion antibody	8(50)	36(68)	44(64)
Antigenuria	24(96)	116(98)	140(98)
Antigenemia	16(84)	62(78)	78(80)

Abbreviations: N/(), number(%).
Source: From Ref. 39.

hemophagocytic syndrome may be seen. Meningitis may be associated with CSF lymphocytosis and hypoglycorrachia, or in patients with HIV, relatively normal findings. The erythrocyte sedimentation rate and C-reactive protein levels tend to be elevated, though these are not specific.

African Histoplasmosis

African histoplasmosis, caused by *H. capsulatum* var. *duboisii*, is endemic to Central and Western Africa between the latitudes 15°N and 10°S, roughly between the Sahara and Kalahari deserts; the majority of cases have been reported from Nigeria. The ecology of the var. *duboisii* is not well known, but it has been found in bat caves (68). Although the lungs are the initial portal of infection in African histoplasmosis, pulmonary manifestations are not prominent and the disease more commonly attacks the bone, skin, and soft tissue (2).

Clinical Clues to Diagnosis

There are two clinical forms of African histoplasmosis: localized and disseminated. In the more common localized form, there is regional lymphadenopathy, and cutaneous and osseous lesions. Cutaneous involvement manifests as papules or nodules that may evolve into abscesses and ulcers. Osteomyelitis occurs in one-third of patients and is characterized by osteolysis and involvement of adjacent joints. The cranium, ribs, sternum, scapula, vertebrae, and long bones are the most common sites of bony involvement. Multiple bones may be involved simultaneously, and there may be overlying abscesses and draining sinus tracts.

Untreated, local intestinal involvement may occur (2). The disseminated form has been reported in patients with AIDS (69,70). The clinical manifestations of the African histoplasmosis may mimic cancer or tuberculosis (71–75).

Laboratory Clues to Diagnosis

Microbiology: At 25°C, the mycelial forms of both varieties of *Histoplasma* develop on standard media within one to three weeks. At 37°C on enriched media, both *Histoplasma* varieties grow as the yeast forms. Macroscopically and microscopically, the mycelial and yeast forms of the two varieties of *Histoplasma* cannot be distinguished (76).

Histopathology: In histopathologic specimens from patients with *H. c.* var. *duboisii* infection, the spherical to oval organism has thick, doubly-contoured walls, and may show chain formation and "hour-glass" or "figure-eight" budding (2). The organism elicits a granulomatous reaction, in which abundant yeast cells are within cytoplasm of epithelioid histiocytes and giant cells. The giant cell reaction may be particularly pronounced, with enormous giant cells containing 20 or more yeast forms. The granulomas may be accompanied by focal necrosis and fibrosis (2).

Histopathologic differential diagnosis: In tissue specimens, the yeast forms of *H. c.* var. *duboisii* is easily distinguished from *H. c.* var. *capsulatum* by their larger size, "double-cell" budding (two attached yeast cells of nearly identical size), and the presence of the enormous giant cells. Differentiation from *B. dermatitidis* may be more difficult. However. *B. dermatitidis* displays broad-based budding instead of the double-cell budding of *H. c.* var. *duboisii*. Also, *B. dermatitidis* is multinucleated, whereas *H. c.* var. *duboisii* is uninucleate. The diagnosis can be confirmed by either culture or immunofluorescence staining of tissue sections (2).

BLASTOMYCOSIS

Epidemiologic Clues to Diagnosis

B. dermatitidis is endemic to the region around and to the north of the Mississippi and Missouri rivers, but it also extends into the Carolinas and Alabama (Fig. 13) (3,7,77). Thus there is some overlap with the zone of *H. capsulatum*. However, *B. dermatitidis* does not extend south of the U.S. border, but does extend further north than *H. capsulatum*, indeed well up into the province of Manitoba, Canada and as far west as Colorado (6,78). Sporadic cases may be seen on other continents, such as Africa (79,80). Blastomycosis begins with inhalation and pulmonary infection. Patients tend to be exposed via outdoor activities, such as hunting and fishing (7), especially if the activities are close to waterways (81). The organism has been rarely recovered from wood piles and river banks (82). There have been far fewer epidemics and more scattered individual cases than for

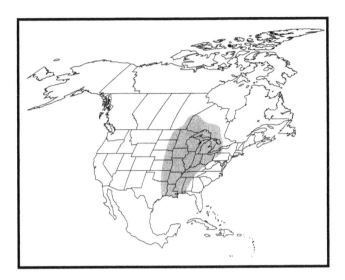

Blastomyces dermatitidis
North American blastomycosis

Figure 13 Geographic range of *Blastomyces dermatitidis*. *Source*: From Ref. 77.

histoplasmosis. However, in mini-outbreaks, several members of a family have been exposed at the same time, suggesting a point *Source* for infection (7). This suggests areas of hyperendemicity within the broader geographic range for *B. dermatitidis*. Dogs are also susceptible to *B. dermatitidis*, and may be sentinels for high-risk localities (80). Some cases have been associated with exposure to infected dogs and others have been associated with exposure to beaver dams (7,82–84). However, the specific association to beavers has been disputed (85). Although some cases of severe disease have been reported in patients with AIDS, in general, blastomycosis is not strongly associated with immunodeficiency. Smoking (30%) and diabetes (13%) were the most commonly associated conditions in one series (7). Outbreaks have tended to occur in the winter months.

Clinical Clues to Diagnosis

Overwhelming exposure or severe T-cell immunodeficiency may cause the development of severe pneumonia with acute respiratory distress syndrome, indistinguishable from bacterial sepsis (86–89). However, the usual course of pneumonitis is much less severe, may resolve spontaneously, and may only be discovered as a slowly resolving or non-resolving pneumonia (Fig. 14) (3,90,91). Blastomycosis is rarely considered in the initial differential diagnosis. With its myriad clinical presentations, the diagnosis of blastomycosis is often delayed, even in its endemic areas. In a series of 132 patients from Mississippi, in only 18% of cases was blastomycosis correctly suspected at the initial patient

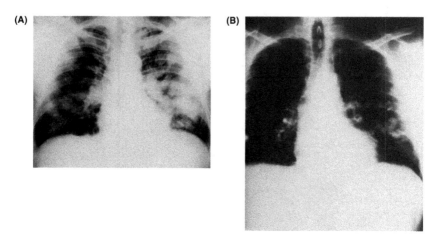

Figure 14 (**A**) Primary blastomycotic pneumonia, symptomatic, showing bilateral nodular infiltrates. (**B**) Same patient as (**A**), radiograph two months later showing incomplete resolution. *Source*: From Ref. 91.

evaluation (92). Pneumonia, with copious mucopurulent sputum, is far the most common manifestation, being the only locus of disease in 77% of one series (Table 4) (7). As with histoplasmosis, chronic nodular pulmonary infiltrates and cavitary disease may be long-term sequelae (Fig. 15) (91,93–96). Occasionally, acute pulmonary blastomycosis may be associated with rheumatologic manifestations, such as erythema nodosum (97).

Like histoplasmosis, *B. dermatitidis* may spread from the lungs hematogenously to appear focally in other sites (3,5,93). Focal cutaneous lesions appear

Table 4 Clinical Findings in 73 Patients with Blastomycosis

Symptoms	
Cough	85%
Fever	65%
Night sweats	61%
Pleuritic pain	58%
Weight loss	58%
Myalgias	34%
Hemoptysis	17%
Foci of disease	
Pulmonary	77%
Skin only	4%
Bone only	3%
Disseminated[a]	15%

[a] Active disease ≥2 organ systems.
Source: From Ref. 7.

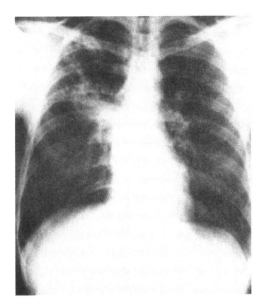

Figure 15 Chest radiograph showing chronic fibronodular blastomycotic pneumonia. *Source*: From Ref. 91.

as nodules and abscesses which may initially be mistaken for skin cancer (Fig. 16) (98). Focal bone lesions may occur in 25% of those with disseminated disease, commonly in the spine as lytic lesions (Fig. 17) (80,99–101). Prostatic involvement may be occult or appear as mass lesions. Meningitis may occur, but is uncommon (4% of patients with disseminated disease), as is adrenal gland involvement (102). These lesions tend to be chronic, with the diagnosis often made by biopsy for suspicion of cancer.

Laboratory Clues to Diagnosis

Microbiology: The bases of diagnosis of blastomycosis are direct exam of sputa, culture, and histopathology. Direct examination of the sputum by potassium hydroxide (KOH) has been very helpful in the rapid diagnosis of suspicious cases, and may be lifesaving in the critically ill patient (Fig. 18) (91). It is easy to do and organisms are readily seen. The organisms grow as mycelium on Sabouraud's agar, and are distinguished by the absence of tuberculate macroconidia. They may be converted to the yeast phase by culture at 37°C, or identified directly by nucleic acid probes.

Histopathology

B. dermatitidis yeast cells are larger than *H. capsulatum*, and have broader based single buds as daughter cells. Like *Histoplasma*, they are not encapsulated and are readily stained with GMS and PAS. In general they are readily identified

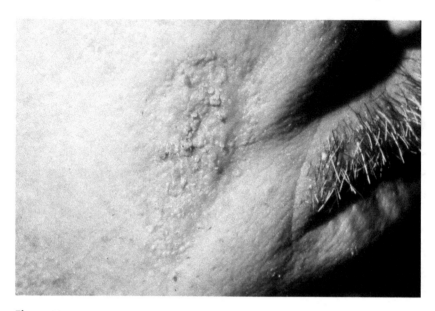

Figure 16 Verrucous blastomycotic skin lesion. *Source*: Courtesy of J. R. Graybill.

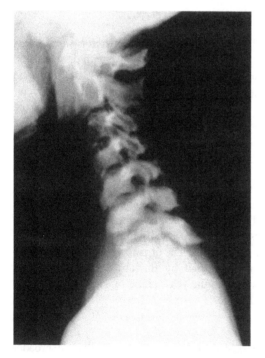

Figure 17 Vertebral lytic lesion caused by *Blastomyces dermatitidis*. *Source*: From Ref. 80.

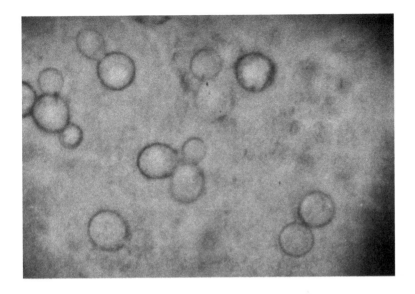

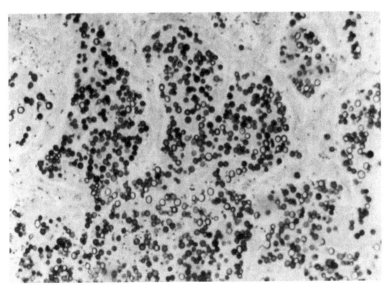

Figure 18 Potassium hydroxide (KOH) smear (**A**) and Gomori's methenamine silver stain (**B**) of tracheal secretions in a patient with adult respiratory distress syndrome caused by overwhelming blastomycosis. Note broad-based buds of dividing organisms in KOH smear. *Source*: From Ref. 89.

in tissue biopsy specimens. Children may require lung biopsy to establish the diagnosis, whereas adults are more likely to yield positive sputa.

One clue favoring *B. dermatitidis* in histopathological specimens, especially of skin lesions, is the characteristic pyogranulomatous reaction, with both granulomas and microabscesses filled with abundant polymorphonuclear leukocytes (3,91). This is to be distinguished from *H. capsulatum*, in which strong immune response manifests as well-formed granulomas and ultimately caseous necrosis with very few organisms. Conversely, in severe immunosuppressed patients, such as those with AIDS or on corticosteroid therapy, there are poorly formed granulomas and masses of organisms, but less necrosis.

Serodiagnosis

Like all of the endemic mycoses, antibodies are raised against *B. dermatitidis* during the course of infection. However, the complement fixation and immunodiffusion tests are not positive as regularly seen as with *C. immitis* and *H. capsulatum* infection, and tests for blastomycosis also are strongly cross-reactive with *H. capsulatum* (103). An ELISA assay, using the A antigen, appears more sensitive and specific than prior methods (104,105). Antibody testing is helpful in outbreaks where patients had culture negative sputa (81). Additional cases may be identified by antibody testing of asymptomatic visitors to an endemic area (83). An ELISA titer positive at 1:32 identified 18 subjects, all of who were negative by complement fixation and immunodiffusion tests. *Histoplasma* antigen may give false-positive results in patients with blastomycosis (106). Recently, Miravista Laboratories has marketed a *Blastomyces* antigen test, with a sensitivity of 92% and a specificity of 79%, using normal controls. Unfortunately, there is cross-reactivity in 96% patients with histoplasmosis, the disease from which it is in most need of being differentiated (107). It is not yet clear whether this test will enjoy the popularity of the *Histoplasma* antigen test. There are as yet no PCR-based methods for diagnosis of blastomycosis.

COCCIDIOIDOMYCOSIS

Epidemiologic Clues to Diagnosis

Coccidioidomycosis is an infection caused by dimorphic fungi of the genus *Coccidioides*. These soil-dwelling fungi have an endemic range that encompasses semiarid to arid life zones principally in the southwestern United States and northern Mexico (108). *Coccidioides* is also found in parts of Argentina, Brazil Columbia, Guatemala, Honduras, Nicaragua, Paraguay, and Venezuela (Fig. 19) (77,109). Hyperendemic areas include Kern County in the San Joaquin Valley of California and Pima, Pinal, and Maricopa Counties in Arizona. Major cities within these hyperendemic areas include Bakersfield, California, and Phoenix and Tucson, Arizona (109). Residence in or travel to these areas provides an important clue to the diagnosis. Persons with occupations that have soil exposure,

(A)

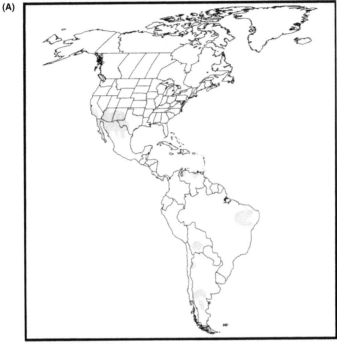

Coccidioides immitis

☐ Coccidiodomycosis

(B)

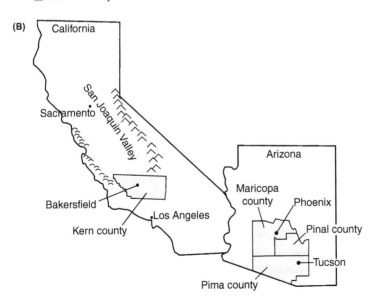

Figure 19 (**A**) Endemic area of coccidioidomycosis. (**B**) Hyperendemic areas for coccidioidomycosis. *Source*: (**A**) From Refs. 77, 191–193.

such as agricultural workers, excavators, military personnel, and archeologists, are at the greatest risk to acquire coccidioidomycosis (109–111).

Until the advent of the HIV epidemic, coccidioidomycosis was considered an infection primarily of the immunocompetent host, with fewer than half of those exposed developing symptoms, and very few developing progressive disease. There has been a greatly increased risk of progressive infection associated with AIDS (12). The major risk factor for developing active coccidioidomycosis in patients with HIV infection is a CD4 lymphocyte count less than 250 μL (12,13,112).

Recently described risk groups for coccidioidomycosis include organ transplant recipients who received *Coccidioides*-infected organs, patients being treated with tumor necrosis factor antagonists, and travelers to the southwestern United States and Mexico (113–116). Careless handling of cultures has caused a number of human infections in laboratory workers (117). Outbreaks of coccidioidomycosis may also follow natural events that result in atmospheric soil dispersion, such as dust storms, earthquakes, and droughts (118,119). Also, there may be common-source outbreaks among persons who participated together in an activity that caused disruption of the soil, such as an archaeological dig. Often those affected were not from the endemic area and thus have no prior immunity. Also, these patients may have extensive pulmonary infiltrates, due to the intense exposure to the fungus in a confined area (110).

Clinical Clues to Diagnosis

In immunocompetent persons, more than 60% of infections with *Coccidioides* are asymptomatic, and the majority of the remainder of patients has nonspecific complaints including fever, pleuritic substernal chest pain, cough, malaise, anorexia, or chills. This illness may be attributed to the "flu," and medical attention is often not sought (120).

Pulmonary infiltrates can take multiple forms, are commonly associated with hilar adenopathy, and may also occur with pleural effusions. Up to 25% of men and 4% of women have immune complex-mediated manifestations, including erythema nodosum or erythema multiforme, or both. Arthralgias may also occur, as well as eosinophilia, ranging up to 20% of the leukocyte count. Untreated, pneumonia usually resolves within six to eight weeks. About 5% of patients develop chronic pulmonary lesions, which may include thin-walled residual cavities, nodules, abscesses, or infiltrates, which may wax and wane. The course and rate of evolution from primary infection is highly variable. Pulmonary foci may coalesce into nodules that persist, resolve slowly, or undergo necrosis to form cavities. Cavities may persist for months or even years, may slowly resolve, or may rupture into the pleural space, causing pneumothorax, empyema, or both (121). Hemoptysis or rarely severe pulmonary hemorrhage may also occur. In a case-control study conducted in Kern County, California, risk factors for severe pulmonary disease were diabetes mellitus, recent history of smoking, low income, and older age (122). Dissemination, when it occurs, often presents within a few months of the primary infection. In its disseminated form, coccidioidomycosis may involve nearly any organ of the body; the most common sites of involvement are the lungs, skin and soft tissue, bones, joints, and meninges (Figs. 20–22) (110). Other sites that have reported include the liver and spleen, peritoneum, pericardium, prostate, epididymis, urethra, and female genital tract (110). With its diverse clinical presentations, coccidioidomycosis has been called "the great imitator" disease (123). In contrast to histoplasmosis and tuberculosis, in coccidioidomycosis, the gastrointestinal tract is usually spared. Ocular disease is also rare (110). Pregnancy, particularly the third trimester, is also risk factor for dissemination (124).

Filipinos, African-Americans, and Hispanics are also at increased risk of dissemination. Patients with a deficient cell-mediated immune response may have miliary pulmonary infiltrates and widespread extra-pulmonary infection with abscesses draining purulent material with many spherules, many neutrophils, and few lymphocytes. This disseminated infection is associated with a negative skin test and high complement fixation antibody titers. In contrast, the patient with partially competent cell-mediated immunity may have a few

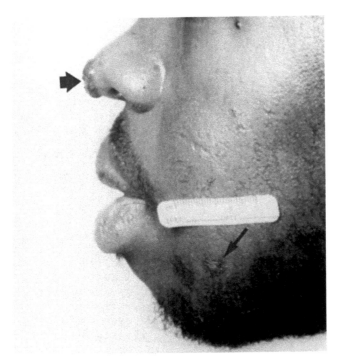

Figure 20 Skin lesions on the face and nose in disseminated coccidioidomycosis. *Source:* From Ref. 77.

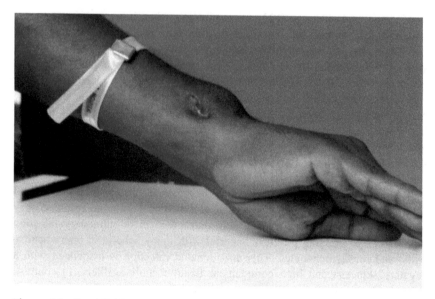

Figure 21 Coccidioidomycosis involving the wrist joint. *Source*: Courtesy of J. R. Graybill.

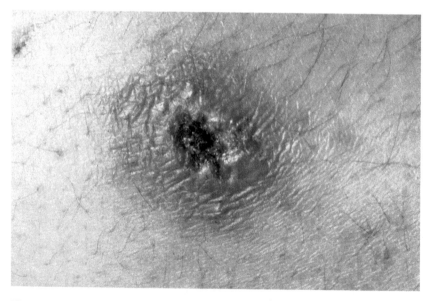

Figure 22 Skin lesion on the elbow in disseminated coccidioidomycosis. *Source*: Courtesy of J. R. Graybill.

granulomas in the skin, or scattered lung foci, with a few spherules seen trapped within multinucleated giant cells. In patients with AIDS, the infection has a more aggressive course, which inversely correlates with the CD4 count (12). Pulmonary cavitation is rather uncommon in patients with AIDS and coccidioidomycosis (125). For HIV patients on highly active antiretroviral therapy (HAART), one might anticipate a much more benign course, but few data are available (112).

In coccidioidal meningitis, the cerebrospinal fluid is characterized by lymphocytic pleocytosis, low glucose, elevated protein, and culture positivity in up to half of the patients (126). Eosinophilia may occur in the CSF of up to 70% of patients with coccidioidal meningitis (127). There is also associated focal vasculitis, but some series report remarkably few clinically apparent focal lesions (128,129). In one series of 15 patients autopsied with disseminated disease, 8 had central nervous system (CNS) involvement. Of these, 8 had meningitis; 7, encephalitis; 5, parenchymal abscesses and granulomas; 4, endarteritis obliterans; 2, infarcts; and 1, radiculitis. Associated clinical findings included headache, confusion, seizures, nuchal rigidity, each in a minority of patients; none had focal neurologic findings (128). A larger series of 25 patients reported headache, vomiting, and meningismus in multiple patients, but none of the patients suffered focal neurologic deficits (130). Banuelos et al. reported six patients with coccidioidal brain abscesses (131). About one-third of patients with brain abscesses have no associated meningitis, and these patients may have negative CSF serology, thus increasing the difficulty of making a diagnosis.

Dissemination to the bones occurs most often in the vertebrae and other weight-bearing joints, such as the knee, though any joint may be involved (Figs. 23 and 24). Arthritis is associated with synovial thickening and fluid accumulation. Paraspinous abscesses may occur (132).

Laboratory Clues to Diagnosis

Microbiology

Obtaining positive cultures of *Coccidioides* from clinical specimens is usually not difficult. At 25°C to 30°C, the organism converts to the mycelial form and readily grows on most culture media (Sabouraud's agar, brain heart infusion agar, blood agar), appearing within 7 to 10 days. The colonies are usually white, but may be tan, brown, pink, purple, or yellow. The hyphae are thin and septate and the branches produce distinctive unicellular barrel-shaped arthroconidia ($30–4 \times 3–6$ μm) alternating with empty disjunctor ("ghost") cells (Fig. 25) (133).

Although the mycelial morphology of *Coccidioides* spp. is unique, other genera also produce hyphae and arthroconidia, such as *Malbrachea*, *Arthroderma*, *Geotrichum*, and *Geomyces*. Definitive identification is most rapidly done by nucleic acid probes (Gen-Probe Inc., San Diego, California), but some labs still use the exoantigen test (Immuno-Mycologics, Inc., Norman, Oklahoma) (133). Bronchoscopy with bronchoalveolar lavage and pulmonary biopsy may yield

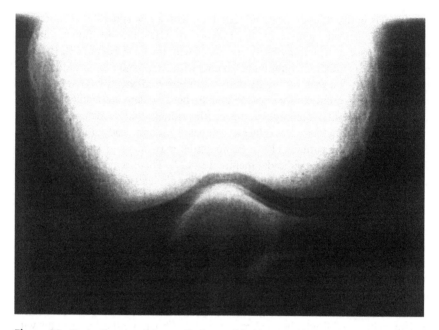

Figure 23 Lytic disease of the patella in coccidioidomycosis. *Source*: Courtesy of J. R. Graybill.

diagnostic cultures when routine sputum cultures fail to grow the organism (134). Needle biopsy of lung nodules may also yield the diagnosis (135).

Recovery of organisms from the CSF is less predictable, though McGinnis has noted that 76% of cases have positive cultures and 8% may have spherules identified (136). *C. immitis* can be recovered from synovial biopsies more readily than from joint fluid in coccidioidal arthritis.

Histopathology

The observation of the characteristic spherules (20–60 μm) with multiple endospores (2–4 μm) in histologic sections is pathognomonic of coccidioido-mycosis (Fig. 26). In active disease, these can typically be seen in hematoxylin-eosin-stained specimens. In resolving and residual lesions with fewer organisms, GMS stain is preferable. In response to released endospores, a suppurative reaction is seen, whereas spherules elicit a granulomatous response. An active lesion tends to have a central area of suppuration with surrounding granulo-matous reaction (137). Mycelial forms of *Coccidioides* may also occur in cytologic and histologic specimens (Fig. 27).

A few other organisms have morphologic forms in histologic specimens that may superficially resemble the spherules of *C. immitis*. *Rhinosporidium seebri* is a protozoan that produces a spherical sporangium that has a diameter of 100 to 200 μm and contains many small immature sporangiospores (1–2 μm).

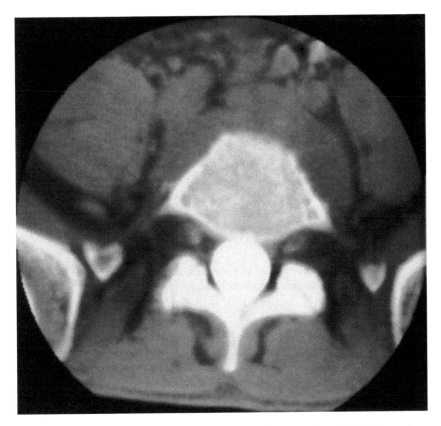

Figure 24 Coccidioidal lytic lesions in lower lumbar vertebra. Lytic lesions give a moth-eaten appearance to the centrum. *Source*: Courtesy of J. R. Graybill.

The sporangiospores are arranged as a crescentic mass at one pole and also peripherally along the wall of the sporangium. As the sporangiospores mature, they enlarge and migrate centrally (138). This internal arrangement is much different from the uniform size and distribution of the endospores seen within the spherule in coccidioidomycosis. *Chrysosopium parvum* var. *crescens* is a fungus that produces large thick-walled spherical arthroconidia (200–400 μm in diameter) in tissue. These structures are usually empty; this feature and the much larger size should clearly distinguish it from *Coccidioides* (139).

　　Protheca wickerhamii and *Protheca zopfii* are achlorophyllous algae that display endosporulating sporangia in tissue that stain with GMS and PAS; in the former species, the internal sporangiospores of the sporangia are symmetrically arranged, whereas in *P. zopfii*, the distribution of sporangiospores is random (140). In neither species does the sporangium resemble the spherule of *Coccidioides* with its many small endospores.

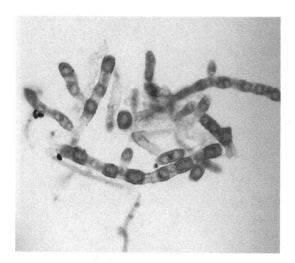

Figure 25 Arthroconidia of *Coccidioides immitis* with alternating empty disjunctor cells (Lactophenol cotton blue preparation; ×520). *Source*: From Ref. 133.

Serodiagnosis

Serodiagnosis is a very useful indirect method for both diagnosis and following the course of coccidioidomycosis. IgM antibodies are present soon after infection or relapse, but then wane; they are not helpful in the diagnosis of meningitis, and quantification does not correlate with severity of disease. The IgM antibodies have been assayed by a variety of methods over the years. Originally, the tube

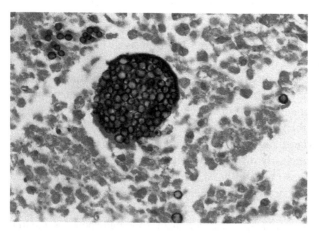

Figure 26 A large endosporulating spherule of *Coccidioides* spp., with released endospores (GMS-H&E; ×160). *Source*: From Ref. 137.

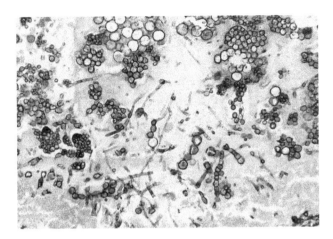

Figure 27 Miliary pulmonary coccidioidomycosis. The center of a necrotic nodule showing immature and endosporulating spherules, septate hyphae, and arthroconidia (GMS-H&E; ×40). *Source*: From Ref. 137.

precipitin test was used, in which the serum was combined with a soluble antigen to form a precipitate. If the test was performed as diffusion assay using agar, it was termed the immunodiffusion tube precipitin (IDTP) test. More recently, an enzyme immunoassay (EIA) to detect anticoccidioidal IgM antibodies has become commercially available.

The anti-coccidial IgG antibody converts to positive later than the IgM antibody, and generally remains positive for months. The IgG antibodies are able to fix complement when combined with coccidioidal antigen, and can be detected by immunodiffusion techniques. Rising titers of IgG are associated with progressive disease, while declining titers are associated with resolution. Patients with immunodiffusion complement fixation (IDCF) titers of ≥1:16 are more likely to have disseminated disease. In the CSF, a positive IDCF of any titer is considered diagnostic of coccidioidal meningitis. ELISA is now replacing the IDCF assay. For additional details on the serologic diagnosis of coccidioidomycosis, the reader is referred to the chapter on serodiagnosis of fungal infections in this volume (40). The PCR has been advocated for early diagnosis (prior to serologic conversion), using serum or CSF as the specimen, though it is not yet generally available (141).

PENICILLIOSIS MARNEFFEI

Epidemiologic Clues to Diagnosis

Penicilliosis marneffei is a fungal infection that occurs primarily in AIDS patients and is endemic to southeast Asia (Thailand, Vietnam, Myanmar, Hong Kong, Indonesia, Laos, Malaysia, Singapore, Taiwan, the Manipur state of India,

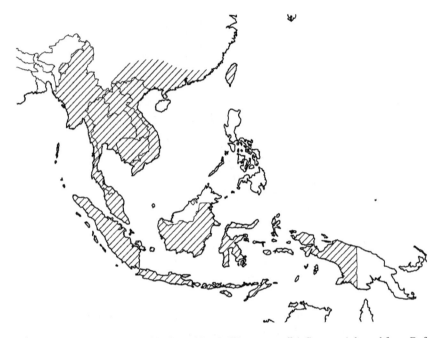

Figure 28 Geographic distribution of *Penicillium marneffei*. *Source*: Adapted from Refs. 19, 21, 142.

and the Guangxi province of China) (Fig. 28) (21,142–146). Residence in or travel to these areas is an essential clue to the diagnosis. The infection typically occurs in immunocompromised hosts. It was very rare prior to the advent of the AIDS epidemic, but in Northern Thailand it is the fourth most common opportunistic infection in AIDS patients, after tuberculosis, pneumocystosis, and cryptococcosis (19). Patients with AIDS with disseminated penicilliosis marneffei usually have CD4 counts less than 100 cells/μL (145). A case-control study conducted in Northern Thailand that compared AIDS patients with and without the infection found that the main risk factor for penicilliosis marneffei was occupational soil exposure during the rainy season (Table 5) (144,147). The disease has a definite seasonality; the incidence doubles in the rainy season. Although bamboo rats (genera *Rhizomys* and *Cannomys*) are reservoirs of this fungus, there is no epidemiologic association between penicilliosis marneffei and the consumption of these rats (148). The soil of rodent burrows also represents a natural source of the fungus (149).

Clinical Clues to Diagnosis

Clinical manifestations of penicilliosis marneffei are nonspecific, including fever, chills, prostration, weight loss, cough, dyspnea, anemia, lymphadenopathy,

Table 5   Signs and Symptoms in 80 HIV-infected Patients with Disseminated
Penicilliosis marneffei in Northern Thailand

Symptom or sign	%
Fever	93
Skin lesions	68
Cough	49
Diarrhea	31
Wasting	76
Anemia	78
Generalized lymphadenopathy	58
Hepatomegaly	51
Splenomegaly	16
Genital ulcer	6

Source: From Ref. 19.

arthritis, and hepatomegaly (19). Hepatic involvement is revealed by elevated transaminases and alkaline phosphatase (Table 4). The signs and symptoms of usually develop over weeks, but may be more acute (19).

The clinical presentation may mimic tuberculosis, melioidosis, leishmaniasis, histoplasmosis, or cryptococcosis (149). In the AIDS patient, frequently there are diffuse papular skin lesions with central necrosis or umbilication, resembling molluscum contagiosum (Fig. 29) (150). Other cutaneous manifestations of penicilliosis marneffei include maculopapular rash, pustules, and subcutaneous nodules. Mucocutaneous ulcers, including at genital sites, may be chronic or recurrent. Chest radiographic findings include diffuse reticulonodular,

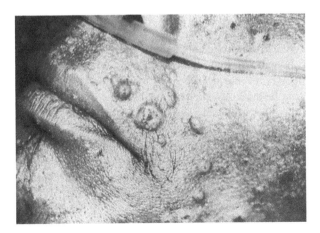

Figure 29   Molluscum contagiosum-like lesions in a patient with penicilliosis marneffei.
Source: From Ref. 19.

localized interstitial, or alveolar infiltrates. Arthritis can be monoarticular or polyarticular, with no specific joint predominance (150,151).

Laboratory Clues to Diagnosis

Microbiology

In disseminated disease, the organism can typically be cultured from bone marrow and lymph nodes, with a sensitivity approaching 100%. In HIV patients infected with *P. marneffei*, the organism has been recovered from blood cultures in 76% of cases (151). The organism can also be cultured from skin lesions, liver, bone, synovial fluid, lung, and occasionally urine. The use of Sabouraud's dextrose agar and an incubation temperature of 30°C are the culture conditions of choice. The fungus grows rapidly within two to five days in its mycelial form, producing gray to white colonies that have yellowish-green to olive drab to brown to yellowish-brown areas. The colonies are flat and velvety with radial folds. The organism produces a characteristic soluble red pigment, which diffuses throughout the agar. The globose conidia become elliptical, occur in tangled chains, and are 3–4×6–7 µm. At 37°C, the organism grows as a yeast (152). The mycelia/yeast dimorphism of *P. marneffei* is unique among the members of its genus (149). An exoantigen test can also be used to identify the organism.

Histopathology

Histopathologic exam is considered to be the most rapid and reliable method of diagnosis (152). Three histopathologic patterns have been described: granulomatous, suppurative, and necrotizing. The granulomatous and suppurative patterns are seen in patients with greater immunocompetence, whereas the necrotizing form is seen in immunocompromised hosts (21). In tissue sections, *P. marneffei* is seen within histiocytes as an oval yeast-like form 2.5 to 5 µm in size. Extracellular yeast forms are longer (about 8 µm), with rounded ends. In specimens stained with hematoxylin and eosin, the cytoplasm is retracted from the unstained walls, thus giving the impression of an unstained capsule (Fig. 30). With GMS staining, the fungal call wall is intensely stained and there is no pseudocapsular effect (Fig. 31). *P. marneffei* bears a morphologic resemblance to *H. capsulatum*, and it can be difficult to distinguish between them. However, *P. marneffei* tends to form more elongated yeast cells with no budding and divides by central septate fission rather than budding (152).

Pathologic diagnosis can be more difficult in immunocompetent patients in whom granulomatous inflammation may be the only finding, with negative fungal stains (21). More recently, specific fluorescent antibody examination of tissue samples has been described (149,151).

Serodiagnosis

With the high diagnostic yield of culture and histopathologic exam, serologic methods for the diagnosis of penicilliosis marneffei have not achieved

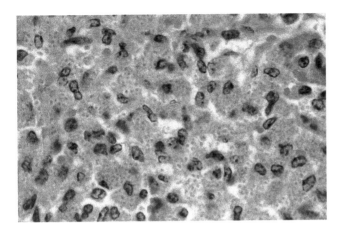

Figure 30   Yeast forms of *Penicillium marneffei* in a hepatic granulomas. The cytoplasm of the fungal cells is retracted from their unstained walls, producing a halo or pseudocapsular effect (H&E; ×250). *Source*: From Ref. 151.

widespread use. A few serological techniques for the diagnosis of penicilliosis marneffei have been described, including immunodiffusion for antibody detection and an indirect immunofluorescent antibody test; however, these tests need further evaluation to be used in clinical practice (153,154,155), Problems with the serologic diagnosis of penicilliosis marneffei are the depressed antibody response in HIV patients and cross-reactivity with other fungal pathogens (156), Nevertheless, with the inherent delay in awaiting culture results, there has been an interest in the development of rapid antigen detection assays. Desakorn and

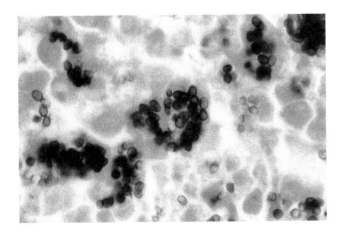

Figure 31   Septate and non-septate yeast forms of *Penicillium marneffei* within histiocytes. With Gomori's methenamine silver staining, there is intense staining of the fungal cell walls. (×400). *Source*: From Ref. 151.

coworkers developed an ELISA, a dot blot ELISA, and a latex agglutination test for detecting *P. marneffei* antigenuria using a rabbit polyclonal antibody raised against killed whole-fission-form arthroconidia of *P. marneffei*. The latex agglutination test was highly sensitive (100%), specific (99.3%), and was simple and quick to perform (157), The diagnostic sensitivity and specificity of the test were 92.5% and 97.5%, respectively. Thus, antigen detection may offer a rapid and sensitive means for the diagnosis of penicilliosis marneffei; it is uncertain at this stage of development if the these tests will also prove useful for following the course of infection or the detection of relapsed disease. Antibody and antigen detection methods for penicilliosis marneffei are described in more detail in the chapter on serodiagnosis in this volume (40), Sensitive PCR-based assays for the detection of *P. marneffei* have also been described, but only one of these has been applied to clinical specimens (158–160), Prariyachatigul and coworkers devised a one-tube nested PCR technique using three primers based on 18S rRNA gene sequences (158), The detection limit was 250 yeast cells. The specificity of the technique was verified by using 52 strains of 16 species of medically important fungi and 22 strains of 21 species of bacteria as negative controls. The test was 100% sensitivity and specificity for the direct detection of *P. marneffei* in blood samples of AIDS patients, but only 19 patients were investigated and only two of these had penicilliosis marneffei. The use of PCR does hold promise as a sensitive and rapid diagnostic test for the diagnosis of penicilliosis marneffei. However, in the underdeveloped regions of the world in which this disease is endemic, antigen testing may be less technologically demanding than PCR.

PARACOCCIDIOIDOMYCOSIS

Epidemiologic Clues to Diagnosis

Paracoccidioidomycosis (PCM) is a chronic or subacute, granulomatous systemic fungal infection caused by the thermally dimorphic fungus *P. brasiliensis*. The disease was first described by Adolpho Lutz, in São Paulo (Brazil) in 1908. Subsequently, it was identified in other parts of Brazil and South America. This systemic mycosis occurs endemically in the humid subtropics of Latin America, with a higher incidence in Brazil, Venezuela, Colombia, Argentina and Ecuador (Fig. 32) (161,162). Thus far, no cases have been reported in Nicaragua, Chile, and the Antilles. Sporadic cases have been observed in the United States, Europe, and Japan in individuals who came from endemic areas in Latin America. Therefore, PCM should be also regarded as a disease of travelers or immigrants who had lived for extended times in endemic areas (163). Some epidemiologic aspects of PCM are less well understood than those of other systemic mycoses. It is thought that *P. brasiliensis*, like *C. immitis*, *B. dermatitidis* and *H. capsulatum*, exists as a saprobe in the soil, where it produces propagules that can infect humans and other animals (164). Although the fungus has been occasionally recovered from soil samples and frequently from armadillos, in the endemic

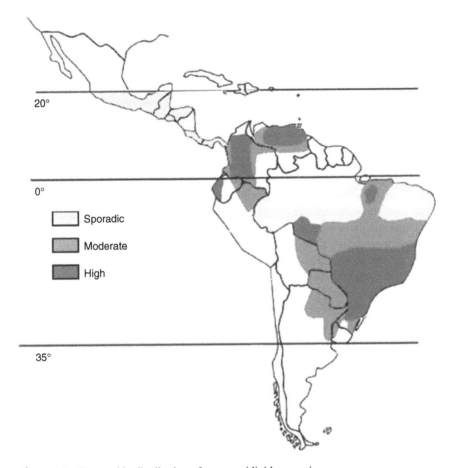

Figure 32 Geographic distribution of paracoccidioidomycosis.

areas, its ecological niche remains uncertain (165). The lack of outbreaks and the long period between infection and the development of disease hinder in the determination of probable infection *Source*. The clinical forms of the disease have mostly been observed in humans, but sporadic cases in domestic animals have been reported (166). On the other hand, skin surveys with paracoccidioidin shows a high percentage of reactors, including humans, sheep, cows, and horses. As expected, the disease is observed predominantly from rural areas, where individuals are more exposed to the causative agent. In adults with the chronic form, it is clearly prevalent among men between the ages of 30 and 60 years with rates of incidence ranging from 10 to 70 men for each woman (161,165,167). Females seem to be protected from the disease, but not from the infection, by the presence of β-estradiol, based on intradermal test surveys. In addition, the difference of prevalence between genders is not reported among prepubescent individuals who may present with the acute or juvenile clinical form. These epidemiologic characteristics are supported by experiments showing that β-estradiol inhibits the transition of conidia-mycelial propagules to the yeast form, a critical step in the pathogenesis of the disease (161,165,167). It is also believed that both conidia and yeast cells of *P. brasiliensis* are capable of producing melanin-like pigments, which may also contribute to the virulence of this species (168). Most of the patients are or were rural workers, with ages ranging from 30 to 60 years old. The consumption of alcohol and tobacco may also play a role in the development of the chronic form of PCM. The risk of becoming ill may be 14 times greater among smokers and 3.6 times greater among individuals with an alcohol intake of more than 50 g/day.

After infection, the progression to clinically apparent disease may be related to the strain virulence, inoculum size, and the status of the host defense mechanisms. In an immunocompetent host, fungal growth and spread is blocked in a pulmonary lymph node complex, and resolution of the infection usually occurs without any signs or symptoms (169–171). In this situation, scars formed at the primary and metastatic foci may contain viable quiescent forms of the fungus. After a long period of time, following changes in the host-parasite balance, the infection may progress and give rise to the chronic form of the disease. Less frequently, the disease also may arise directly from a primary focus, without a latency period, or by re-infection of the host in an endemic area. Once established, acute or chronic clinical forms may develop. Untreated, the natural evolution of disease usually results in death (163).

Paracoccidioidomycosis and AIDS

PCM occurs in patients with advanced AIDS who are not receiving prophylaxis for pneumocystosis with trimethoprim-sulfamethoxazole, which is also effective against *P. brasiliensis*. Despite a critical role for cell-mediated immunity, PCM has been scarcely reported among AIDS patients, transplant recipients, and cancer patients (165,169). However, as of the year 2000, only 54 cases of co-infection with *P. brasiliensis* and AIDS were reported (172). Initially, the scarcity of reported cases was explained by the use of trimethoprim-sulfamethoxazole as prophylaxis for pneumocystosis and the fact that the AIDS epidemic had been limited to medium-sized and large-sized urban centers, which were somewhat removed from rural areas in which PCM is endemic (173). However, the true incidence of *P. brasiliensis* infection among HIV-positive patients may be underestimated and there are probably more cases than have been reported. This was supported by the low rates of trimethoprim-sulfamethoxazole use, combined with the under-diagnosis of HIV-infection in a population with low socioeconomic level, and the difficulty in diagnosing clinically unsuspected PCM. With the progressive spread of the HIV epidemic in Brazil to small urban areas, which are close to rural areas in which PCM is endemic, there was an increase in the number of case reports of PCM-HIV co-infection.

Clinical Clues to Diagnosis

Primary Infection

The primary infection is almost always asymptomatic, and it is recognized by a positive paracoccidioidin intradermal test or by finding *P. brasiliensis* in partially calcified lesions from patients with no clinical evidence of this mycosis. According to skin test surveys carried out in the endemic areas, human hosts may present commonly with subclinical infection or nonspecific symptoms of respiratory infection with noteworthy radiological findings (174,175). The majority of the infected population evolves to cure but carry latent viable yeast forms of *P. brasiliensis*.

Acute/Subacute Form

This is also called the "juvenile form" and represents 5% to 10% of all cases of PCM involving children, youths, and young adults under 30 years of age. In prepubertal subjects both sexes are equally affected but after puberty, females are less affected. Signs and symptoms of PCM rapidly progress and within weeks to a few months the patient's general condition is seriously impaired. The reticuloendothelial system involvement is the predominant clinical feature, but any organ system may be affected. The most common clinical manifestation is generalized lymphadenopathy, including superficial and deep lymph node enlargement (Fig. 33). This clinical scenario is may be accompanied by fever, weight loss, hepatosplenomegaly, and bone marrow suppression. Gastrointestinal

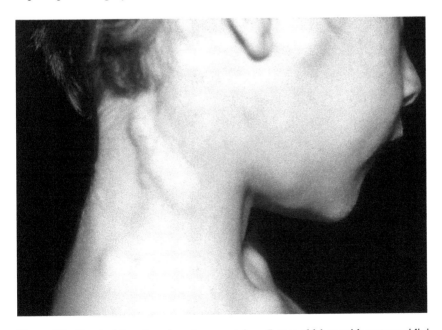

Figure 33 Cervical lymph node enlargement in a 7-year-old boy with paracoccidioidomycosis. *Source*: Courtesy of F. Queiroz-Telles.

involvement may cause abdominal pain, masses, and chronic diarrhea. Protein-losing enteropathy may lead to edema and ascites. Some patients may present several types of skin lesions resulting from fungemia and/or osteoarticular involvement mimicking arthritis or osteomyelitis (Figs. 34 and 35). Solitary or multiple osteolytic lesions can be also observed. In contrast with the chronic form, lung or mucous membrane involvement is rarely seen (161,163,165,176).

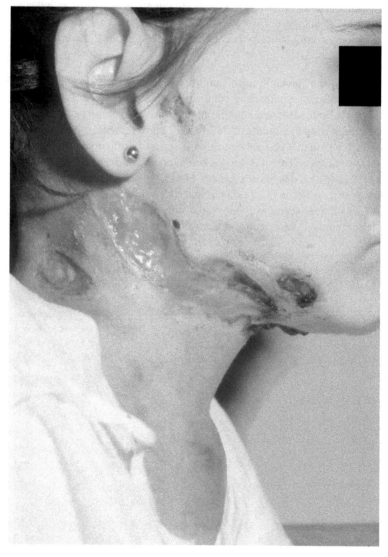

Figure 34 Ulcerated skin lesions and abscess in a 7-year-old girl with paracoccidioi-domycosis. *Source*: Courtesy of F. Queiroz-Telles.

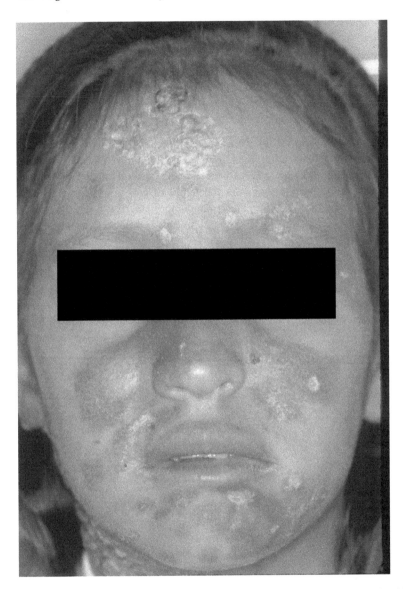

Figure 35 Verrucous and plaque cutaneous lesions in a 12-year-old girl with paracoccidioidomycosis. *Source*: Courtesy of F. Queiroz-Telles.

Paracoccidioidomycosis and AIDS

Most AIDS patients (77%) present with clinical features compatible with the acute form of PCM, although the illness likely represents reactivation of a latent infection, making classification as typical acute or chronic disease inappropriate. Clinical manifestations include prolonged fever, weight loss, generalized lymphadenopathy, splenomegaly, hepatomegaly, and skin rash. In HIV-positive patients there is uncontrolled proliferation of the fungus from reactivated quiescent foci rather than from an acute or subacute infection, as is usual in normal hosts with the acute form of the disease. Patients with HIV disease that present with PCM usually have CD4 cell counts less than 200 cells/μL (172).

Chronic Paracoccidioidomycosis

The chronic or adult form results from a reactivation of a quiescent pulmonary lesion and mostly affects adult men. Signs and symptoms usually progress slowly, and the patients do not seek medical care until several months of the onset of the disease. Although the lungs are the portal of entry, frequently there is dissemination to the oral mucosa. This prompts the patient to seek medical or dental consultation (Figs. 36 and 37). Symptoms may be related to a single organ or system (unifocal) or to several organs (multifocal). *P. brasiliensis* can disseminate to any part of the body by the hematogenous or lymphatic routes or invade adjacent tissues, turning chronic PCM into a polymorphic disease (161,163,165). Significant weight loss is often noted. In contrast to the acute form, fever is infrequent, unless a co-infection, such as tuberculosis, is present. Twenty to 40% of the patients may present with the chronic pulmonary form,

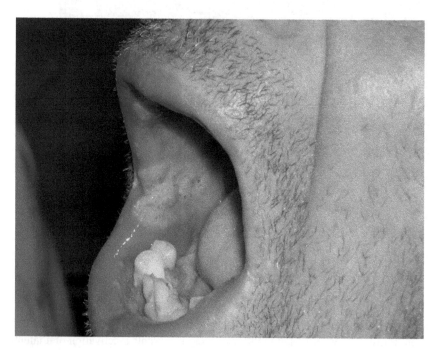

Figure 36 Granulomatous lesions of the gingiva, resembling cancer in a patient with paracoccidioidomycosis. *Source*: Courtesy of F. Queiroz-Telles.

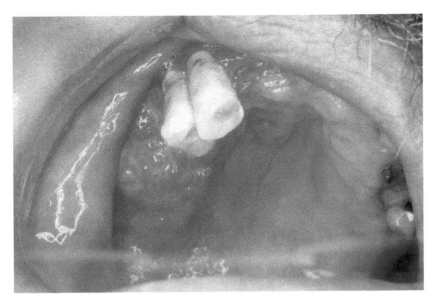

Figure 37 Mulberry stomatitis in a patient with paracoccidioidomycosis. *Source*: Courtesy of F. Queiroz-Telles.

which usually runs a course of a continuous or recurrent respiratory infection with cough, mucoid or purulent sputum, and dyspnea. Many of the radiographic findings are nonspecific, including diffuse micronodular infiltrates, mass lesions, and cavitations. However, mixed infiltrates distributed in the median zone (butterfly wing image) is strongly suggestive (Figs. 38 and 39) (177,178). In several clinical series, the chronic disseminated form of PCM is found in 60% to 80% of the subjects. All of them have pulmonary involvement in addition to lesions elsewhere. Lesions occurring in the oropharyngeal mucous membranes may begin as an unspecific gingivitis, with local bleeding and loose teeth. With time, typical painful granulomas, "mulberry-like" lesions, may appear and may extend to lips, tongue, gums, and hard and soft palate (Fig. 37). The larynx and vocal chords may present the same pattern of lesions leading to dysphonia or even aphonia. There are several types of cutaneous lesions resulting from blood or lymphatic dissemination. They vary from papules to verruciform lesions or tumors and must be differentiated from other infectious and non-infectious diseases (Figs. 40 and 41). Cervical and submandibular lymphadenopathy are frequently associated with oral lesions, but any other lymph node chains may be involved. Initially, lymph nodes are small with an elastic consistency but later they may enlarge and suppurate. Deep lymphadenomegaly may compress internal structures such the intestines, the biliary tract, or the upper mediastinum, which can lead to intestinal occlusion, jaundice, or superior cava vein syndrome, respectively. Adrenal involvement is frequently documented in this systemic

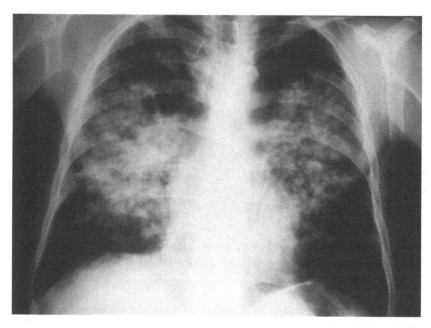

Figure 38 Butterfly wing image in a chest radiograph of a patient with chronic paracoccidioidomycosis. *Source*: Courtesy of F. Queiroz-Telles.

mycosis. Postmortem studies report adrenal abnormalities in 40% to 80% of PCM patients. However, hypoadrenalism manifests only when significant destruction of the adrenal gland has occurred. Adrenal insufficiency has been reported as a common sequela of PCM. In some cases, it may be the only clinical evidence of this infection (179,180). Central nervous system lesions have been reported in up to 20% of PCM patients in necropsy or radiographic studies. However, less than 5% of patients in clinical series have central nervous system manifestations. Neuroparacoccidioidomycosis is usually associated with the systemic form of the illness, but predominant involvement of CNS with only neurological symptoms may occur. The most common presentation is the pseudotumoral form, with single or multiple lesions with mass effect causing sensory or motor deficits, seizures, mental status changes, and intracranial hypertension. Involvement of brain stem, cerebellum and spinal cord are less frequently reported than hemispheric lesions (181–183). Other neurologic presentations include chronic meningitis, meningoencephalitis, and meningoradiculitis.

Microbiologic Clues

When appropriate collection and preparation methods are used, it is straight-forward to demonstrate *P. brasiliensis* in its parasitic form, using light

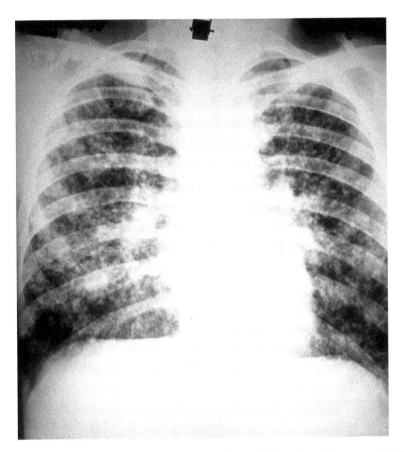

Figure 39 Micronodular radiologic pattern in an adult patient with paracoccidioidomycosis. *Source*: Courtesy of F. Queiroz-Telles.

microscopy. Cultures may be easily obtained if adequate material is sampled. In addition, several non-microbiologic tests can be employed. However, most of these indirect methods have not yet been standardized.

Direct Examination

The easiest way to confirm a suspected diagnosis of PCM is visualization of the yeast cells of *P. brasiliensis* in clinical specimens, including sputum, abscess or lymph nodes aspirates, tissue samples, urine, and bone marrow. Routine methods include KOH or calcofluor for wet mounts and GMS stain or PAS for smears. Digested and concentrated sputum can be positive in 60% to 70% of the subjects with the pulmonary or disseminated chronic form (184). In endemic countries, it is recommended that respiratory secretions should be also stained

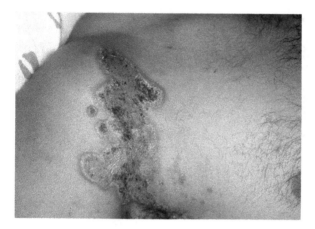

Figure 40   Verrucous and ulcerative cutaneous involvement with satellite lesions of the shoulder in a patient with paracoccidioidomycosis. *Source*: Courtesy of F. Queiroz-Telles.

by the Ziehl-Nielsen methods due to the high rate (10–15%) of tuberculosis co-infection. The yeast cells have a thick mucopolysaccharide cell wall, which under the light-microscopy may look bi-refringent, with the characteristic multi-budding yeast, resembling a "pilot wheel" or a "floating mine" (Fig. 42A). Mother cells presenting two buds may look like a "Mickey-mouse head" (Fig. 42B) (185).

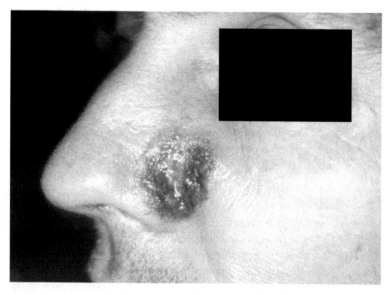

Figure 41   Ulcerative skin lesion resembling basal cell carcinoma in a patient with paracoccidioidomycosis. *Source*: Courtesy of F. Queiroz-Telles.

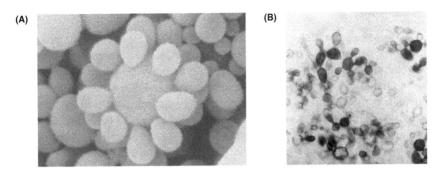

Figure 42 (**A**) Scanning electron microscopy of *Paracoccidioides brasiliensis* showing multiple narrow *P. brasiliensis* parasitic cells in pilot wheel configuration. (**B**) *P. brasiliensis* in tissue, Gomori methenamine silver stain. Narrow based budding cells give "Mickey Mouse" appearance to mother and daughter cells. *Source*: Courtesy of F. Queiroz-Telles.

Histopathology

Tissue sections can be stained by hematoxylin-eosin, GMS stain or PAS. The tissue reaction is similar to those of other systemic mycosis: granulomatous or mixed granulomatous and suppurative. *P. brasiliensis* yeast cells are usually large, ranging from 6 to 12 μm in diameter, with a refringent cell wall with intra-cytoplasmic organelles. Unlike *B. dermatitidis*, yeasts are multi-budded and have daughter cells with thin necks. Sometimes *P. brasiliensis* predominantly produces minute forms in its tissue phase. These elements may not show the typical multi-budding aspect and may be mistaken as the yeast cells of *H. capsulatum*, *B. dermatitidis*, or *Sporothrix schenckii*, the endospores of *C. immitis*, or capsule-deficient *Cryptococcus neoformans*. This situation requires the confirmation by culture and or by non-microbiologic methods.

Culture

Considered the gold standard for the diagnosis, the isolation of *P. brasiliensis* from clinical specimen material requires up to four weeks for the mycelial phase and 8 to 10 days for the yeast phase. Sterile biological specimens, such as tissue samples and lymph node aspirates, are preferred. Subjects with severe forms of the diseases may have positive blood or bone marrow cultures. As the fungus is slow growing in vitro, contaminated samples such as respiratory secretions or abscess fluid may yield only bacteria, yeasts, and rapidly growing commensal molds. Samples may be inoculated in Sabouraud's agar or yeast extract agar containing chloramphenicol and cycloheximide at room temperature. As the mycelial form is not characteristic, conversion to the yeast form is necessary to establish the identity. A rapid immunologic method was developed to identify *P. brasiliensis* in its filamentous form using cell-free soluble exoantigens.

Serology

Sometimes the microbiological documentation of PCM is not feasible, such as in occasional patients with the chronic pulmonary PCM who present with minimal expectoration and have negative findings with bronchoalveolar lavage and lung biopsy. In these cases, the detection of specific antibodies in serum has also been a diagnostic tool. More commonly, serologic evaluation is used to monitor the evolution of the disease and its response to treatment (24). Many different serologic tests and antigens have been employed for the diagnosis and treatment outcome, including double-immunodiffusion, immuno-enzymatic assays, and counter-immunoelectrophoresis. It has been shown that 90% of those with untreated PCM have measurable specific antibodies. The agar gel double immunodiffusion technique employing the gp43-glycoprotein exoantigen is the most widely used serologic test in clinical practice, because it is simple, specific, and readily available; it has a sensitivity of 90% and a specificity of 100%. A positive double diffusion test indicates active lesions of PCM even when clinical manifestations are not yet detected. However, the serodiagnosis of PCM can be problematic because of the cross-reactivity observed with other mycoses, mainly histoplasmosis and lobomycosis.

The histoplasmin antigen test supplied by Miravista Laboratories cross-reacts extensively with patients with PCM (59). Thus, the histoplasmin urine antigen test is of limited value in distinguishing these two diseases. In contrast, the detection of *P. brasiliensis* gp43 circulating antigen by inhibition enzyme-linked immunosorbent assay may afford a more practical approach to the rapid diagnosis of the disease, providing high specificity and sensitivity using sera, cerebrospinal fluid, and bronchoalveolar lavage fluid of patients with active PCM (186). Usually patients with severe forms of PCM have higher antibody titers. However, in the most disseminated cases, the excess of circulating antigen may produce false-negative results. The lack of reactivity of sera from PCM patients in immunodiffusion assays may also be related to the production of low-avidity IgG antibodies directed against carbohydrate epitopes (187). Antibody levels are used in conjunction with clinical, radiographic, and mycological parameters to determine when therapy for PCM can be discontinued. After a median time of six months of continuous itraconazole or 24 months of continuous trimethoprim-sulfamethoxazole, the antibodies titers tend to be negative or stabilized at low levels (188). Antigen detection is also a valuable tool in the diagnosis and prognosis of patients with *P. brasiliensis* infection. Although serological diagnosis might be a helpful tool it should not be used as the single method of diagnosis of PCM. In immunocompromised subjects, especially HIV-positive patients, B-cell dysfunction can be responsible for the false-negative serologic tests, and when the result is positive it normally shows low titers of antibodies. PCR assay may be a promising diagnostic tool for these patients (173). An experimental nested PCR assay for the detection of *P. brasiliensis* DNA has been evaluated, using a sequence of the immunogenic gp43 gene as a target. The authors demonstrated that this non-microbiological assay for the detection of *P. brasiliensis* in tissues of mice had high sensitivity and specificity. The assay may be useful for diagnosis of PCM in human tissue samples (189). Preliminary data also demonstrate that PCR assay based on oligonucleotide primers derived from the sequence of the gene coding for the 43,000-Da gp43 antigen may detect *P. brasiliensis* DNA in sputa, detecting 10 fungal cells/mL of sputum (190).

REFERENCES

1. Wheat LJ. Histoplasmosis. Infect Dis Clin N Amer 1988; 2:841–59.
2. Chandler F, Ajello L. Histoplasmosis duboisii. In: Connor D, Chandler F, Manz H, Schwartz D, Lack E, eds. Pathology of Infectious Diseases. Stamford, CT: Appleton and Lange, 1997:1017–22.
3. Bradsher RW. Blastomycosis. Clin Infect Dis 1992; 14(Suppl. 1):S82–90.
4. Pappas PG, Pottage JC, Powderly WG, et al. Blastomycosis in patients with acquired immunodeficiency syndrome. Ann Intern Med 1992; 116:847–53.
5. Assaly RA, Hammersley JR, Olson DE, et al. Disseminated blastomycosis. J Am Acad Dermatol 2003; 48:123–7.
6. Crampton TL, Light RB, Berg GM, et al. Epidemiology and clinical spectrum of blastomycosis diagnosed at Manitoba hospitals. Clin Infect Dis 2002; 34:1310–6.
7. Baumgardner DJ, Buggy BP, Mattson BJ, Burdick JS, Ludwig D. Epidemiology of blastomycosis in a region of high endemicity in north central Wisconsin. Clin Infect Dis 1992; 15:629–35.
8. Londero AT, Severo LC. The gamut of progressive pulmonary paracoccidioido-mycosis. Mycopathologia 1981; 75:65–74.
9. Greer DL, Restrepo A. La epidemiologia de la paracoccidioidomicosis. Bol Sanit Panama 1977; 83:428–45.
10. Golgani LZ, Sugar AM. Paracoccidioidomycosis and AIDS: an overview. Clin Infect Dis 1995; 21:1275–81.
11. Galgiani JN. Coccidioidomycosis: a regional disease of national importance—rethinking approaches for control. Ann Intern Med 1999; 130:293–300.
12. Fish DG, Ampel NM, Galgiani JN, et al. Coccidioidomycosis during human immunodeficiency virus infection. Medicine (Baltimore) 1990; 69:394–8.
13. Ampel NM, Dols CL, Galgiani JN. Coccidioidomycosis during human immuno-deficiency virus infection: results of a prospective study in a coccidioidal endemic area. Am J Med 1993; 94:235–40.
14. Woods CW, McRill C, Plikaytis BD, et al. Coccidioidomycosis in human immunodeficiency virus-infected persons in Arizona, 1994–1997: incidence, risk factors, and prevention. J Infect Dis 2000; 181:1428–34.
15. Pappagianis D. Epidemiology of coccidioidomycosis. In: Stevens DA, ed. Coccidioidomycosis: A Text. New York: Plenum, 1980:63–85.
16. Borelli D. Prevalence of systemic mycoses in Latin America. In: Pan American Health Organization, editor. Proceedings of an International Symposium on Mycoses. Publication No. 205. Washington, DC: Pan American Health Organization, 1970:28–38.

17. Posadas A. Un nuevo caso de micosis fungoidea con psorospermias. An Circ Med Argent 1892; 15:585–97.
18. Bialek R, Kern J, Herrmann T, et al. PCR assays for identification of *Coccidioides posadasii* based on the nucleotide sequence of the antigen 2/proline-rich antigen. J Clin Microbiol 2004; 42:778–83.
19. Supparatpinyo K, Khamwan C, Baosoung V, Nelson KE, Sirisanthana T. Disseminated *Penicillium marneffei* infection in Southeast Asia. Lancet 1994; 344:110–3.
20. Duong TA. Infection due to *Penicillium marneffei*, an emerging pathogen: review of 155 reported cases. Clin Infect Dis 1996; 23:125–30.
21. Deng Z, Ribas J, Gibson DW, Connor DH. Infections caused by *Penicillium marneffei* in China and Southeast Asia. Review of 18 published cases and report of four more cases. Rev Infect Dis 1988; 10:640–52.
22. Goodwin RA, Nickell JA, Dez Prez RM. Mediastinal fibrosis complicating healed histoplasmosis and tuberculosis. Medicine (Baltimore) 1972; 51:227–32.
23. Goodwin RA, Owens FT, Snell JD, et al. Chronic pulmonary histoplasmosis. Medicine (Baltimore) 1976; 55:413–52.
24. Goodwin RA, Shapiro JL, Thurman GH, Thurman SS, Des Prez RM. Disseminated histoplasmosis: clinical and pathologic correlations. Medicine (Baltimore) 1980; 59:1–33.
25. Edwards LB, Acquaviva FA, Livesay VT, Cross FW, Palmer CE. An atlas of sensitivity to tuberculin, PPD-B, and histoplasmin in the United States. Am Rev Respir Dis 1969; 99(Suppl.):1–132.
26. Silverman FN, Schwarts J, Lahey ME, Carson RP. Histoplasmosis. Am J Med 1955; 19:410–59.
27. McKinsey DS, Spiegel RA, Hutwagner L, et al. Prospective study of histoplasmosis in patients infected with human immunodeficiency virus: incidence, risk factors, and pathophysiology. Clin Infect Dis 1997; 24:1195–203.
28. Sigrest ML, Lummus FL, Campbell GD, Busey JF, Allison FJ. Effect of diagnostic skin testing on antibody levels for histoplasmosis. N Engl J Med 1963; 269:390–4.
29. Hajjeh RA. Disseminated histoplasmosis in persons infected with human immunodeficiency virus. Clin Infect Dis 1995; 21(Suppl. 1):S108–10.
30. Ashford DA, Hajjeh RA, Kelley MF, Kaufman L, Hutwagner L, McNeil MM. Outbreak of histoplasmosis among cavers attending the National Speleological Society Annual Convention, Texas, 1994. Am J Trop Med Hyg 1999; 60:899–903.
31. Wheat LJ. Histoplasmosis in Indianapolis. Clin Infect Dis 1992; 14:591–9.
32. Wheat LJ, Slama TG, Eitzen HE, Kohler RB, French MLV, Biesecker JL. A large urban outbreak of histoplasmosis: clinical features. Ann Intern Med 1981; 94:331–7.
33. Wheat J. Histoplasmosis: recognition and treatment. Clin Infect Dis 1994; 19(Suppl. 1):S19–27.
34. Goodwin RA, Snell JD, Jr. The enlarging histoplasmoma. Am Rev Respir Dis 1969; 100:1–12.
35. Feigin DS, Eggleston JC, Siegelman SS. The multiple roentgen manifestations of sclerosing mediastinitis. Johns Hopkins Med J 1979; 144:1–8.
36. Loyd JE, Tillman BF, Atkinson JB, Des Prez RM. Mediastinal fibrosis complicating histoplasmosis. Medicine (Baltimore) 1988; 297:295–310.

37. Rubin H, Furculow ML, Yates JL, Bradsher CA. The course and prognosis of histoplasmosis. Am J Med 1959; 27:278–88.

38. Ongkosuwito JV, Kortbeek LM, Van der Lelij A, et al. Aetiological study of the presumed ocular histoplasmosis syndrome in the Netherlands. Br J Ophthalmol 1999; 83:535–9.

39. Wheat LJ, Chetchotisakd P, Williams B, Connolly P, Shutt K, Hajjeh R. Factors associated with severe manifestations of histoplasmosis in AIDS. Clin Infect Dis 2000; 30:877–81.

40. Warnock D, Morrison C. Serodiagnosis: antibody and antigen detection. In: Maertens J, Marr K, eds. Diagnosis of Fungal Infections. New York: Informa Healthcare, 2007:65–120.

41. Warnock DW. Amphotericin B: an introduction. J Antimicrob Chemother 1991; 28:27–38.

42. Wheat LJ. Current diagnosis of histoplasmosis. Trends Microbiol 2003; 11:488–94.

43. Wheat LJ, French MLV, Kohler RB. The diagnostic laboratory tests for histoplasmosis: analysis of experience in a large urban outbreak. Ann Intern Med 1982; 97:680–5.

44. Waite RT, Woods GL. Evaluation of BACTEC MYCO/F Lytic Medium for recovery of mycobacteria and fungi from blood. J Clin Microbiol 1998; 36:1176–9.

45. Klatt EC, Cosgrove M, Meyer PR. Rapid diagnosis in disseminated histoplasmosis in tissues. Arch Pathol Lab Med 1986; 110:1173–5.

46. Patino MM, Graybill JR, Hansen JT. Immunocytochemical staining of *Histoplasma capsulatum* at the electron microscopic level. Mycopathologia 1986; 94:157–61.

47. Graybill JR, Patino MM, Ahrens J. In situ localization of antigens of *Histoplasma capsulatum* using colloidal gold immune electron microscopy. Mycopathologia 1988; 104:181–8.

48. Bauman DS, Smith CD. Comparison of immunodiffusion and complement fixation tests in the diagnosis of histoplasmosis. J Clin Microbiol 1975; 2:77–80.

49. Bullock WE. *Histoplasma capsulatum*. In: Mandell GL, Bennett JE, Dolin R, eds. Principles and Practice of Infectious Diseases. New York: Churchill-Livingston, 1994:2340–53.

50. Pine L, Bradley G, Gross M, Gray SB. Evaluation of purified H and M antigens of Histoplasmin as reagents in the complement fixation test. Sabouraudia 1978; 16:257–69.

51. Wheat LJ, Kohler RB, French MLV, et al. Immunoglobulin M and G histoplasmal antibody response in histoplasmosis. Am Rev Respir Dis 1983; 128:65–70.

52. Williams B, Fojtasek M, Connolly-Stringfield P, Wheat J. Diagnosis of histoplasmosis by antigen detection during an outbreak in Indianapolis, Ind. Arch Pathol Lab Med 1994; 118:1205–8.

53. Kaufman L, Kovacs JA, Reiss E. Clinical immunomycology. In: Rose NR, deMacario EC, Folds JD, Lane HC, Nakamura RM, eds. Manual of Clinical and Laboratory Immunology. Washington, DC: American Society of Microbiology, 1997:559–76.

54. Guimaraes AJ, Pizzini CV, Guedes HLM, et al. ELISA for early diagnosis of histoplasmosis. J Med Microbiol 2004; 53:509–14.

55. Pizzini CV, Zancope-Oliviera RM, Reiss E, Hajjeh R, Kauffman L, Peralta JM. Evaluation of a Western blot test in an outbreak of acute pulmonary histoplasmosis. Clin Diagn Lab Immunol 1999; 6:20–3.

56. Wheat LJ, Kohler RB, Tewari R. Diagnosis of disseminated histoplasmosis by detection of *Histoplasma capsulatum* antigen in serum and urine specimens. N Engl J Med 1986; 314:83–8.

57. Durkin MM, Connolly PA, Wheat LJ. Comparison of radioimmunoassay and enzyme-linked immunoassay methods for detection of *Histoplasma capsulatum* var *capsulatum* antigen. J Clin Microbiol 1997; 35:2252–5.

58. Wheat LJ, Garringer T, Brizendine E, Connolly P. Diagnosis of histoplasmosis by antrigen detection based on experience at the histoplasmosis reference laboratory. Diagn Microbiol Infect Dis 2002; 43:29–37.

59. Wheat LJ, Wheat H, Connolly P, et al. Cross-reactivity in *Histoplasma capsulatum* variety *capsulatum* antigen assays of urine samples from patients with endemic mycoses. Clin Infect Dis 1997; 24:1169–71.

60. Wheart LJ, Kohler RB, Tewari RP, Garten M, French MLV. Significance of *Histoplasma* antigen in the cerebrospinal fluid of patients with meningitis. Arch Intern Med 1989; 149:302–4.

61. Wheat LJ, Connolly-Stringfield P, Blair R, et al. Effect of successful treatment with amphotericin B on *Histoplasma capsulatum* variety *capsulatum* polysaccharide antigen levels in patients with AIDS and histoplasmosis. Am J Med 1992; 92:153–60.

62. Wheat LJ, Cloud G, Johnson PC, et al. Clearance of fungal burden during treatment of disseminated histoplasmosis with liposomal amphotericin B versus itraconazole. Antimicrob Agents Chemother 2001; 45:2354–7.

63. Wheat LJ, Connolly-Stringfield P, Kohler RB, Frame PT, Gupta MR. *Histoplasma capsulatum* polysaccharide antigen detection in diagnosis and management of disseminated histoplasmosis in patients with acquired immunodeficiency syndrome. Amer J Med 1989; 87:396–400.

64. Gomez BL, Figueroa JI, Hamilton AJ, et al. Detection of the 70-kilodalton *Histoplasma capsulatum* antigen in serum of histoplasmosis patients: correlation between antigenemia and therapy during followup. J Clin Microbiol 1999; 37:675–80.

65. Bialek R, Ernst F, Dietz K, et al. Comparison of staining methods and a nested PCR assay to detect *Histoplasma capsulatum* in tissue sections. Am J Clin Pathol 2002; 117:597–603.

66. Bialek R, Feucht A, Aepinus C, et al. Evaluation of two nested PCR assays for detection of *Histoplasma capsulatum* DNA in human tissue. J Clin Microbiol 2002; 40:1644–7.

67. Corcoran GR, Al-Abdely H, Flaners CD, Geimer J, Patterson TF. Markedly elevated serum lactate dehydrogenase levels are a clue to the diagnosis of disseminated histoplasmosis in patients with AIDS. Clin Infect Dis 1997; 24:942–7.

68. Gugnani HC, Muotoe-Okafor FA, Kaufman L, Dupont B. A natural focus of *Histoplasma capsulatum* var. *duboisii* is a bat cave. Mycopathologia 2004; 127:151–7.

69. Carme B, Ngaporo AI, Ngolet A, Ibara JR, Ebikili B. Disseminated African histoplasmosis in a Congolese patient with AIDS. J Med Vet Mycol 1992; 30:245–8.

70. Arendt V, Coremans-Pelseneer J, Bril T, Bujan-Boza W, Fondu P. African histoplasmosis in a Belgian AIDS patient. Mycoses 1991; 34:59–61.

71. Onwuasoigwe O, Gugnani HC. African histoplasmosis: osteomyelitis of the radius. Mycoses 1998; 41:105–7.

72. Arlet JB, Furco-Mazzantini A, Huerre M, Neuville S, Molina JM. African histoplasmosis infection with peritoneal involvement. Eur J Clin Microbiol Infect Dis 2004; 23:342–4.

73. Sanguino JC, Rodrigues B, Baptista A, Quina M. Focal lesion of African histoplasmosis presenting as a malignant gastric ulcer. Hepatogastroenterology 1996; 43:771–5.

74. Olasoji HO, Pindiga UH, Adeosun OO. African oral histoplasmosis mimicking lip carcinoma: case report. East Afr Med J 1999; 76:475–6.

75. Musoke F. Spinal African histoplasmosis simulating tuberculous spondylitis. Afr Health Sci 2001; 1:28–9.

76. Ajello L. Histoplasmosis. A dual entity: histoplasmosis capsulati and histoplasmosis duboisii. Ig Mod 1983; 79:3–30.

77. Anstead GM, Graybill JR. Histoplasmosis, blastomycosis, coccidioidomycosis, and cryptococcosis. In: Guerrant RL, Walker DH, Weller PF, eds. Tropical Infectious Diseases. Principles, Pathogens, and Practice. 2nd ed. Philadelphia, PA: Elsevier, 2006:903–17.

78. De Groote MA, Bjerke R, Smith H, Rhodes LV, III. Expanding epidemiology of blastomycosis: clinical features and investigation of 2 cases in Colorado. Clin Infect Dis 2000; 30:582–4.

79. Keon AF, Blumberg LH. North American blastomycosis in South Africa simulating tuberculosis. Clin Radiol 1999; 54:260–2.

80. Baily GG, Robertson VJ, Neill P, Garrido P, Levy LF. Blastomycosis in Africa: clinical features, diagnosis, and treatment. Rev Infect Dis 1991; 13:1005–8.

81. Klein BS, Vergeront JM, DiSalvo AF, Kaufman L, David JP. Two outbreaks of blastomycosis along rivers in Wisconsin. Am Rev Respir Dis 1987; 136:1333–8.

82. Klein BS, Vergeront JM, Weeks RJ. Isolation of *Blastomyces dermatitidis* in soil asociated with a large outbreak of blastomycosis in Wisconsin. N Engl J Med 1986; 314:529–34.

83. Baumgardner DJ, Burdick JS. An outbreak of human and canine blastomycosis. Rev Infect Dis 1991; 13:898–905.

84. Armstrong CW, Jenkins SR, Kaufman L, Kerkering TM, Rouse BS, Miller GB. Common source outbreak of blastomycosis in hunters and their dogs. J Infect Dis 1987; 155:568–9.

85. Bradsher RW. Water and blastomycosis: don't blame beaver. Am Rev Respir Dis 1987; 136:1324–6.

86. Ahkee S, Huang A, Raff MJ, Ramirez JA. Acute miliary blastomycosis in an AIDS patient. J Ky Med Assoc 1994; 92:450–2.

87. Tan G, Kaufman L, Peterson EM, De la Maza LM. Disseminated atypical blastomycosis in two patients with AIDS. Clin Infect Dis 1993; 16:107–11.

88. Herd AM, Greenfield SB, Thompson GW. Miliary blastomycosis and HIV infection. Can Med Assoc J 1990; 143:1329–30.

89. Meyer KC, McManus EJ, Maki DG. Overwhelming pulmonary blastomycosis associated with the adult respiratory distress syndrome. N Engl J Med 1993; 329:1231–6.

90. Sriram PS, Knox KS, Busk MF, Sarosi GA, Mastronarde JG. A 19-year-old man with nonresolving pneumonia—pulmonary blastomycosis. Chest 2004; 125:330–3.

91. Sarosi GA, Davies SF. Blastomycosis. Am Rev Respir Dis 1979; 120:911–38.

92. Lemos LB, Baliaga M, Guo M. Blastomycosis: the great pretender can also be an opportunist. Initial clinical diagnosis and underlying diseases in 123 patients. Ann Diagn Pathol 2002; 6:194–203.

93. Bradsher RW. Histoplasmosis and blastomycosis. Clin Infect Dis 1996; 22(Suppl. 2): S102–11.

94. Wallace J. Pulmonary blastomycosis—A great masquerader. Chest 2002; 121: 677–9.

95. Martynowicz MA, Prakash UBS. Pulmonary blastomycosis—an appraisal of diagnostic techniques. Chest 2002; 121:768–73.

96. Alkrinawi S, Reed MH, Pasterkamp H. Pulmonary blastomycosis in children: findings on chest radiographs. Am J Roentgenol 1995; 165:651–4.

97. Smith JR, Harris JS, Conant NF, Smith JT. An epidemic of North American blastomycosis. JAMA 1951; 158:641–5.

98. Woofter MJ, Cripps DJ, Warner TF. Verrucous plaques on the face—North American blastomycosis. Arch Dermatol 2000; 136:547–50.

99. Blackledge FA, Newlands SD. Blastomycosis of the petrous apex. Otolaryngol Head Neck Surg 2001; 124:347–9.

100. Veligandla SR, Hinrichs SH, Rupp ME, Lien EA, Neff JR, Iwen PC. Delayed diagnosis of osseous blastomycosis in two patients following environmental exposure in nonendemic areas. Am J Clin Pathol 2002; 118:536–41.

101. Hardjasudarma M, Willis B, Black-Payne C, Edwards R. Pediatric spinal blastomycosis: case report. Neurosurgery 1995; 37:534–6.

102. Chowfin A, Tight R, Mitchell S. Recurrent blastomycosis of the central nervous system: case report and review. Clin Infect Dis 2000; 30:969–71.

103. Bradsher RW, Pappas PG. Detection of specific antibodies in human blastomycosis by enzyme immunoassay. South Med J 1995; 88:1256–9.

104. Klein BS, Kuritsky HN, Chappell WA. Comparison of the enzyme immunoassay, immunodiffusion, and complement fixation tests in determining antibody in human sera to the A antigen of *Blastomyces dermatitidis*. Am Rev Respir Dis 1986; 133:144–8.

105. Klein BS, Vergeront JM, Kaufman L, et al. Serological tests for blastomycosis: assessments during a large point-source outbreak in Wisconsin. J Infect Dis 1987; 155:262–8.

106. Garner JA, Kernodle D. False-positive *Histoplasma* antigen test in a patient with pulmonary blastomycosis. Clin Infect Dis 1995; 21:1054.

107. Durkin M, Witt J, LeMonte A, Wheat B, Connolly P. Antigen assay with the potential to aid in the diagnosis of blastomycosis. J Clin Microbiol 2004; 42:4873–5.

108. Stevens DA. Current concepts: coccidioidomycosis. N Engl J Med 1995; 332:1077–82.

109. Fisher FS, Bultman MW, Pappagianis D. Operational guidelines for geological fieldwork in areas endemic for coccidioidomycosis (Valley fever). Reston, VA: U.S. Geological Survey, 2000 (open-file report 00-348).

110. Ampel NM. Coccidioidomycosis. In: Dismukes W, Pappas P, Sobel J, eds. Clinical Mycology. New York: Oxford University Press, 2003:311–27.

111. Perera P, Stone S. Coccidioidomycosis in workers at an archeologic site—Dinosaur National Monument, Utah, June–July 2001. Ann Emerg Med 2002; 39(5):566–9.

112. Ampel NM. Coccidioidomycosis among persons with human immunodeficiency virus infection in the era of highly active antiretroviral therapy (HAART). Sem Respir Infect 2001; 16:257–62.

113. Wright PW, Pappagianis D, Wilson M, et al. Donor-related coccidioidomycosis in organ transplant recipients. Clin Infect Dis 2003; 37:1265–9.

114. Bergstrom L, Yocum DE, Ampel NM, et al. Increased risk of coccidioidomycosis in patients treated with tumor necrosis factor-α antagonists. Arthrit Rheum 2004; 50:1959–66.

115. Panackal AA, Dahlman A, Keil KT, et al. Outbreak of invasive aspergillosis among renal transplant recipients. Transplantation 2003; 75:1050–3.

116. Panackal A, Hajjeh R, Cetron M, Warnock D. Fungal infections among returning travelers. Clin Infect Dis 2002; 35:1088–95.

117. Collins C, Kennedy DA. Laboratory-Acquired Infections. Boston, MA: Butterworth-Heinemann, 1999.

118. Flynn N, Hoeprich P, Kawachi M, et al. An unusual outbreak of windborne coccidioidomycosis. N Engl J Med 1979; 301:358–61.

119. Schneider E, Hajjeh R, Spiegel R, et al. A coccidioidomycosis outbreak following Northridge, Calif, earthquake. JAMA 1997; 277:904–8.

120. Drutz D. Coccidioidal pneumonia. In: Pennington J, ed. Respiratory Infections: Diagnosis and Management. New York: Raven Press, 1983:353–73.

121. Hyde L. Coccidioidal pulmonary cavitation. Dis Chest 1968; 54(Suppl. 1):273–6.

122. Rosenstein N, Emery K, Werner S, et al. Risk factors for severe pulmonary and disseminated coccidoidomycosis: Kern County, California, 1995–1996. Clin Infect Dis 2001; 32:708–15.

123. Huntington RW, Jr. Coccidioidomycosis—a great imitator disease. Arch Pathol Lab Med 1986; 110:182.

124. Peterson CM, Schuppert K, Kelly PC, Pappagianis D. Coccidioidomycosis and pregnancy. Obstet Gynecolog Surv 1993; 48:149–56.

125. Gallant J, Ko A. Cavitary pulmonary lesions in patients infected with human immunodeficiency virus. Clin Infect Dis 1996; 22:671–82.

126. Kelly PC. Coccidioidal meningitis. In: Stevens DA, ed. Coccidioidomycosis: a text. New York: Plenum, 1980:163–93.

127. Ragland AS, ARSURA E, Ismail Y, Johnson R. Eosinophilic pleocytosis in coccidioidal meningitis: frequency and significance. Am J Med 1993; 95:254–7.

128. Mischel PS, Vinters HV. Coccidioidomycosis of the central nervous system: neuropathological and vasculopathic manifestations and clinical correlates. Clin Infect Dis 1995; 20:400–5.

129. Williams PL, Johnson R, Pappagianis D, et al. Vasculitic and encephalitic complications associated with *Coccidioides immitis* infection of the central nervous system in humans: report of 10 cases and review. Clin Infect Dis 1992; 14:673–82.

130. Vincent T, Galgiani JN, Huppert M, Salkin D. The natural history of coccidioidal meningitis: VA-armed forces cooperative studies, 1955–1958. Clin Infect Dis 1993; 16:247–54.

131. Banuelos AE, Williams PL, Johnson RH, et al. Central nervous system abscesses due to *Coccidioides* species. Clin Infect Dis 1995; 22:240–50.

132. Kushwaha V, Shaw B, Gerardi J, Oppenheim WL. Musculoskeletal coccidioido-mycosis. A review of 25 cases. Clinical Orthopedics 1996; 332:190–9.

133. Walsh T, Larone D, Schell W. *Histoplasma, Blastomyces, Coccidioides*, and other dimorphic fungi causing systemic mycoses. In: Murray P, Baron E, Pfaller M, Jorgensen J, Yolken R, eds. Manual of Clinical Microbiology. Washington, DC: ASM Press, 2003.

134. Wallace J, Catanzaro A, Moser K, Ashburn W. Flexible fiberoptic bronchoscopy for diagnosing pulmonary coccidioidomycosis. Am Rev Respir Dis 1981; 123:286–90.

135. Forseth J, Rohwedder B, Levine B, Sarbolle M. Experience with needle biopsy for coccidioidal lung nodules. Arch Intern Med 1986; 146:319–20.

136. McGinnis M. Detection of fungi in cerebrospinal fluid. Am J Med 2004; 75:129–38.

137. Pappagianis D, Chandler F. Coccidioidomycosis. In: Connor DH, Chandler W, Manz H, Schwartz D, Lack E, eds. Pathology of Infectious Diseases. Stamford, CT: Appleton and Lange, 1997:977–87.

138. Watts J, Chandler FW. Rhinosporidosis. In: Connor D, Chandler F, Manz H, Schwartz D, Lack E, eds. Pathology of Infectious Diseases. Stamford, CT: Appleton and Lange, 1997:1085–8.

139. Watts J, Chandler F. Adiaspiromycosis. In: Connor D, Chandler F, Manz H, Schwartz D, Lack E, eds. Pathology of Infectious Diseases. Stamford, CT: Appleton and Lange, 1997:929–32.

140. Ramsay E, Chandler F, Connor D. Protothecosis. In: Connor D, Chandler F, Manz H, Schwartz D, Lack E, eds. Pathology of Infectious Diseases. Stamford, CT: Appleton and Lange, 1997:1067–72.

141. Johnson S, Simmons K, Pappagianis D. Amplification of coccidioidal DNA in clinical specimens by PCR. J Clin Microbiol 2004; 42:1982–5.

142. Ranjana K, Singh T, Priyokamar K. Disseminated *Penicillium marneffei* infection among HIV-infected patients in Manipur State, India. J Infect 2002; 45:268–71.

143. Singh PN, Ranjana K, Singh YI, et al. Indigenous disseminated *Penicillium marneffei* infection in the state of Manipur, India: Report of four autochthonous cases. J Clin Microbiol 1999; 37:2699–702.

144. Chariyalertsak S, Sirisanthana T, Suppuratpinyo K. A case control study of risk factors for *Penicillium marneffei* infections in human immunodeficiency virus-infected patients in Northern Thailand. Clin Infect Dis 1997; 24:1080–6.

145. Chariyalertsak S, Supparatpinyo K, Sirisanthana T, Nelson KE. A controlled trial of itraconazole as primary prophylaxis for systemic fungal infections in patients with advanced human immunodeficiency virus infection in Thailand. Clin Infect Dis 2001; 34:277–84.

146. Hilmarsdottir I, Meynard J, Rogeaux O. Disseminated *Penicillium marneffei* infection associated with human immunodeficiency virus: a report of two cases and review of 35 published cases. J Acquir Immune Defic Syndr 1993; 6:466–71.

147. Chariyalertsak S, Suppuratpinyo K, Sirisanthana T, Nelson KE. Seasonal variation of disseminated *Penicillium marneffei* infection in northern Thailand: a clue to the reservoir. J Infect Dis 1996; 173:1490–3.

148. Chariyalertsak S, Vanittanakom P, Nelson KE, Sirisanthana T, Vanittanakom N. *Rhizomys sumatrensis* and *Cannomys badius*, new natural animal hosts of *Penicillium marneffei*. J Med Vet Mycology 1996; 34:105–10.

149. Perea S, Patterson T. Endemic mycoses. In: Anaissie E, McGinnis M, Pfaller M, eds. Clinical Mycology. New York: Churchill Livingston, 2003.

150. Louthrenoo W, Thamprasert K, Sirisanthana T. Osteoarticular penicilliosis marneffei: a report of eight cases and review of the literature. Br J Rheumatol 2004; 33:1145–994.

151. Borradori L, Schmit JC, Stetzhowski M, Dussoix P, Surat JH, Filthuth I. Penicilliosis marneffei in AIDS. J Am Acad Dermatol 1994; 31:843–6.

152. McGinnis M, Chandler F. Penicillosis marneffei. In: Connor D, Chandler F, Manz H, Schwartz D, Lack E, eds. Pathology of Infectious Diseases. Stamford, CT: Appleton and Lange, 1997.

153. Kaufman L, Standard P, Anderson S, Jalbert M, Swisher B. Development of specific fluorescent-antibody test for tissue form of *Penicillium marneffei*. J Clin Microbiol 1995; 33:2136–8.

154. Sekhon A, Li J, Grag A. Penicilliosis marneffei: serological and exoantigens studies. Mycopathologia 1982; 77:51.

155. Yuen K, Wong SS, Tsang DN, Chau P. Serodiagnosis of *Penicillium marneffei* infection. Lancet 1994; 344:444–5.

156. Chaiyaroj SC, Chawengkirttikul R, Sirisinha S, Watkins P, Srinoulprasert Y. Antigen detection assay for identification of *Penicillium marneffei* infection. J Clin Microbiol 2003; 41:432–4.

157. Desakorn V, Simpson A, Wuthiekanun V. Development and evaluation of rapid urinary antigen detection tests for the diagnosis of penicilliosis marneffei. J Clin Microbiol 2002; 40:3179–83.

158. Prariyachatigul C, Geenkajorn K. Development and evaluation of a one-tube semi-nested PCR assay for the detection and identification of *Penicillium marneffei*. Mycoses 2003; 46:447–54.

159. LoBuglio KF, Taylor JW. Phylogeny and PCR identification of the human pathogenic fungus *Penicillium marneffei*. J Clin Microbiol 1995; 33:85–9.

160. Vanittanakom N, Merz W, Sittisombut N, Khamwan C, Nelson KE, Sirisanthana T. Specific identification of *Penicillium marneffei* by a polymerase chain reaction/hybridization technique. Med Mycol 1998; 36:169–75.

161. Blotta MH, Mamoni RL, Oliveira SJ, et al. Endemic regions of paracoccidioidomycosis in Brazil: a clinical and epidemiologic study of 584 cases in the southeast region. Am J Trop Med Hyg 1999; 61:390–4.

162. Wanke B, Londero AT. Epidemiology and paracoccidioidomycosis infection. In: Franco M, ed. Paracoccidioidomycosis. Boca Raton, FL: CRC Press, 1994:109–20.

163. Colombo A, Kauffmann CA, Queiroz-Telles F. Paracoccidioidomycosis. In: Mandell GD, ed. Atlas of Fungal Infectious, 2nd ed. Philadelphia, PA: Springer, 2007:53–67.

164. McEwen JG, Bedoya V, Patino MM, Salazar MA, Restrepo A. Experimental murine paracoccidioidomycosis induced by the inhalation of conidia. J Med Vet Mycol 1987; 25:165–75.

165. Brummer E, Castaneda E, Restrepo A. Paracoccidioidomycosis: an update. Clin Microbiol Rev 1993; 6:89–117.

166. Ricci G, Mota FT, Wakamatsu A, Serafim RC, Borra RC, Franco M. Canine paracoccidioidomycosis. Med Mycol 2004; 42:379–83.

167. Aristizabal BH, Clemons KV, Stevens DA, Restrepo A. Morphological transition of *Paracoccidioides brasiliensis* conidia to yeast cells: in vivo inhibition in females. Infect Immun 1998; 66:5587–91.

168. Gomez BL, Diez S, Youngchim S, et al. Detection of melanin-like pigments in the dimorphic fungal pathogen *Paracoccidioides brasiliensis* in vitro and during infection. Infect Immun 2001; 69:5760–7.

169. Negroni R. Paracoccidioidomycosis (South American blastomycosis, Lutz's mycosis). Int J Dermatol 2005; 32:847–59.

170. Restrepo A, Robledo M, Giraldo R, et al. The gamut of paracoccidioidomycosis. Am J Med 1976; 61:33–42.

171. Severo LC, Geyer GR, Londero AT, Porto NS, Rizzon CF. The primary pulmonary lymph node complex in paracoccidioidomycosis. Mycopathologia 1979; 67:115–8.

172. Bernard G, Duarte AJS. Paracoccidioidomycosis: a model for evaluation of the effects of human immunodeficiency virus infection on the natural history of endemic tropical diseases. Clin Infect Dis 2000; 31:1032–9.

173. Goldani LZ, Sugar AM. Paracoccidioidomycosis and AIDS: an overview. Clin Infect Dis 1995; 21:1275–81.

174. Bethlem NM, Lemle A, Bethlem E, Wanke B. Paracoccidioidomycosis. Sem Respir Med 1991; 12:81–6.

175. Ramos CD, Londero AT, Gal MC. Pulmonary paracoccidioidomycosis in a nine year old girl. Mycopathologia 1981; 74:15–8.

176. Pereira RM, Bucaretchi F, Barison E, Hessel G, Tresoldi AT. Paracoccidioidomycosis in children: Clinical presentation, follow-up and outcome. Rev Inst Med Trop Sao Paulo 2004; 46:127–31.

177. Londero AT, Severo LC. The gamut of progressive pulmonary paracoccidioidomycosis. Arch Med Res 1995; 26:305–6.

178. Funari M, Kavakama J, Shikanai-Yasuda MA, et al. Chronic pulmonary paracoccidioidomycosis (South American blastomycosis): High-resolution CT findings in 41 patients. Am J Roentgenol 1999; 173:59–64.

179. Colombo AL, Faical S, Kater CE. Systematic evaluation of the adrenocortical function in patients with paracoccidioidomycosis. Mycopathologia 1994; 127:89–93.

180. Leal AMO, Magalhaes PKR, Martinez R, Moreira AC. Adrenocortical hormones and interleukin patterns in paracoccidioidomycosis. J Infect Dis 2003; 187:124–7.

181. De Almeida SM, Queiroz-Telles F, Teive HA, Ribeiro CE, Werneck LC. Central nervous system paracoccidioidomycosis: clinical features and laboratory findings. J Infect 2004; 48:193–8.

182. Elias JJ, Dos Santos AC, Carlotti CG, Jr., et al. Central nervous system paracoccidioidomycosis: diagnosis and treatment. Surg Neurol 2005; 63(Suppl. 1):S13–21.

183. De Castro CC, Benard G, Ygaki Y, Shikanai-Yasuda M, Cerri GG. MRI of head and neck paracoccidioidomycosis. Br J Radiol 1999; 72:717–22.

184. Restrepo A, Cano LE. Recovery of fungi from seeded sputum samples: effect of culture media and digestion procedures. Rev Inst Med Trop Sao Paulo 1981; 23:178–84.

185. Queiroz-Telles F. *Paracoccidioides brasiliensis.* Ultrastructural findings. In: Franco M, ed. Paracoccidioidomycosis. Boca Raton, FL: CRC Press, 1994:27–47.

186. Marques da Silva SH, Colombo AL, Blotta MHSL, Lopes JD, Queiroz-Telles F, Pires de Camargo Z. Detection of circulating gp43 antigen in serum, cerebrospinal fluid, and bronchoalveolar lavage fluid of patients with paracoccidioidomycosis. J Clin Microbiol 2003; 41:3675–80.

187. Neves AR, Mamoni RL, Pires de Camargo Z, Blotta MHSL. Negative immuno-diffusion test results obtained with sera of paracoccidioidomycosis patients may be related to low-avidity immunoglobulin G2 antibodies directed against carbohydrate epitopes. Clin Diagn Lab Immunol 2003; 10:802–7.

188. Queiroz-Telles F, Colombo AL, Nucci M. Comparative efficacy of cotrimoxazole and itraconazole in the treatment of paracoccidioidomycosis. In: 38th Interscience Conference on Antimicrobial Agents and Chemotherapy 38, 1998 (Abstract J-142).

189. Bialek R, Ibricevic A, Aepinus C, Najvar LK, Fothergill A, Graybill JR. Detection of *Paracoccidioides brasiliensis* in tissue samples by a nested PCR assay. J Clin Microbiol 2000; 38:2940–2.

190. Gomes GM, Cisalpino PS, Taborda CP, De Camargo ZP. PCR for diagnosis of paracoccidioidomycosis. J Clin Microbiol 2000; 38:3478–80.

191. Wanke B, Lazera M, Monteiro PC. et al. Investigation of an outbreak of endemic coccidiomycosis in Brazil's north eastern state of Piani with a review of the occurence and distribution of *Coccidiodes Immitis* in three other Brazilian states. Mycopathologia 1999; 148:57–67.

192. Cordeiro RA, Brilhante RS, Rocha MF, et al. Phenotypic characterization and ecological features of *Coccidiodes* spp. from Northeast Brazil. Med Mycol 2006; 44(7):631–9.

193. Cordeiro RA, Brilhante RS, Rocha MF, et al. In vitro activities of caspofungin, amphotericin B and a zoles against *Coccidioides posadasii* strains from Northeast Brazil. Mycopathologia 2006; 161(1):21–6.

Hypersensitivity and Allergic Fungal Manifestations: Diagnostic Approaches

Taruna Madan[†]

Molecular Biochemistry and Diagnostics, Institute of Genomics and Integrative Biology, Delhi, India

INTRODUCTION

Sensitivity to a variety of fungi is known to be a factor in allergic rhinitis, allergic fungal sinusitis (AFS), allergic bronchopulmonary mycoses (ABPMs), hypersensitivity pneumonitis, and asthma. Currently prevalent diagnostic tools and novel diagnostic approaches being developed for hypersensitivity and allergic fungal manifestations are reviewed here. Testing to determine the presence of IgE for specific fungi may be a useful component of a complete clinical evaluation in the diagnosis of illnesses that can be caused by immediate hypersensitivity such as allergic rhinitis and asthma. Detection of IgG for specific fungi has been used as a marker of exposure to fungi that may be diagnostically relevant in hypersensitivity pneumonitis and ABPMs. However, the ubiquitous nature of many fungi and the lack of specificity of fungal antigens limit the usefulness of these types of tests in the evaluation of fungal allergies. At present, more than 70 fungal allergens have been cloned and sequenced, and the recombinant forms of several of these are commercially available. Measurement of IgE antibodies to these commercially available recombinant allergens and nanotechnology-based diagnostic probes could provide the tools useful for development of sensitive and specific diagnostic tests. The knowledge of IgE-binding epitopes of the major fungal allergens may be of importance for increasing the specificity and

---

[†] Currently at the National Institute for Research in Reproductive Health, Parel, Mumbai, India

Table 1   Genera of Fungi Frequently Associated with Allergy

Alternaria	*Drechslera*	*Phoma*
Aspergillus	*Epicoccum*	*Saccharomyces*
Aureobasidium	*Epidermophyton*	*Scopulariopsis*
Botrytis	*Fusarium*	*Stachybotrys*
Beauveria	*Gliocladium*	*Stemphylium*
Candida	*Helminthosporium*	*Trichoderma*
Cephalosporium	*Merulius*	*Trichophyton*
Chaetomium	*Mucor*	*Trichothecium*
Cladosporium	*Paecilomyces*	*Ulocladium*
Curvularia	*Penicillium*	

sensitivity of diagnostic tests by designing model allergens representing such epitopes.

The prevalence of respiratory allergy to fungi is estimated at 20% to 30% among atopic individuals and up to 6% in the general population (1). The major allergic manifestations induced by fungi are asthma, rhinitis, sinusitis, ABPMs, and hypersensitivity pneumonitis (2,3). These diseases can result from exposure to fungal spores, vegetative cells, or metabolites. Small size of the fungal spores (usually less than 10 μm) enables them to penetrate the lower airways of the lung and mediate allergic reactions. The site of deposition of spores depends on their size and nature as individual propagules or as aggregates (2,3). Additionally, there is now evidence that secondary dispersal of allergens, i.e., on other, smaller particles, possibly spore fragments, may serve as a vehicle for allergens.

Of the estimated number of more than one million different fungal species, approximately 80 fungi have been connected with respiratory allergy (Table 1) (2,4). Some of these fungi, *Aspergillus fumigatus*, *Alternaria alternata*, and *Cladosporium herbarum* have been investigated systematically for their role in causing allergy (5,6).

IMMUNE RESPONSE TO ALLERGENIC FUNGI

Exposure to fungal antigens can elicit both humoral and cellular immune responses. Humoral response to allergenic fungi is polyclonal in nature and is characterized by type I and type III hypersensitivity reactions. Type 1 (immediate) hypersensitivity reaction involves the release of mediators from mast cells or basophils caused by the bridging of IgE antibodies on the surface of these cells. Clinical manifestations of this type of reaction include rhinitis and asthma. Type III hypersensitivity (immune complex-mediated) owes its origin to formation of large quantities of soluble antigen–antibody complexes in the blood. These antigen–antibody complexes lodge in the capillaries between the endothelial cells and the basement membrane. The antigen–antibody complexes activate the classical complement pathway and complement proteins and attract leukocytes to the area. The leukocytes then discharge their killing agents and promote massive inflammation. This leads to tissue death and hemorrhage. Clinical manifestations of this type of reaction include allergic bronchopulmonary aspergillosis (ABPA) with extensive pulmonary tissue damage.

CLINICAL MANIFESTATIONS OF ALLERGENIC FUNGI

Allergic Rhinitis

Hay fever (allergic rhinitis or pollinosis) is an allergy characterized by sneezing, itchy and watery eyes, a runny nose, and a burning sensation of the palate and throat. It is usually caused by allergies to airborne substances such as dust, molds, pollens, animal fur, and feathers. Elevation in total and specific IgE antibodies have been observed in patients that initiate the type I hypersensitivity reaction mediated clinical symptoms.

Allergic Fungal Sinusitis

AFS is an increasingly recognized form of hypersensitivity disease, now reported throughout the world. It is probably the most frequently occurring fungal rhinosinusitis disorder. AFS is clinically analogous to ABPA as suggested by histopathology, immunopathology, and the clinical response to oral corticosteroid treatment. Patients with AFS tend to have elevated total serum IgE and fungal-specific IgG at diagnosis but not fungal-specific IgE or precipitins (7).

Allergic Bronchopulmonary Mycosis

Allergic syndromes to fungi, mainly *A. fumigatus* (ABPA) and rarer organisms, such as *Penicillium, Candida, Curvularia, Helminthosporium* spp., or, recently reported, *Saccharomyces cerevisiae* (8), occurring in asthmatic patients as eosinophilic pneumonia are termed ABPMs. ABPA is one of the well-studied ABPMs, which is an immunological disease and depicts the immune mechanisms similar to that of asthma. The presence of *A. fumigatus* growing in the bronchial lumen provokes an allergic response in the airways and parenchyma. Types I and III (and possibly type IV) hypersensitivity reactions are involved in pathogenesis. Central bronchiectasis, fleeting pulmonary shadows, bronchial asthma, immediate skin reactivity to *Aspergillus*, elevated levels of total IgE, specific IgE and IgG antibodies, peripheral and pulmonary eosinophilia, and precipitins against *A. fumigatus* (Af) antigens are characteristic features for diagnosis of ABPA patients. However, often there is difficulty to differentially diagnose ABPA from tuberculosis, pneumonia, bronchiectasis, lung abscess, and bronchial asthma (9–11). Early diagnosis of ABPA is important to prevent irreversible damage of the bronchi and the lungs.

Hypersensitivity Pneumonitis

Exposure to specific fungi, in both the indoor and agricultural environments, has been associated with hypersensitivity pheumonitis (HP) (12,13). HP is thought to be the result of a combination of immune complex and cell-mediated responses to inhaled antigens (14). In hypersensitivity pneumonitis, pulmonary abnormalities are restrictive rather than obstructive, and eosinophilia is rare in comparison to ABPM. Evaluation of elevated levels of precipitins or IgG antibodies is of diagnostic relevance, although their clinical significance in the pathogenesis of disease is not very clear.

Fungus-Induced Asthma

Asthma is one of the atopic diseases strongly associated with allergy. High aeroallergen exposure has been associated with higher risk of sensitization and chronic asthma. In patients with asthma and/or atopy, exposure to fungal biomass might result in age-dependent sensitization and asthmatic reactions, and association of fungus-induced airway obstruction with more severe asthma is documented (15). The association of sensitization to *Alternaria*, *Cladosporium*, *Aspergillus*, *Penicillium*, *Helminthosporium*, *Botrytis*, *Alternaria*, *Curvularia*, *Nigrospora*, and *Fusarium* with severe asthma has been reported.

LABORATORY DIAGNOSTIC TESTS FOR HYPERSENSITIVITY AND ALLERGIC FUNGAL MANIFESTATIONS

Diagnosis of allergic disease is mainly based on clinical symptoms of the patients, mycologic culture and direct microscopic examination, skin test reaction, detection of total IgE in serum, allergen-specific serum IgE antibodies radioallergosorbent test (RAST), enzyme-linked immunosorbent assay (ELISA) allergen specific serum IgG antibodies, and, in some cases, provocative inhalation challenge test (16). The process of reaching the diagnosis of allergic fungal rhinosinusitis and ABPA may require the CT and histopathologic examination.

Mycologic Culture and Direct Microscopic Examination

The patients' tissue specimen or lavage can be directly examined or may be transferred to relevant media for culture. Fungal identification is based frequently on spore morphology such as color, septation, and different methods of spore production. The distinct chemical compositions of the cell walls of different fungi are also helpful in their classification and determining their role in causing allergic responses in patients. The cell walls of yeasts are mostly composed of a chitin–glucan combination, in contrast to the predominantly chitin cell walls in mycelial fungi. Other aspects of vegetative morphology commonly used for identification purposes are color of colony, diffusible pigments, metabolites, and mycelial structures. Most of the spores produced by the imperfect fungi vary in shape, size, texture, color, number of cells, thickness of the cell wall, and methods by which they are attached to each other and to their conidiophores. However, the identification of the common fungi is at times difficult, as the fungal colony characteristics and even microscopic characteristics vary according to the medium in which the fungus is grown, temperature of incubation, and variation in strains and pleomorphic nature of the spores (17).

Skin Testing

Two types of skin reactions can be observed in allergic patients. Type I (immediate) reactivity consists of a "wheal and flare" within 5 to 20 minutes of antigen challenge. The type III reaction (Arthus reaction) is an induration usually developed within four to eight hours after skin testing. Two methods commonly used to diagnose allergies are prick and intradermal skin testing. Skin-prick testing (SPT), a widely accepted clinical method of determining the presence of specific IgE to a given substance, provides a biologically relevant immediate-type hypersensitivity response in the skin (18). Patients are regarded as being sensitive to a particular antigen preparation if the immediately developing wheal diameter is greater than 4 mm. SPT is simple, provides results within minutes, and is inexpensive.

Contraindications to SPT include generalized skin disease or the inability to discontinue antihistamine use; in these cases, in vitro assays for specific IgE may be useful. Although highly sensitive, SPT is not 100% sensitive or specific; SPTs can produce false-positive or false-negative results (19). The American Academy of Allergy, Asthma, and Immunology states that some patients who have a strong history of systemic reactions may have negative skin test results for IgE to suspected allergens (20). Until recently, crude fungal antigens have been used for skin-testing patients; however, the results of these reactions are not always satisfactory. In recent years, purified recombinant allergens from *Aspergillus*, *Alternaria*, and *Cladosporium* have been used with considerable success (21). The late skin response has been associated with ABPA (17).

Serological Testing for Total IgE, and Allergen-Specific IgE and/or IgG Antibodies

Indirect ELISA

ELISA has been demonstrated to be a sensitive, reliable, and quantitative diagnostic tool for allergic disorders. Although the sensitivity of the conventional ELISA system depends on many variables, the nature and type of antigens used and their ability to bind to polystyrene plates are the most important decisive factors. Currently, a mixture of diagnostically relevant antigens of Af is being used in ELISA-based detection for specific IgG and IgE antibodies (22,23) (*A. fumigatus*-specific IgA/IgG/IgM ELISA by IBL Immuno-biological

Laboratories, Hamburg, Germany) (Table 2). Total IgE antibodies in the circulation are also estimated by ELISA using monoclonal antibodies raised against human IgE antibodies (Human IgE ELISA quantitation kit, BETHYL Laboratories, Texas, U.S.A.).

RAST

The RAST is an in vitro test designed to measure the circulating allergen-specific IgE antibodies of a patient. The RAST is generally considered less sensitive than skin testing, although a RAST conducted with partially purified fungal allergens can be comparable to skin tests in both sensitivity and specificity (24,25). However, use of radiolabeled reagents limits its use.

Automated Antibody Determination Assay (Pharmacia immunoCAP System)

For estimation of specific IgE antibodies, an immunoCAP® (pharmacia Diagnostics AB, Uppsala, Sweden) assay has been designed, which is used to measure specific IgE antibodies to rAsp f 1 (26). For IgE antibody estimations, this commercially available immunofluor assay was calibrated against the World Health Organization standard for IgE and allows quantitative expression of total or allergen-specific IgE. The results are expressed as kilo units of allergen specific IgE per liter (KUA/L). The antigens are immobilized on cap-like structures made of spongy matrix, which capture the specific IgE antibodies from the patient sera.

Multiple Allergosorbent Chemiluminescent Assay

Multiple allergosorbent chemiluminescent assay (MAST) is a highly sensitive commercially available assay for specific IgE determination based on chemiluminescent detection and ELISA (27).

Halogen Immunoassay

Halogen immunoassay (HIA) is a new method for the detection of sensitization to fungal allergens that overcomes the variability in allergens in fungal extracts. The assay uses allergens expressed by freshly germinated spores that are bound to protein binding membranes (PBM). For HIA, spores from reference cultures are germinated on PBM, laminated, and then probed with patient serum. Green et al. reported that HIA correlates significantly with CAP and to a lesser extent with SPT. The significance of this derives from the unique ability of the HIA to measure IgE antibodies to the non-degraded allergens that are actively secreted by germinating conidia and hyphae (28).

Precipitin Testing

Precipitins are found in 95% of cases involving a fungus ball (e.g., aspergilloma) (29). About half of hypersensitivity pneumonitis cases have been reported to show precipitins (30). It is one of the diagnostic criteria for ABPA patients, and an immunodiffusion-based test is commercially available (Table 2) (31).

Detection of antibody by precipitin testing is a commonly used means of confirming exposure to a suspected antigen source, but it is not clear if the antibody detected is related to the pathogenesis of the illness. Precipitin assays are relatively insensitive, generally only detecting larger concentrations of specific IgG. Newer, more sensitive assays, such as IgG-specific ELISAs, can also be used to detect exposure to suspect antigens.

LIMITATIONS OF THE CURRENTLY AVAILABLE SERODIAGNOSTIC METHODS

Development of serologic methods for detection of fungi-specific antibodies is especially problematic because of the lack of standardized fungal extracts (32).

Any fungal species can make several allergens, which are produced variably, depending on the strain cultured and the conditions of growth (including the substrate) (33). With some fungi it is almost impossible to grow two consecutive cultures with similar antigenic profiles (34,35). Factors contributing to the variability of commercial and laboratory-made extracts are (*i*) variability of stock cultures used to prepare allergenic extracts and their proper identification, (*ii*) the use of mycelial-rich material as the source of allergens, (*iii*) conditions under which molds are grown and extracts prepared, (*iv*) the stability of the extracts, and (*v*) the quality control measures employed to ascertain comparability of extracts. The standardization of commercial fungi extracts results are extremely

Table 2 Commercially Available Assays for Diagnosing Fungal Allergy

Name	Assay	Manufacturer
Platelia candida antigen detection enzyme immunoassay	*Aspergillus fumigatus* IgA/IgG/IgM	IBL Immuno-Biological Laboratories, Hamburg, Germany
HALISA	Anti-*A. fumigatus* IgG	HAL Allergy Group, Haarlem, The Netherlands
SERION ELISA	Classic *Aspergillus fumigatus* IgG, IgM, IgA/quant	Serion Immunodiagnostica, Germany
An immunodiffusion test, test reagents for serodiagnosis of aspergillosis	Precipitins, anti- *A. fumigatus* IgG	Gibson laboratories, Lexington, U.S.A.
RIDA® AllergyScreen	A new panel strip test for specific IgE	R-Biopharm, Marshall, Michigan, U.S.A.
The Imutest system	In vitro diagnostic self test kits to detect total and allergen specific IgE	Clinical Diagnostic Chemicals Ltd., U.K.

important as diagnostic procedure as well as to decide an efficacious and safe immunotherapy. Ruiz Reyes et al. have reviewed important methodological steps in the standardization of fungi extracts and, finally, the clinical use of these extracts (36). It is now possible to grow allergenic fungi in synthetically defined media rather than in complex media containing no macromolecules. These allergenic extracts show less variability and demonstrate specific reactivity with patients (35,37). Two- to three-week-old cultures are a rich source of culture filtrate antigens, while reliable mycelial antigens for immunoassay can be obtained from short-term fungal growth of aerated culture (37). Integrity of allergenic extracts can be preserved by including a stabilizer such as human serum albumin, glycerol, phenol, or ε-aminocaproic acid (38). Substantial cross-reactivity among allergens of various fungal species and genera, often, leads to erroneous diagnosis (39).

Challenge Testing

Challenge testing (e.g., bronchoprovocation, nasal provocation) may be the most clinically relevant test available to demonstrate causation by a specific allergen. However, its use is problematic due to the clinical and ethical issues raised by such testing and questions raised about the clinical relevance of non-natural exposure protocols.

DIAGNOSTICALLY RELEVANT ALLERGENS

In recent years, considerable attention has been paid to obtaining purified relevant allergens from fungi associated with allergy (39). Using molecular biology techniques, a number of mold allergens have been obtained by cloning the genes encoding the allergens. A recent survey of fungal allergens shows that the best studied fungi may have up to 20 known well-characterized allergens (in the case of *A. fumigatus*, *C. herbarum*, and *A. alternata*), between 27 and 60 other less well-characterized IgE binding proteins as determined by IgE binding to phage displayed allergen libraries, and another 20 proteins predicted to be allergen orthologues by virtue of close homology to allergens known in other species (40). Thus an estimated 0.5% to 1% of proteins in a given fungal proteome may be allergens (40). The known fungal allergens appear to occur as functional groups, such as serine proteases, heat shock proteins, or thioredoxins or orthologues of proteins such as Mn superoxide dismutase or enolase. Alkaline/vacuolar serine proteases comprise a major group of panfungal allergens from several prevalent airborne fungal species. A further group of allergens containing the major allergens Asp f 1, Alt a 1, and Cla h 1 have only been found in fungi from particular genera. Currently, about 70 fungal allergens have been approved by the International Allergen Nomenclature Committee (41). However, not many of these allergens have been analyzed for their diagnostic specificity and sensitivity.

Alternaria species

A. alternata, a member of the *Deuteromycetes* class, is one of the most important allergenic fungi, and Alt a 1 is the most frequently recognized allergen, binding to IgE in more than 80% of asthmatic patients with *Alternaria* allergy. A sensitive two-site ELISA has been recently developed for measurement of the major *A. alternata* allergen Alt a 1 with a detection limit lower than 0.5 ng/mL and a practical working range of 0.5 to 50 ng/mL (42). A specific double monoclonal antibody based assay was developed for Alt a 1 by Portnoy et al. with a sensitivity of 0.2 μg/mL (43). Various isoelectric variants and isoforms of Alt a 1 have also been reported (5,44). Saenz-de-Santamaria et al. recently reported phosphatase and esterase activities in Alt a 1 (45). Other *Alternaria* allergens identified include a heat-stable glycoprotein allergen of 31 kDa, a 53-kDa aldehyde dehydrogenase (ALDH), a 22-kDa allergen, and an 11-kDa ribosomal P2 protein. Schneider et al. recently reported that NADP-dependent mannitol dehydrogenase (Alt a 8) is an important fungal allergen of *A. alternata* (46). In IgE-ELISA and immunoblots, mannitol dehydrogenase (MtDH) is recognized by 41% of *A. alternata*-allergic patients. In vivo immunoreactivity of the recombinant MtDH was verified by SPT (46). Portnoy et al. reported a double monoclonal antibody-based assay for the 70-kD Alternaria allergen GP70 that was sensitive to GP70 concentrations as low as 0.2 μg/mL and was highly specific for the allergen (47).

Cladosporium herbarum

C. herbarum is one of the major sources of inhalant fungal allergens in cooler climates (5). At least 60 antigens from *C. herbarum* have been detected by counter immuno-electrophoresis and 36 of them have been shown to be allergenic by crossed radioimmunoelectrophoresis (34). Various diagnostically relevant allergens that have been purified and characterized from this fungi include Cla h 1 (Ag 32) (13-kDa) with five isoforms (pI 3.4–4.4), Cla h 2 (Ag 54) (23-kDa, pI 5.0, and a glycoprotein with 80% carbohydrates), hsp 70, Cla h 8, Cla h 3 (11.1. kDa, ribosomal P2 protein), Cla h 6, (48 kDa, enolase), and HCh-1 (hydrophobin, a cell wall component) (48–51).

Aspergillus fumigatus

A. fumigatus secretes a plethora of allergens/antigens with biological activities, and many of them have been evaluated for their diagnostic relevance. An acidic glycoprotein with an isoelectric point (pI) of 5.2 to 5.6 and 4 polypeptide chains of molecular weight 45 kDa was isolated from cell sap and detected specific antibodies in 75% of sera of patients of ABPA (52). An IgE antibody mediated response to Asp f 1, a major allergen/antigen/cytotoxin, has been reported in 85% of the patients with *A. fumigatus*-induced allergic disorders (53). Immunoreactivity of the purified 45 kDa glycoprotein antigen with the sera of ABPA and aspergilloma patients was observed by immunodiffusion, Western blot, and

ELISA (54). Teshima et al. reported another diagnostically relevant glycoprotein allergen/antigen, gp 55, from *A. fumigatus* (55).

Some of the recombinant proteins showed specific binding to IgE antibodies from asthmatic and ABPA patients. Asp f 1 was found to be an important allergen with respect to immunoreactivity and skin testing with patients of allergic asthma sensitized to *A. fumigatus* (56). Diagnostic relevance of Asp f 2, a glycoprotein of molecular weight 37 kDa with N-terminal homology to gp 55, has been recently demonstrated (57).

In an ELISA, serum IgE antibody reactivity to rAsp f 3 could be detected in 72% of 89 individuals sensitized to *A. fumigatus*, demonstrating that the protein represents a major allergen of the mold (58). A secreted ribotoxin (rAsp f 1) and a peroxisomal protein (rAsp f 3) were recognized by sera from *A. fumigatus*-sensitized cystic fibrosis (CF)-patients with or without ABPA, while an intracellular manganese superoxide dismutase (rAsp f 6) and rAsp f 4, a protein with unknown function, were recognized exclusively by IgE antibodies from sera of CF patients with ABPA. Therefore, rAsp f 4 and rAsp f 6 represent specific markers for ABPA and allow a sensitive, fully specific diagnosis of the disease (59). rAsp f 4 and rAsp f 6 were able to facilitate discrimination between ABPA and *A. fumigatus* sensitization with high specificity (100%) and sensitivity (90%) (59,60). In contrast to fungal extracts, rAsp f 4 and rAsp f 6 allergens were observed to be suitable for an automated serologic diagnosis of ABPA, facilitating their introduction in clinical practice (59,61). Recombinant *Aspergillus* allergens Asp f 1, f 2, f 3, f 4, and f 6 were studied for their specific binding to IgE antibodies in the sera of ABPA patients, *A. fumigatus* SPT-positive asthmatics, and normal controls. The results demonstrate that Asp f 2, f 4, and f 6 can be used in the serodiagnosis of ABPA, while IgE antibody binding to Asp f 1 and f 3 was not specific (60). High levels of serum IgE antibodies to Asp f 16, a 43 kDa protein, were observed in 70% of patients with ABPA, whereas in patients with allergic asthma, *Aspergillus* SPT-positive asthmatics without clinical evidence of ABPA and normal controls failed to show Asp f 16 specific IgE binding by ELISA (62).

Some of these allergens are highly specific for ABPA and allow serologic discrimination between ABPA and *A. fumigatus* allergy with a specificity of 100%. Recently, Bowyer et al. examined the IgE antibody response to crude and recombinant allergen tests (Asp f 1, Asp f 2, Asp f 4, and Asp f 6) in individuals with allergic conditions ABPA, severe asthma with fungal sensitization and chronic cavitary aspergillosis (63). However, none of these recombinant allergens from *A. fumigatus* showed a sensitivity of 100%, suggesting that a combination of well characterized recombinant allergens and synthetic epitopes needs to be identified to facilitate diagnosis of ABPA with optimal sensitivity and specificity.

Aspergillus flavus

The 34-kDa alkaline serine proteinase, Asp fl 13, has been identified as a major allergen of *A. flavus* (64).

Aspergillus niger

Glucoamylase, cellulase, and hemicellulase from *A. niger* have been shown to be allergenic by SPT, specific serum IgE response, and reactivity in immunoblots. In addition, xylosidase (Asp *n* 14) from *A. niger* causes sensitization in 4% of symptomatic bakers (65). The vacuolar serine proteinase (Asp *n* 18) has also been identified as a major allergen in *A. niger*, analyzed by immunoblotting using sera from asthmatic patients (60).

Aspergillus oryzae

α-amylase of *A. oryzae* has been recognized as an important occupational allergen in baker's asthma, and Baur et al. showed that 14 out of 43 (32%) were sensitized to the isolated baking additive α-amylase from *A. oryzae* (66). In addition, the 34-kDa alkaline serine proteinase (Asp o 13) has also been identified as a major allergen in *A. oryzae* (67).

Penicillium spp.

Shen et al. showed that, among the allergens of *Penicillium* species, the 32 to 34-kDa alkaline and/or vacuolar serine proteinases were the major allergens of *Penicillium citrinum*, *Penicillium brevicompactum*, *Penicillium notatum*, and *Penicillium oxalicum* (68). These allergens showed cross-reactivity with other major allergens from different *Penicillium* and *Aspergillus* species (67). In addition, the purified Pen *n* 13 demonstrated positive immediate skin test reactivity in asthmatic patients and showed histamine release from the peripheral leukocytes of asthmatic patients. Furthermore, an 18-kDa peroxisomal membrane protein (Pen c 3) having IgE cross-reactivity with recombinant Asp f 3 has also been reported (68).

Fusarium spp.

A 65-kDa major allergen and a 45-kDa allergen have been purified and characterized from *Fusarium solani* (69,70).

Candida albicans

Ishiguro and associates investigated various components of *C. albicans* by Western blot analysis and reported the specific IgE-binding to enolase (46 kDa), phosphoglycerate kinase (43 kDa), and aldolase (36 kDa) in the sera of patients who showed IgE to *C. albicans* (71). The alcohol dehydrogenase and mannan polysaccharide have also been identified as allergens from *C. albicans*.

Saccharomyces cerevisiae

The most important protein allergen of *S. cerevisiae* appears to be the enolase enzyme with a molecular weight of 48 to 52 kDa (72).

Trichophyton spp.

A 30-kDa, hydrophobic major allergen of *Trichophyton tonsurans* (Tri t 1) was purified, and two MAbs that recognize distinct epitopes on Tri t 1 were prepared (73).

Calvatia spp.

Cal c Bd 9.3 (16 kDa) and Cal c Bd 6.6 are the two diagnostically relevant allergens isolated and purified (74,75).

Psilocybe cubensis

Reese et al. have prepared MAbs to a 48-kDa allergen, which, for the first time, will allow structural analysis of a basidiomycete allergen (76). A cDNA clone that codes for the 16-kDa allergen with homology to cyclophilin has been isolated (77).

Rhizopus nigricans

Two allergens, Rhiz 3b (12 kDa; pI 4.8) and Rhiz 6b (14 kDa; pI 3.6) have been purified and were more potent in skin testing than the crude *R. nigricans* extract (78).

Beauveria bassiana

Entomopathogenic fungi such as *B. bassiana* are considered promising biological control agents for a variety of arthropod pests. *Beauveria* species, however, have the potential to elicit allergenic reactions in humans, and recently four putative allergens were identified to be Bb-Eno1, with similarity to fungal enolases: Bb-f2, similar to the *A. fumigatus* major allergen, Asp f 2, and to a fibrinogen binding mannoprotein; Bb-Ald, similar to ALDHs; and Bb-Hex, similar to *N*-acetyl-hexosaminadases (79).

SYNTHETIC EPITOPES FOR DIAGNOSIS

Application of recombinant DNA technology to fungal allergens provided scope for better understanding on molecular nature of the fungal allergens and identification of immunodominant epitopes. The knowledge of IgE-binding epitopes of the major fungal allergens may be of importance for increasing the specificity and sensitivity of diagnostic tests for designing model allergens representing such epitopes for in vitro tests. Advances made in epitope mapping of major antigens of pathogenic microbes resulted in the rapid development of diagnostic technologies and products. Availability of the deduced amino acid sequences of a few major allergens/antigens and partial sequencing of several other allergens/antigens have now provided opportunity to analyze regions both by algorithms and by experiment (by chemical/enzymatic cleavage of allergenic/antigenic proteins). Identified peptide fragments can be synthesized and evaluated for their potential in immunodiagnosis. Synthesis of overlapping peptides spanning the whole protein is one of the approaches for development of peptide-based diagnostics for infectious diseases. Another approach is based on the recombinant expression of the epitopic sequences.

Few antigens of *A. fumigatus*, Asp f 1, gp55, Asp f 2, and Asp f 13, have been studied with respect to immune responses to their peptides. Evaluation of synthetic peptides from the N-terminal of Asp f 1 suggested their diagnostic relevance by ELISA, dot-blot, lymphoproliferation, cytokine analysis, and histamine release assays (80). The eleven amino acid synthetic peptide (P1) significantly inhibited both IgG binding (89.10$\pm$4.45%) and IgE binding (77.32$\pm$3.38%) of the standardized diagnostic antigen, SDA (well-defined pool of diagnostically relevant allergens/antigens of *A. fumigatus*). With a panel of sera of ABPA patients, allergic patients with skin test negativity to *A. fumigatus* and normals, P1 showed a higher diagnostic efficiency than SDA [specific IgG (100%)] and specific IgE (98.3%). The same peptide was characterized with respect to structure-function relationship and it was observed that tryptophan residue plays an important role in the immunoreactivity of this peptide (81). The carboxy-terminal region of Asp f 1, representing amino acid residues 115 to 149, as an epitope was involved in both humoral and cell-mediated immune responses in ABPA was patients (82).

Evaluation of synthetic decamer peptides of Asp f 2 on derivatized cellulose membranes showed that either the N- or C-terminal region of Asp f 2 is involved in binding to specific IgE antibodies (83). Several epitopes of Asp f 13 were found to react with rabbit anti-Asp f 13 antiserum. Three of these immunodominant epitopes, near the C-terminal region of the protein, bound to IgE antibodies from *A. fumigatus*-sensitive patients (84). Seven linear IgE-binding regions were identified on Asp f 3 (85). Ramachandran et al. reported that an Asp f 4 mutant with deletion of cysteines at the C-terminal showed IgE reactivity with fewer patients suggesting that C-terminal with cysteines is an IgE binding epitope (86).

Epitope mapping of allergens of other fungi has been very limited. A twenty-amino-acid peptide representing the N-terminus of a major allergen, Alt a I, of *A. alternata* reacted with both human IgE and rabbit anti-Alt a I IgG in ELISA (87). Kurup et al. synthesized overlapping peptides spanning the whole sequence of Alt a I and identified four IgE-binding linear regions with sera from patients with *Alternaria*-induced allergy (88). Two of these regions K41-P50 and Y54-K63 showed consistent reactivity with all four patients studied. An epitopic peptide, peptide IV-1, has been identified from the 65 kDa major allergen of *F. solani* and showed IgE binding but could not evoke intradermal response in *Fusarium*-sensitive patients, demonstrating its potential use in diagnosis and immunotherapy of *Fusarium*-allergic patients (89).

Epitopes have been mapped for alkaline/vacuolar serine proteases of various airborne allergens, and a monoclonal antibody raised against these panfungal allergens is recognized by a linear epitope encompassing 9 amino acids from Pen ch 18 and Rho m 2 (90).

CONCLUDING REMARKS

For diagnosis of fungal hypersensitivity and allergens, the current need is for a panel of well-defined, sensitive, and specific diagnostic reagents, which could be a combination of recombinant allergens and/or synthetic epitopes. So far, the development in serodiagnostic tests is the use of sensitive detection systems with ELISA. Application of nanotechnology-based probes such as cantilevers for detection of specific antibodies could lead to an ultra-rapid and sensitive diagnosis for allergic diseases induced by fungi.

REFERENCES

1. Wuethrich B. Epidemiology of allergic diseases: are they really on the increase. Int Arch Allergy Appl Immunol 1989; 90:3–10.
2. Kurup VP, Fink JN. Fungal allergy. In: Murphy JW, Friedman H, Bendinelli M, eds. Fungal Infection and Immunity Responses. New York: Plenum Press, 1993:393–404.
3. Kurup VP. Hypersensitivity pneumonitis due to sensitization with thermophilic actinomycetes. Immunol Allergy Clin North Am 1989; 9:285–306.
4. Burge HA. Airborne-allergenic fungi. Immunol Allergy Clin North Am 1989; 9:307–19.
5. Achatz G, Oberkofler H, Lechenauer E, et al. Molecular cloning of major and minor allergens of *Alternaria alternata* and *Cladosporium herbarum*. Mol Immunol 1995; 32:213–27.
6. Kurup VP, Kumar A. Immunodiagnosis of aspergillosis. Clin Microbiol 1991; 4:439–59.
7. Schubert MS, Goetz DW. Evaluation and treatment of allergic fungal sinusitis. I. Demographics and diagnosis. J Allergy Clin Immunol 1998; 102:387–94.
8. Ogawa H, Fujimura M, Tofuku Y. Allergic bronchopulmonary fungal disease caused by *Saccharomyces cerevisiae*. J Asthma 2004; 41:223–8.
9. Behera D, Guleria R, Jindal SK, Chakrabarti A, Panigrahi D. Allergic bronchopulmonary aspergillosis: a retrospective study of 35 cases. Indian J Chest Dis Allied Sci 1994; 36:173–9.
10. Al-Moudi OS. Allergic bronchopulmonary aspergillosis mimicking pulmonary Tuberculosis. Saudi Med J 2001; 22:708–13.
11. Kothari K, Singh VR, Sharma R, Khandelwal R. Diagnostic dilemma: aspergillosis. J Assoc Physicians India 2000; 48:445–7.
12. Yoshida K, Ando M, Sakata T, Araki S. Prevention of summer-type hypersensitivity pneumonitis: effect of elimination of *Trichosporon cutaneum* from the patients' homes. Arch Environ Health 1989; 44:317–22.

13. Yocum MW, Saltzman AR, Strong DM, et al. Extrinsic allergic alveolitis after *Aspergillus fumigatus* inhalation. Evidence of a type IV immunologic pathogenesis. Am J Med 1976; 61:939–45.

14. McSharry C, Anderson K, Bourke SJ, Boyd G. Takes your breath away—the immunology of allergic alveolitis. Clin Exp Immunol 2002; 128:3–9.

15. Kauffman HF. Interaction of environmental allergens with airway epithelium as a key component of asthma. Curr Allergy Asthma Rep 2003; 3:101–8.

16. Trout DB, Seltzer JM, Page EH, et al. Clinical use of immunoassays in assessing exposure to fungi and potential health effects related to fungal exposure. Ann Allergy Asthma Immunol 2004; 92:483–91.

17. Kurup VP, Shen HD, Banerjee B. Respiratory fungal allergy. Microbes Infect 2000; 2:1101–10.

18. Hamilton RG, Adkinson NF, Jr. Clinical laboratory assessment of IgE-dependent hypersensitivity. J Allergy Clin Immunol 2003; 111(Suppl. 2):687–701.

19. McCann WA, Ownby DR. The reproducibility of the allergy skin test scoring and interpretation by board-certified/board-eligible allergists. Ann Allergy Asthma Immunol 2002; 89:368–71.

20. American Academy of Allergy, Asthma, and Immunology. The Allergy Report: Volume 1: Diagnostic Testing. Arlington Heights, IL: American Academy of Allergy, Asthma, and Immunology, 2000:31–40.

21. Kurup VP. Fungal allergens. Curr Allergy Asthma Rep 2003; 3:416–23.

22. Banerjee B, Chetty A, Joshi AP, Sarma PU. Identification and characterisation diagnostically relevant antigens of *Aspergillus fumigatus*. Asian Pac J Allergy Immunol 1990; 18:13–8.

23. Sharma GL, Sarma PU. ELISA based diagnosis for aspergillosis. Indian J Clin Biochem 1997; 12:107–10.

24. Anonymous. Skin testing and radioallergosorbent testing (RAST) for diagnosis of specific allergens responsible for IgE-mediated diseases. J Allergy Clin Immunol 1983; 72:515–7.

25. Koivikko A, Viander M, Lanner A. Use of the extended Phadebas RAST panel in the diagnosis of mould allergy in asthmatic children. Allergy 1991; 46:85–91.

26. Crameri R, Lidholm J, Gronlund H, Stuber D, Blaser K, Menz G. Automated specific IgE assay with recombinant allergens: evaluation of the recombinant *Aspergillus fumigatus* allergen I in the Pharmacia Cap System. Clin Exp Allergy 1996; 26:1411–9.

27. Tang RB, Shen HD, Chen SJ, Lee CY. Detection of IgE reactivity to fungus antigens by immunoblotting in allergic diseases in children. J Chin Med Assoc 2003; 66:453–9.

28. Green BJ, Yli-Panula E, Tovey ER. Halogen immunoassay, a new method for the detection of sensitization to fungal allergens; comparisons with conventional techniques. Allergol Int 2006; 55:131–9.

29. Garros Garay J, Ruiz de Gordejuela E, Vara Quadrado F. Pulmonary aspergillomas. Analysis of 31 patients. Arch Bronconeumol 1994; 30:424–32.

30. Lacasse Y, Selman M, Costabel U, et al. Clinical diagnosis of hypersensitivity pneumonitis. Am J Respir Crit Care Med 2003; 168:952–8.

31. Rosenberg M, Patterson R, Roberts M, Wang J. The assessment of immunologic and clinical stages occurring during corticosteroid therapy for ABPA. Am J Med 1978; 64:599–607.

32. Esch RE. Manufacturing and standardizing fungal allergen products. J Allergy Clin Immunol 2004; 113:210–5.

33. Turner KJ, Stewart GA, Sharp AH, Czarny D. Standardization of allergen extracts by inhibition of RAST, skin test and chemical composition. Clin Allergy 1980; 10:441–50.

34. Aukrust L. Cross radioimmunoelectrophoretic studies of distinct allergens in two extracts of *Cladosporium herbarum*. Int Arch Allergy Appl Immunol 1979; 58:375–90.

35. Kim SJ, Chaparas SD. Characterization of antigens from *Aspergillus fumigatus*. I. Preparation of antigens from organism grown in completely synthetic medium. Am Rev Respir Dis 1978; 118:547–51.

36. Ruiz Reyes H, Rodriguez Orozco AR. Allergic fungi: importance of the standardization of fungal extracts and their application on clinical practice. Rev Alerg Mex 2006; 53:144–9.

37. Kurup VP, Fink JN, Scribner GH, Falk J. Antigenic variability of *Aspergillus fumigatus* strains. Microbios 1977; 19:191–204.

38. Weber RW. Allergen immunotherapy and standardization and stability of allergen extracts. J Allergy Clin Immunol 1989; 84:1093–5.

39. Horner WE, Helbling A, Salvaggio JE, Lehrer SB. Fungal allergens. Clin Microbiol Rev 1995; 8:161–79.

40. Bowyer P, Denning DW. Genomic analysis of allergen genes in *Aspergillus* spp.: the relevance of genomics to everyday research. Med Mycol 2007; 45:17–26.

41. Yasueda H, Takeuchi Y. Molecular cloning of fungal allergens and clinical applications of recombinant allergens in fungal allergy. Nippon Ishinkin Gakkai Zasshi 2004; 45:71–6.

42. Asturias JA, Arilla MC, Ibarrola I, Eraso E, Gonzalez-Rioja R, Martinez A. A sensitive two-site enzyme-linked immunosorbent assay for measurement of the major *Alternaria alternata* allergen Alt a 1. Ann Allergy Asthma Immunol 2003; 90:529–35.

43. Portnoy J, Brothers D, Pacheco F, Landuyt J, Barnes C. Monoclonal antibody-based assay for Alt a 1, a major *Alternaria* allergen. Ann Allergy Asthma Immunol 1998; 81:59–64.

44. Paris S, Debeaupuis JP, Prevost MC, Casotto M, Latge JP. The 31 kDa major allergen, Alt a I1563, of *Alternaria alternata*. J Allergy Clin Immunol 1991; 88:902–8.

45. Saenz-de-Santamaria M, Guisantes JA, Martinez J. Enzymatic activities of *Alternaria alternata* allergenic extracts and its major allergen (Alt a 1). Mycoses 2006; 49:288–92.

46. Schneider PB, Denk U, Breitenbach M, et al. *Alternaria alternata* NADP-dependent mannitol dehydrogenase is an important fungal allergen. Clin Exp Allergy 2006; 36:1513–24.

47. Portnoy J, Pacheco F, Upadrashta B, Barnes C. A double monoclonal antibody assay for the Alternaria allergen GP70. Ann Allergy 1993; 71:401–7.

48. Sward-Nordmo M, Paulsen BS, Wold JK. Immunological studies of the glycoprotein allergen Ag-54 (Cla h II) in *Cladosporium herbarum* with special attention to the carbohydrate and protein moieties. Int Arch Allergy Appl Immunol 1989; 90:155–61.

49. Sward-Nordmo M, Wold JK, Paulsen BS, Aukrust L. Purification and partial characterization of the allergen Ag-54 from *Cladosporium herbarum*. Int Arch Allergy Appl Immunol 1985; 78:249–55.
50. Breitenbach M, Simon B, Probst G, et al. Enolases are highly conserved fungal allergens. Int Arch Allergy Immunol 1997; 113:114–7.
51. Weichel M, Schmid-Grendelmeier P, Rhyner C, Achatz G, Blaser K, Crameri R. Immunoglobulin E-binding and skin test reactivity to hydrophobin HCh-1 from *Cladosporium herbarum*, the first allergenic cell wall component of fungi. Clin Exp Allergy 2003; 33:72–7.
52. Calvanico NJ, Dupont BL, Huang CJ, Patterson R, Fink JN, Kurup VP. Antigens of *Aspergillus fumigatus* 1. Purification of cytoplasmic antigens reactive with sera of patients with *Aspergillus* related diseases. Clin Exp Immunol 1981; 45:662–71.
53. Arruda LK, Mann BJ, Chapman MD. Selective expression of a major allergen and cytotoxin, Asp f I, in *Aspergillus fumigatus*. Implications for the immunopathogenesis of *Aspergillus*-related diseases. J Immunol 1992; 149:3354–9.
54. Banerjee B, Madan T, Sharma GL, Prasad HK, Nath I, Sarma PU. Characterisation of 45 kDa glycoprotein antigen of *A. fumigatus*. Serodiag Immunother Infect Dis 1995; 7:147–52.
55. Teshima R, Ikebuchi H, Sawada J, et al. Isolation and characterisation of a major allergenic component gp 55 of *Aspergillus fumigatus*. J Allergy Clin Immunol 1993; 92:698–706.
56. Moser M, Crameri R, Menz G, et al. Cloning and expression of recombinant *A. fumigatus* allergen I/a:(rAsp f I/a) with IgE binding and type I skin test activity. J Immunol 1992; 149:454–60.
57. Banerjee B, Kurup VP, Greenberger PA, Hoffman DR, Nair DS, Fink JN. Purification of a major allergen, Asp f 2 binding to IgE in allergic bronchopulmonary aspergillosis, from culture filtrate of *Aspergillus fumigatus*. J Allergy Clin Immunol 1997; 99:821–7.
58. Hemmann S, Ismail C, Blasé K, Menz G, Crameri R. Skin-test reactivity and isotype-specific immune responses to recombinant Asp f 3, a major allergen of *Aspergillus fumigatus*. Clin Exp Allergy 1998; 28:860–7.
59. Crameri R, Hemmann S, Ismail C, Menz G, Blaser K. Disease-specific recombinant allergens for the diagnosis of allergic bronchopulmonary aspergillosis. Int Immunol 1998; 10:1211–6.
60. Kurup VP, Banerjee B, Hemmann S, Greenberger PA, Blaser K, Crameri R. Selected recombinant *Aspergillus fumigatus* allergens bind specifically to IgE in ABPA. Clin Exp Allergy 2000; 30:988–93.
61. Nikolaizik WH, Weichel M, Blaser K, Crameri R. Intracutaneous tests with recombinant allergens in cystic fibrosis patients with allergic bronchopulmonary aspergillosis and *Aspergillus* allergy. Am J Respir Crit Care Med 2002; 165:916–21.
62. Banerjee B, Kurup VP, Greenberger PA, Johnson BD, Fink JN. Cloning and expression of *Aspergillus fumigatus* allergen Asp f 16 mediating both humoral and cell-mediated immunity in allergic bronchopulmonary aspergillosis (ABPA). Clin Exp Allergy 2001; 31:761–70.
63. Bowyer P, Blightman O, Denning DW. Relative reactivity of Aspergillus allergens used in serological tests. Med Mycol 2006; 44:23–8.

64. Yu CJ, Chiou SH, Lai WY, Chiang BL, Chow LP. Characterization of a novel allergen, a major IgE-binding protein from *Aspergillus flavus*, as an alkaline serine protease. Biochem Biophys Res Commun 1999; 261:669–75.

65. Sander I, Raulf-Heimsoth M, Siethoff C, Lohaus C, Meyer HE, Baur X. Allergy to *Aspergillus*-derived enzymes in the baking industry: identification of beta-xylosidase from *Aspergillus niger* as a new allergen (Asp *n* 14). J Allergy Clin Immunol 1998; 102:256–64.

66. Baur X, Chen Z, Sander I. Isolation and denomination of an important allergen in baking additives: alpha-amylase from *Aspergillus oryzae* (Asp o II). Clin Exp Allergy 1994; 24:465–70.

67. Shen HD, Lin WL, Tam MF, et al. Alkaline serine proteinase: a major allergen of *Aspergillus oryzae* and its cross-reactivity with *Penicillium citrinum*. Int Arch Allergy Immunol 1998; 116:29–35.

68. Shen HD, Lin WL, Tam MF, et al. Characterization of allergens from *Penicillium oxalicum* and *P. notatum* by immunoblotting and N-terminal amino acid sequence analysis. Clin Exp Allergy 1999; 29:642–51.

69. Verma J, Pasha S, Gangal SV. Purification and characterization of Fus sI3596*, a 65 kDa allergen of *Fusarium solani*. Mol Cell Biochem 1994; 131:157–66.

70. Verma J, Singh BP, Sridhara S, Gaur SN, Arora N. Purification and characterization of a cross-reactive 45-kDa major allergen of *Fusarium solani*. Int Arch Allergy Immunol 2003; 130:193–9.

71. Ishiguro A, Homma M, Torii S, Tanaka K. Identification of *Candida albicans* antigens reactive with immunoglobulin E antibody of human sera. Infect Immun 1992; 60:1550–7.

72. Baldo BA, Baker RS. Inhalant allergies to fungi: reactions to bakers' yeast (*Saccharomyces cerevisiae*) and identification of bakers' yeast enolase as an important allergen. Int Arch Allergy Appl Immunol 1988; 86:201–8.

73. Deuell B, Arruda LK, Hayden ML, Chapman MD, Platts-Mills TA. *Trichophyton tonsurans* allergen. I. Characterization of a protein that causes immediate but not delayed hypersensitivity. J Immunol 1991; 147:96–101.

74. Horner WE, Ibanez MD, Lehrer SB. Immunoprint analysis of *Calvatia cyathiformis* allergens. I. Reactivity with individual sera. J Allergy Clin Immunol 1989; 83:784–92.

75. Horner WE, Lopez M, Salvaggio JE, Lehrer SB. Basidiomycete allergy: identification and characterization of an important allergen from *Calvatia cyathiformis*. Int Arch Allergy Appl Immunol 1991; 94:359–61.

76. Reese G, Tracey D, Daul CB, Lehrer SB. IgE and monoclonal antibody reactivities to the major shrimp allergen Pen a 1 (tropomyosin) and vertebrate tropomyosins. Adv Exp Med Biol 1996; 409:225–30.

77. Horner WE, Reese G, Lehrer SB. Identification of the allergen Psi c 2 from the basidiomycete *Psilocybe cubensis* as a fungal cyclophilin. Int Arch Allergy Immunol 1995; 107:298–300.

78. Sridhara S, Gangal SV, Joshi AP. Immunochemical investigation of allergens from *Rhizopus nigricans*. Allergy 1990; 45:577–86.

79. Westwood GS, Huang SW, Keyhani NO. Molecular and immunological characterization of allergens from the entomopathogenic fungus *Beauveria bassiana*. Clin Mol Allergy 2006; 4:12.

80. Madan T, Priyadarsiny P, Vaid M, et al. Use of a synthetic peptide epitope of Asp f 1, a major allergen or antigen of *Aspergillus fumigatus*, for improved immunodiagnosis of allergic bronchopulmonary aspergillosis. Clin Diagn Lab Immunol 2004; 11:552–8.

81. Kamal N, Chowdhury S, Madan T, et al. Tryptophan residue is essential for immunoreactivity of a diagnostically relevant peptide epitope of *A. fumigatus*. Mol Cell Biochem 2005; 275:223–31.

82. Kurup VP, Banerjee B, Murali P, et al. Immunodominant peptide epitopes of allergen, Asp f 1 from the fungus *Aspergillus fumigatus*. Peptides 1998; 19:1469–77.

83. Banerjee B, Greenberger PA, Fink JN, Kurup VP. Conformational and linear B-cell epitopes of Asp f 2, a major allergen of *Aspergillus fumigatus*, bind differently to immunoglobulin E antibody in the sera of allergic bronchopulmonary aspergillosis patients. Infect Immun 1999; 67:2284–91.

84. Chow LP, Liu SL, Yu CJ, Liao HK, Tsai JJ, Tang TK. Identification and expression of an allergen Asp f 13 from *Aspergillus fumigatus* and epitope mapping using human IgE antibodies and rabbit polyclonal antibodies. Biochem J 2000; 346:423–31.

85. Ramachandran H, Jayaraman V, Banerjee B, et al. IgE binding conformational epitopes of Asp f 3, a major allergen of *Aspergillus fumigatus*. Clin Immunol 2002; 103:324–33.

86. Ramachandran H, Banerjee B, Greenberger PA, Kelly KJ, Fink JN, Kurup VP. Role of C-terminal cysteine residues of *Aspergillus fumigatus* allergen Asp f 4 in immunoglobulin E binding. Clin Diagn Lab Immunol 2004; 11:261–5.

87. Zhang L, Curran IH, Muradia G, De Vouge MW, Rode H, Vijay HM. N-terminus of a major allergen, Alt a I, of *Alternaria alternata* defined to be an epitope. Int Arch Allergy Immunol 1995; 108:254–9.

88. Kurup VP, Vijay HM, Kumar V, Castillo L, Elms N. IgE binding synthetic peptides of Alt a 1, a major allergen of *Alternaria alternata*. Peptides 2003; 24:179–85.

89. Verma J, Sridhara S, Singh BP, Pasha S, Gangal SV, Arora N. *Fusarium solani* major allergen peptide IV-1 binds IgE but does not release histamine. Clin Exp Allergy 2001; 31:920–7.

90. Lee LH, Tam MF, Chou H, Tai HY, Shen HD. Lys, Pro and Trp are critical core amino acid residues recognized by FUM20, a monoclonal antibody against serine protease pan-fungal allergens. Int Arch Allergy Immunol 2007; 143:194–200.

—————————————— **14** ——————————————

Molecular Mycology and Emerging Fungal Pathogens

David N. Fredricks

Program in Infectious Diseases at the Fred Hutchinson Cancer Research Center, and Division of Allergy and Infectious Diseases, Department of Medicine, University of Washington, Seattle, Washington, U.S.A.

INTRODUCTION

Advances in molecular biology have created new opportunities for the detection and classification of fungi and the diagnosis of fungal infections. Molecular targets have been characterized (e.g., fungal rDNA and cytochrome b sequences) and methods have been refined for detecting these targets [e.g., polymerase chain reaction (PCR)]. These advances are needed because conventional diagnostic assays for fungi, such as standard histology and laboratory cultivation, have low sensitivity or specificity for some infections (1,2). The population of immuno-compromised subjects has grown with the continued spread of human immunodeficiency virus, increased use of solid organ and hematopoietic cell transplantation, and the expanding armamentarium of drugs that dismantle the human immune response such as cancer chemotherapy and anti-tumor necrosis factor monoclonal antibodies (e.g., infliximab). The population of immunocom-promised hosts is increasingly being exposed to antifungal medications used for prophylaxis, empiric therapy, or directed treatment, practices that are likely to change the spectrum of fungal infections that we encounter by selecting for resistant pathogens (3). Immunocompetent hosts are also susceptible to unusual fungal infections through factors such as travel and traumatic inoculation. The confluence of these factors is likely to foster the emergence of novel, previously unrecognized, or heretofore-rare fungal pathogens that will challenge our diagnostic capabilities.

Several issues are raised at the intersection of molecular biology and mycology: (*i*) the impact of new molecular sequence data on fungal taxonomy, (*ii*) the notion of a species, (*iii*) the challenges and opportunities associated with detecting uncultivated fungal pathogens with molecular methods, (*iv*) emerging fungal pathogens, and (*v*) the future of fungal diagnostics.

IMPACT OF MOLECULAR SEQUENCE DATA ON FUNGAL TAXONOMY

Several notable taxonomic revisions have resulted from use of molecular sequence data to infer phylogenetic relationships among fungi and related taxa. An organism believed to be a fungus (*Rhinosporidium seeberi*) was re-classified to a protistan parasite on the basis of 18S rDNA sequence, while an organism believed to be a protistan parasite (*Pneumocystis jiroveci*) was re-classified to a fungus. Although these taxonomic revisions can be confusing to physicians and microbiologists, they help to clarify the sometimes-nebulous origins of some organisms. It is particularly challenging to classify organisms based solely on morphological criteria, such as for organisms that are uncultivated. Resolving the evolutionary relationships between microbes can yield unexpected scientific benefits, such as by suggesting optimal culture conditions, identifying likely natural hosts, or suggesting environmental reservoirs for microbes based on the characteristics of microbes with close phylogenetic relationships.

Molecular methods have proven very reliable for inferring evolutionary relationships among microbes. Two microbes may have similar morphologies but very different origins due to convergent evolution. These different evolutionary pathways will be written in their DNA, and several genes are useful for establishing where microbes fall on the evolutionary tree of life.

What makes a gene useful for molecular phylogeny? First, the gene should be present in all organisms under study, and this requirement forces one to select genes with essential cellular functions, such as ribosomal RNA genes. Second, the gene should serve as a molecular clock, with increasing evolutionary time since two organisms shared a common ancestor ticked off as accumulated nucleotide changes in the gene. If two organisms are close evolutionary cousins, then their genes should share a high degree of sequence similarity. If two organisms are distant evolutionary kin, then their genes should have been subjected to additional mutation and selection over this time period, with a resulting lower rate of sequence similarity noted. The application of molecular phylogenetic methods to some long-standing problems in mycology helps to illustrate this point.

The small subunit ribosomal RNA gene, or 18S rDNA in fungi, is one useful molecular chronometer for inferring evolutionary relationships between organisms, though additional targets such as the large subunit rRNA, cytochrome b, beta-tubulin, chitin synthase, and heat shock protein genes have been used. PCR amplification of rDNA from fungi is facilitated by the presence of highly conserved sequences in the 18S rRNA gene. PCR primers targeting these conserved sites can be used to amplify segments of the gene containing more variable and, hence, phylogenetically informative sequences. When these PCR products are sequenced and aligned with known 18S rDNA sequences, phylogenetic trees depicting inferred evolutionary relationships can be generated. One problem with use of a single gene for phylogenetic analysis is that the output reflects the phylogeny of the gene, which may differ from the phylogeny of the organism in the unusual scenario of gene transfer between organisms. The taxonomic position of an organism is bolstered when analysis of several genes in the organism suggests the same phylogeny (4).

R. seeberi: Fungus No More

R. seeberi is a microbe with a confusing taxonomic history that demonstrates that looks can indeed be deceiving. *R. seeberi* causes rhinosporidiosis, a granulomatous disease of humans and animals manifested by slowly growing tumor-like masses of the nasal mucosa (polyps), respiratory tract, or ocular conjunctivae (5). Polyps may lead to nasal obstruction, and bleeding is common from the inflamed hyper-vascular tissue. Surgery can be curative, though relapse is common, and there is no accepted and effective medical therapy. Biopsy of affected tissue typically reveals acute and chronic inflammation with characteristic large, thick-walled, spherical organisms. Microbial cells range in size from a few microns to >300 µm, and the largest cells can be seen as macroscopic white flecks in affected tissue such that the tissue surface may resemble a strawberry. Daughter cells or endospores form in the larger, more mature sporangia, and are released into tissue where they propagate the infection. Sporangia can be visualized with classical fungal stains such as periodic acid Schiff, methenamine silver, and mucicarmine. Cultivation of *R. seeberi* has not been achieved with axenic media, though limited propagation was reported by co-cultivation with rectal epithelial cells in cell culture (6).

Guillermo Seeber saw an Argentinean agricultural worker with a nasal polyp in 1900 and later described this organism. Seeber thought the microbe was a sporozoan parasite and Wernicke proposed the name *Coccidium seeberi* in 1903 (5). Ashworth suggested that this microbe was a fungus related to the *Chytridiales*, and renamed it *R. seeberi* in 1923. The large thick-walled sporangia with endospores seen in rhinosporidiosis (Fig. 1) are similar in morphology to the spherules with endospores seen with the fungus *Coccidioides immitis*. What is the correct taxonomic position for *R. seeberi*, given the low-resolution tool of morphological comparison did not produce a clear answer and phenotypic analysis is difficult without cultivated organisms?

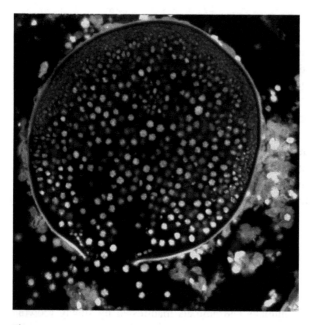

Figure 1 Fluorescence micrograph of *R. seeberi* in nasal polyp tissue. A large spherical sporangium discharges endospores into surrounding tissue through an opening in the cell wall. The endospores are in varying stages of maturity, with the smallest and least developed endospores along the internal cell wall of the sporangium and more mature endospores in the center. Organisms are visualized with YoPro1 nucleic acid stain. The appearance of *R. seeberi* in tissue is similar to that of *C. immitis*; however, these organisms are not closely related (see Fig. 2).

Consensus sequence PCR was used to amplify *R. seeberi* 18S rDNA directly from infected tissue. Phylogenetic analysis of 18S rDNA sequences showed that *R. seeberi* is most closely related to the microbe *Dermocystidium salmonis* and several other fish pathogens (7,8). *D. salmonis* infects fish gills. It is noteworthy that like *R. seeberi*, *D. salmonis* forms large sporangia or cysts up to 400 µm in diameter containing endospores that are released to propagate infection. These organisms belong to a distinct group of microbes that form an evolutionary branch at the animal-fungal divergence that have been called the DRIPs clade [for *D*ermocystidium, *R*osette agent (a.k.a. *Sphaerothecum destruens*), *I*chthyophonus, and *P*sorospermium], the Ichthyosporea (spore-forming fish pathogens), or the *Mesomycetozoea* (meaning between animals and fungi) (9–11). Thus, these data suggest *R. seeberi* is not a fungus, but is a protistan parasite from a newly described clade of microorganisms that are related to both animals and fungi. Figure 2 shows a phylogenetic tree of inferred evolutionary relationships between *R. seeberi* and some selected species. *R. seeberi* is not closely related to *C. immitis* despite some morphological

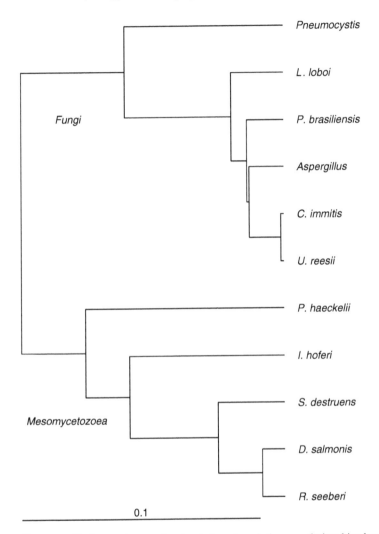

Figure 2 Phylogenetic tree showing inferred evolutionary relationships between several fungal species and organisms in the *Mesomycetozoea* clade of protists. The tree is based on aligned 18S rDNA sequences interpreted with a maximum likelihood algorithm. *R. seeberi* is not a true fungus, despite its morphological similarity to *C. immitis*. *Pneumocystis* spp. form a deeply branching lineage within the fungi. The uncultivated fungus *Lacazia loboi* is most closely related to *P. brasiliensis*. The bar represents 0.1 base changes per nucleotide position.

similarities. *R. seeberi* is the only known human pathogen from microbes in the *Mesomycetozoea* phylum. The lack of response to conventional antifungal therapy in rhinosporidiosis likely reflects the unique metabolic properties of the *Mesomycetozoea*.

Lacazia (*Loboa*) *loboi*: A Fungus Finds Its Place in the Family of Ascomycetes

Lobomycosis is a chronic cutaneous and subcutaneous infection caused by the organism previously known as *Loboa loboi*, now amended to *Lacazia loboi* (12). The disease manifests as slowly growing skin nodules with smooth, veruccoid, or ulcerated surfaces (13). Lobomycosis occurs predominantly in Central and South America and has been noted in dolphins as well as man. Amerindians of the Amazon are most affected. Although the disease can spread contiguously and can be locally destructive, it does not disseminate to visceral organs. The legs, ears, face, and arms are most commonly affected and there is a paucity of acute inflammation or symptoms. Histology of lesions shows chronic inflammatory cells and yeast forms that are about 10 μm in diameter and have a spherical or lemon shape. The yeasts may occur singly or in short chains with tubular bridges connecting the cells. *Lacazia loboi* has not been propagated in culture, but has been propagated in rodents (14). Ketoconazole or itraconazole plus clofazamine have been used to treat lobomycosis, but there is little published evidence suggesting a successful medical therapy (15). Surgical resection of small lesions can be curative.

The inability to cultivate *Lacazia loboi* on artificial media has impeded the proper classification of this organism. The disease was originally reported by Jorge Lobo in 1931 when he described a case of a keloidal skin lesion on the back of a man from the Amazon Valley (13). He believed that the organisms visible in tissue might be related to *Paracoccidioides brasiliensis*, another South American fungus. Rabbits inoculated with *P. brasiliensis* produce antibodies that attach to *Lacazia loboi* in tissue sections, suggesting that there are shared antigens. Consensus sequence PCR was used to amplify portions of the 18S rRNA gene and the chitin synthase-2 gene from tissue harboring *Lacazia loboi* (16). Phylogenetic analysis of the amplified DNA sequences suggests that *Lacazia loboi* is most closely related to the ascomycetous fungi and is a sister taxon to *P. brasiliensis*, thereby validating Jorge Lobo's original suspicion. The close evolutionary relationships between *Lacazia loboi* and *P. brasiliensis*, *Histoplasma capsulatum*, and *Blastomyces dermatitidis* support the hypothesis that *Lacazia loboi* may be a dimorphic fungus. The molecular tools developed to study *Lacazia loboi* taxonomy can be used to study the epidemiology and environmental reservoirs of this fungus, and can also be used to develop diagnostic assays for lobomycosis. Thus, molecular phylogenetic analysis and molecular diagnostics share a common approach.

Pneumocystis carinii and *jiroveci*: Taxonomic Evolution from Protistan Parasites to Fungi

The taxonomic history of *Pneumocystis* has been especially confusing (17). Chagas described *Pneumocystis* in 1909 and thought it was a trypanosome. Later investigators considered *Pneumocystis* a unique protozoan, giving it the designation *P. carinii* in recognition of the work by Carini. *Pneumocystis* can cause an interstitial pneumonia in immunocompromised and malnourished persons and usually responds to treatment with trimethoprim-sulfamethoxazole, pentamidine, atovaquone, or clindamycin–primaquine. *Pneumocystis* has not been propagated in long-term axenic cultures. The protozoan nature of *Pneumocystis* was supported by the morphology of the organism in tissue, the lack of response to antifungal agents, the failure to propagate the organism in culture, and the favorable response to anti-protozoal agents. However, ultrastructural analysis of *Pneumocystis* suggested that it might be a fungus (18,19). *Pneumocystis* contains elongation factor 3, which is only found in fungi. Phylogenetic analysis of rRNA, beta-tubulin, dihydrofolate reductase, and other genes revealed that *Pneumocystis* is a fungus, though a rather strange one (20–22). *Pneumocystis* lacks ergosterol and thus is not sensitive to most antifungal agents. *Pneumocystis* does contain β-1, 3 D-glucan in its cell wall and the cyst form is sensitive to echinocandin antifungals. *Pneumocystis* has been placed in a new fungal phylum, the *Archiascomycetes*, a deeply branching lineage within the Ascomycota (23). The circuitous taxonomic history of *Pneumocystis* shows how far we can stray from the accurate classification of microbes and highlights the clarity that is generated from well-performed molecular phylogenetic studies.

Additional work has shown that most mammals have unique host-restricted species of *Pneumocystis*, and there is significant sequence diversity between and within *Pneumocystis* spp. (24). It has been proposed that the species found in rats should be designated *P. carinii* and the species found in humans should be designated *P. jiroveci* (25). Nucleic acid sequence differences between *P. jiroveci* types have been used to study the epidemiology of pneumocystosis in humans (26). Thus, even without cultivated microbes, molecular microbiological methods allow one to investigate the diversity of fungal pathogens and their epidemiology.

Malassezia: The Expanding Genus

Man and other warm-blooded vertebrates share their skin with basidiomycetous yeasts that are part of the normal flora. These fungi can produce cutaneous disease in some individuals. The factors that lead to disease are not completely known, though immunological mechanisms are suspected. The association between pityriasis versicolor and a cutaneous fungus was first noted in 1846 (27). Malassez described yeasts associated with dandruff in 1874. Later investigators named these species *Pityrosporum ovale* and *Pityrosporum orbiculare*, but these organisms were later considered to be the same fungus, and thus were designated *Malassezia furfur*. *M. furfur* has been linked to rare episodes of invasive disease, such as catheter infections in infants receiving intravenous lipid emulsions. In 1992, there were three known species in the *Malassezia* genus, including *M. furfur*, *Malassezia sympodialis*, and *Malassezia pachydermatis* (28). *M. furfur* and *M. sympodialis* are lipophilic yeasts that colonize human skin. *M. pachydermatis* does not require lipid for growth and colonizes other warm-blooded animals such as dogs and rhinoceroses. In 1996, four additional species were added to the genus based on differences in morphology, ultrastructure, physiology, and rRNA sequence (29). These new species were *Malassezia globosa*, *Malassezia obtusa*, *Malassezia restricta*, and *Malassezia slooffiae*. Subsequently, investigators have proposed adding several additional species to the genus, including *Malassezia japonica*, *Malassezia yamotoensis*, *Malassezia nana*, and *Malassezia dermatis* (30–33).

Sequencing and phylogenetic analysis of large subunit rDNA, internal transcribed spacer sequences (ITS) of rDNA, and chitin synthase-2 genes have confirmed that these different *Malassezia* species are genetically distinct and there is substantial diversity within species (34–36). *M. globosa* has a morphology that corresponds to the original description of *P. orbiculare*. *M. restricta* has a morphology that corresponds to the original description of *P. ovale* (37). Curiously, although *M. furfur* was previously considered to be the dominant fungal species on normal human skin, more recent molecular studies suggest that *M. globosa*, *M. restricta*, and *M. sympodialis* are actually more prevalent (38,39). *M. furfur* is not as fastidious as other *Malassezia* species, and this cultivation bias likely explains previous studies suggesting *M. furfur* dominance. *M. globosa* has been associated with pityriasis versicolor, though the associations between particular *Malassezia* species and cutaneous diseases have thus far not been particularly illuminating. Nevertheless, the increased taxonomic resolution that is generated by molecular sequence data may help link particular fungal species or subspecies to specific diseases. The expanding list of species in the *Malassezia* genus is a trend that is increasingly evident for many fungal genera, as molecular studies reveal previously unappreciated fungal diversity (see below).

The Endemic Mycoses: Molecular Insights into Species Diversity

Sequencing and phylogenetic analysis of fungal genes has revealed that some species can be divided into several distinct groups that are not apparent from conventional phenotypic classification schemes. For instance, the single species *C. immitis* has been considered the cause of coccidioidomycosis (Valley fever) in the southwestern United States, Mexico, and Central and South America. Phylogenetic analysis of several genes in *C. immitis* and typing of strains by PCR amplification of microsatellite loci show there are two genetically isolated populations of *Coccidioides* with different geographic ranges (40,41). One group is found in California and has been designated *C. immitis*. The second group is found outside of California and has now been designated *Coccidioides posadasii*, in honor of Alejandro Posadas who first described coccidioidomycosis in an Argentinean patient. Although *C. immitis* and *C. posadasii* are phylogenetically deeply divergent, the only phenotypic trait distinguishing these species is a trend for *C. posadasii* to grow more slowly on high salt media, and this trait is not very robust or reliable. Human disease produced by these two phylotypes is indistinguishable. The sister taxon to *Coccidioides* based on phylogenetic analysis of several genes is *Uncinocarpus reesii*, a saprobe found in soil that produces arthroconidia like *C. immitis* (42).

H. *capsulatum* causes histoplasmosis with endemic regions on most continents. Three varieties of *H. capsulatum* have been identified, including var. *capsulatum*, var. *duboisii*, and var. *farciminosum*. *H. capsulatum* var. *capsulatum* causes a pulmonary infection in humans and is hyperendemic in the Mississippi and Ohio River valleys of the United States and much of Latin America. Phylogenetic analysis of North American isolates has revealed two genetically isolated clades designated class 1 and class 2 (43). The class 1 *H. capsulatum* var. *capsulatum* clade has been detected mostly in patients with AIDS, whereas the class 2 clade has been detected in normal hosts as well. At least 7 phylogenetic clades have been identified with distinct geographic proclivities, including clades from Africa, Australia, the Netherlands, and 2 clades each from Latin America and North America (44). A separate Eurasian clade is present within the Latin American A clade. The phylogeographic data suggest an origin for *H. capsulatum* in Latin America with radiation to other continents. *H. capsulatum* var. *duboisii* is found in Africa, forms larger yeasts than var. *capsulatum*, and produces more cutaneous and osseous disease than var. *capsulatum*. The *H. capsulatum* var. *duboisii* isolates group together on phylogenetic analysis, suggesting a common evolutionary history that may explain its phenotypic and pathological characteristics. *H. capsulatum* var. *farciminosum* causes cutaneous and lymphangitic disease in horses and mules, mostly in Africa and the Middle East. Unexpectedly, phylogenetic analysis of variety *farciminosum* isolates reveals that this fungus is closely related to *H. capsulatum* var. *capsulatum* isolates from several different clades, and is thus polyphyletic (44). These data suggest that equine histoplasmosis is not caused by a particular variety of *H. capsulatum* (*farciminosum*), but is a syndrome caused by *H. capsulatum* var. *capsulatum* in animals. This example illustrates how molecular phylogenetic analysis can occasionally show novel relationships between fungi that collapse rather than expand the list of fungal taxa.

Cryptococcus neoformans was previously considered to have four serotypes, A–D, and two varieties, var. *neoformans* (serotypes A and D) and var. *gattii* (serotypes B and C). Molecular phylogenetic analysis of *C. neoformans* has revealed that serotype A isolates form a monophyletic cluster, and these organisms have been given the designation var. *grubii*, whereas serotype D isolates form a clearly separate monophyletic group and the moniker var. *neoformans* has been retained (45). In contrast, there is a high degree of genetic diversity among *C. neoformans* var. *gattii* isolates, with at least 3 distinct genogroups noted (46). Genogroup I contains both serotypes B and C. It has been proposed that *Cryptococcus gattii* complex organisms be designated a separate species based on their phenotypic and genetic differences compared to

C. neoformans. The additional taxonomic resolution provided by molecular sequence data creates new opportunities to explore the epidemiology and disease associations for each genetic variant.

MOLECULAR CHALLENGES TO FUNGAL TAXONOMY: WHAT IS A SPECIES?

The rapid accumulation of sequence information for fungal species threatens to burst existing taxonomic conventions. Fungal systematics is based on the description of sexual characteristics of fungi in culture, such as the production of ascospores, basidiospores, or zygospores (47). This classification scheme fails for uncultivated fungi. In addition, molecular sequence data show that many fungi previously thought to be separate species are merely the teleomorph or anamorph of the same fungus, such as with *Pseudallescheria* and *Scedosporium.* Another challenge arises when molecular studies show that a species contains more than one distinct phylogenetic cluster of organisms (cryptic species), such as for *C. immitis, H. capsulatum,* and *C. neoformans* (48). At what point do we call a genetically isolated population of fungi a new species based on molecular sequence data, particularly when there is a paucity of phenotypic and morphological criteria to suggest separate species status (49)? There are many definitions for a species, and one must distinguish between the operational definition of a species and the scientific classification scheme that includes genus and species. The Linnaean system of scientific classification was based on morphological differences between organisms. For bacteria, species designations rest largely on shared metabolic phenotypes, such as carbon source utilization, since morphological differences between microbes yield insufficient power to discriminate. For fungi, greater emphasis has been placed on morphological differences since distinct reproductive structures help to distinguish between species. However, this approach is not optimal for poorly sporulating fungi where reproductive structures are not evident. Furthermore, even for sporulating fungi, this approach may lump genetically distinct fungi with similar spores into a single taxonomic group.

The description of *Aspergillus lentulus* and other *Aspergillus* species as separate species from *Aspergillus fumigatus* provides an example of how molecular methods have been employed to identify cryptic species within the opportunistic fungi. Upon screening 128 clinical isolates of *A. fumigatus* for susceptibility to itraconazole, Balajee and colleagues identified 7 isolates that were resistant to many antifungal agents and were slow to sporulate, producing white colonies on initial incubation (50). Multilocus sequence typing was used to demonstrate that these slowly sporulating isolates were phylogenetically very similar to each other but distinct from *A. fumigatus* (51). In this case, an unusual antifungal susceptibility profile in organisms presumed to be *A. fumigatus* led to phenotypic and genetic patterns that identified a new species, now designated *A. lentulus.* Hong et al. confirmed that *A. lentulus* is a separate species using a polyphasic taxonomic approach (combining genomic and phenotypic characteristics), but also identified two other cryptic species within the *A. fumigatus* group, designated *Aspergillus fumigatiaffinis* and *Aspergillus novofumigatus* (52). These studies demonstrate the synergy that emerges from combining molecular phylogenetic analysis with conventional phenotypic analysis to describe fungal species diversity more completely.

The evolutionary definition of a species is a lineage of organisms descended from a common ancestor that maintains its identity distinct from other lineages. The phylogenetic definition of a species is a cluster of organism with a common ancestor and a shared pattern of descent as revealed by genetic sequence information or polymorphisms. The biological definition of a species is a population of interbreeding organisms that are reproductively isolated from other organisms and thus genetically distinct. For mitosporic fungi, the biological species definition fails because interbreeding has not been observed and presumably cannot occur. Even for meiosporic fungi, mating between different taxonomic groups can be a challenging endeavor to observe in the laboratory, and some fungi cannot be propagated under any laboratory conditions. In these scenarios, we are forced to use a more restricted definition of species, such as a population of reproductively isolated organisms with shared ancestry. One way to measure the reproductive isolation of two organisms is to assess their genetic similarity. For instance, if California and non-California isolates of *Coccidioides* share identical polymorphisms across several genes, this suggests either a recent introduction of *Coccidioides* to California, or a remote introduction with flow of genetic material between populations, such as through airborne dispersal or animal migration. On the other hand, if the California and non-California populations of *Coccidioides* have unique polymorphisms in these genes that segregate by geography, this suggests there is little exchange of genetic information across populations and implies that the organisms share a distant common ancestor (40). Thus, analysis of fungal gene sequences can provide a useful indicator of genetic isolation and hence help define a species. Multilocus sequencing typing is one approach to collect these data, as has been used to assign new species status to the genetic variant *C. posadasii* (4). The case for splitting a currently identified fungal species into two or more separate species is bolstered when molecular phylogenetic data suggest there is genetic isolation of populations, and when there are morphological, phenotypic, or clinical characteristics that distinguish these clusters.

DETECTION OF UNCULTIVATED FUNGAL PATHOGENS: CHALLENGES AND OPPORTUNITIES

Clinicians have been spoiled by the ease with which most bacterial pathogens are cultivated in the laboratory. In contrast, many fungal pathogens are not as pliable to cultivation. For instance, only about half the patients with pulmonary aspergillosis will have an *Aspergillus* species detected on cultivation of bronchoalveolar lavage fluid. Similarly, only about half the patients with hepatosplenic candidiasis will have a blood culture positive for Candida. There are many instances when fungi, such as zygomycetes, can be seen on histopathological examination of tissue, yet no organism is recovered in the microbiology laboratory. The failure to culture fungal pathogens from clinical samples obtained from subjects with fungal infections has fostered the development of diagnostic methods that rely on non-cultivation approaches, such as serology, antigen detection, or PCR.

Why is it so difficult to propagate fungi in the laboratory? For some fungi, such as *Lacazia loboi* and *P. jiroveci*, continuous cultivation on axenic media has not been possible. We clearly have not been able to duplicate in the laboratory the conditions that foster propagation of these fungi in the natural environment. For other fungi, such as *A. fumigatus* and *Candida albicans*, we are able to grow the pathogens in the laboratory, yet cultivation from clinical material remains a challenge. It is possible that fungi that are growing in the human body at 37°C, high carbon dioxide concentration, and low oxygen concentration, do not quickly adapt to laboratory environment. A study of novel cultivation approaches for the diagnosis of invasive aspergillosis suggested that creating simulated tissue conditions in the laboratory with tissue culture media rather than mycological media resulted in a higher rate of recovery of *Aspergillus* from clinical samples and experimentally inoculated animal tissues (53). Efforts to understand why fungi fail to grow from tissue specimens could yield significant benefits if this knowledge increases the rate at which fungal isolates are recovered. Although molecular diagnostic methods have numerous advantages over cultivation, obtaining an isolate allows one to perform antifungal susceptibility testing that is not currently practical with molecular methods.

The difficulties encountered in cultivating clinically significant pathogens can be placed in perspective by considering the more global problem of detecting fungal diversity in the environment. It is thought that only 1% to 10% of bacteria detected by microscopy or molecular methods can be propagated in the laboratory using conventional cultivation methods (54). Similarly, only a fraction of the fungi detected in soil communities by molecular methods are closely related to previously cultivated species (55). For example, investigators used small subunit rRNA gene PCR to identify fungal species present in a grass root community (56). Only 7 of 49 sequence types were closely related to previously cultivated fungi or fungi with known 18S rDNA sequences, demonstrating that most of the fungal species present in this community were novel. Similar findings have been noted in other environmental samples. It is fortunate that most of these environmental fungi are probably not capable of causing human disease, but these findings highlight the fact that many fungi remain unidentified because they fail to jump through the metabolic hoops created by laboratory cultivation.

Molecular diagnostic methods offer the potential to detect all fungi, regardless of their ability to be cultivated. Methods such as consensus sequence PCR of fungal genes is one promising approach that will allow us to determine if novel fungi or previously known but cultivation refractory fungi are responsible for unexplained human disease (57). We likely do not appreciate the true diversity of fungal pathogens that colonize the human host and are capable of causing disease, as has been demonstrated by the recent identification of numerous *Malassezia* species on human skin. Although molecular methods offer the potential to make significant contributions to our diagnostic armamentarium, they also create unique challenges. Fungi are ubiquitous in water, soil, and air, making highly sensitive molecular diagnostic methods prone to false-positive results from environmental contamination. The potential of molecular diagnostic tests can only be realized fully when environmental contamination of reagents and samples is controlled.

EMERGING FUNGAL PATHOGENS

It is estimated there are more than 1 million fungal species present on earth, with only about 70,000 validly described to date, leaving the vast majority of fungi undiscovered. Between 800 and 1500 new species of fungi are described annually (47). Some of these newly described fungi have been found in association with humans, including *Dissitimurus exedrus, Calyptrozyma arxii, Hormographiella* spp., *Onychocola canadensis, Ramichloridium mackenziei, Polycytella hominis, Pyrenochaeta unguis-hominis, Phoma* spp., and *Botryomyces caespitosus*. Some novel fungal species will likely prove to have pathogenic potential as the enlarging population of immunocompromised hosts provides new opportunities for infection. The challenge for clinicians and microbiologists will be sorting out true infection with a novel fungus from laboratory contamination with saprophytic environmental contaminants that may arise in the laboratory or be carried on clinical samples. This task will not be easy, but a strategy combining cultivation, histology, and molecular sequence amplification methods can help bolster the case for identification of a novel pathogen by demonstrating concordance of results.

Although *Candida* and *Aspergillus* species are the most frequent fungi producing nosocomial and iatrogenic infections, the diversity of pathogens continues to expand (58,59). An emerging infectious disease is one marked by (*i*) the appearance of a new pathogen, or (*ii*) a surge in the incidence of infection with a previously recognized pathogen. The increasing incidence of invasive aspergillosis in hematopoietic cell transplant recipients fulfills the second criterion (60). The appearance of novel fungal pathogens is an example of emerging infection due to the first criterion (61,62). There are case reports describing many rare fungal pathogens, such as caused by *Hormographiella aspergillata, Acrophialophora fusispora, Cylindrocarpon lichenicola, Gymnascella hyalinospora, Phomopsis saccardo, Arthographis kalrae, Veronaea botryosa, Chaetomium perlucidum, Thermoascus taitungiacus*, and others. More frequent fungal pathogens to consider in immunocompromised patients include *Zygomycetes, Pneumocystis, Scedosporium, Fusarium, Cryptococcus,* and agents of the endemic mycoses (63). In one review of mold infections in 53 recipients of heart or lung transplants, non-*Aspergillus* molds produced 27% of infections, and these infections were associated with higher rates of dissemination and death (64). Uncommon pathogens include fungi in numerous genera, such as *Trichoderma, Acremonium, Paecilomyces, Rhodotorula, Sporobolomyces, Hansenula, Saccharomyces, Blastoschizomyces, Trichosporon, Malassezia, Alternaria, Curvularia, Bipolaris, Exophiala, Cladophialophora, Phialophora, Scopulariopsis,* and *Ulocladium.* Although this is an extensive list of pathogens, an emerging threat from fungal infections does not occur simply because we are better at recognizing and identifying pathogens.

There are several factors that may be contributing to the emergence of fungal infections caused by species previously considered rare. Zygomycete infections in immunocompromised patients are an example of an emerging disease. Several groups have reported increased rates of zygomycosis in allogeneic hematopoietic cell transplant recipients, and some have linked this surge in cases to the use of voriconazole, an agent that has poor activity against the *Zygomycetes.* At the Fred Hutchinson Cancer Research Center, we reported 13 breakthrough fungal infections in 139 stem cell transplant recipients receiving voriconazole (65). Six of the 13 patients had a Zygomycete infection, though infections with *Candida glabrata, Acremonium* species, and *Scedosporium prolificans* were also noted in more than one patient. Marty et al. described 4 cases of zygomycosis in 124 stem cell transplant patients (3.2%) from Brigham and Women's Hospital over a 9-month period (66). Each of these 4 patients was receiving voriconazole. This rate contrasts with a diagnosis of zygomycosis in 2 of 370 patients (0.54%) in the preceding 32-month period at the same institution. At the University of Iowa, Siwek et al. reported no cases of zygomycosis over a 3-year period, then 4 cases in 45 stem cell transplant recipients (8.9%) receiving voriconazole prophylaxis (67). Others have noted an increase in zygomycosis prior to the use of voriconazole, suggesting that increased susceptibility of patients or greater environmental exposure may be contributing to higher rates of disease as well (68). Nevertheless, a case-control study from one center showed that voriconazole use was an independent risk factor for zygomycosis (odds ratio of 10) based on multivariate analysis (69).

Regardless of the cause, the emergence of zygomycosis as an important fungal disease in stem cell transplant recipients highlights the moving target of fungal infections. Use of fluconazole prophylaxis significantly reduced rates of *Candida* infection in stem cell transplant patients, but we soon noted increasing rates of aspergillosis. Use of voriconazole for directed therapy in aspergillosis has improved outcomes, but use in less focused settings such as for prophylaxis and empiric therapy may lead to the emergence of resistant molds, especially the *Zygomycetes.* As our diagnostic assays improve and as new therapeutic interventions take hold, we are not likely to vanquish fungal infections. Rather, the spectrum of fungal infections is likely to change as new species emerge to occupy vacant human niches. *Scedosporium prolificans*, *Acremonium* species, and azole resistant *Aspergillus* species may become more prominent causes of infection (along with *Zygomycetes*) in patients exposed to voriconazole. Despite a large antibacterial armamentarium, bacteria still manage to overcome high-powered antibiotics to produce ventilator-associated pneumonia and other fatal hospital-acquired infections. We should not be very sanguine that the small quill of antifungal agents currently available will prevent some of the million fungal species in our environment from establishing new niches in immunocompromised humans. The thinking of mycologists will need to change to keep pace with our evolving fungal pathogens, seeking new diagnostic and therapeutic interventions to counter the moves of our more genetically malleable adversaries.

FUNGAL DIAGNOSTICS OF THE FUTURE

The continued use of empiric antifungal therapy in many settings is evidence that current diagnostic tests for fungal infections do not meet clinical needs. Most conventional diagnostic tests are neither rapid, nor sensitive, nor capable of detecting early disease. Hence, clinicians continue to use antifungal therapy in high-risk patients with negative diagnostic tests and unexplained disease. A convergence of advances in molecular biology, microfluidics, nanotechnology, and genomics is likely to change the face of fungal diagnostics in the coming years. It is not unreasonable to consider the possibility that most fungal pathogen genomes will be sequenced in the next decade. Knowledge of the nucleic acid sequences and proteins unique to each pathogen may help direct the development of molecular diagnostic tests. It is clear that nucleic acid sequence information alone cannot readily predict the polysaccharide structure of a fungal cell wall antigen, but PCR and protein antigen assays may be developed from these data. Even without complete genomes, the generation of data on fungal gene sequences from many different taxa can be used to develop better PCR assays. Part of what makes rDNA PCR so useful is the fact that there is already a wealth of sequence information for these gene targets available in public databases that can be used to design PCR assays and identify species based on phylogenetic analysis (70).

Several technologies may play a role in future fungal diagnostics. Detection of fungal nucleic acid sequences by chemical amplification (PCR, nucleic acid sequence-based amplification, ligase chain reaction) or by signal amplification (branched DNA, electronic DNA detection methods, probe-based amplification) may be used to detect fungal DNA or RNA. Use of real-time, quantitative PCR assays for fungal DNA or RNA will rapidly diagnose fungal infections and will provide a measure of fungal burden in tissues or body fluids. The ability to miniaturize reaction vessels, capture target molecules to increase their concentration, and control the flow of reagents with microfluidic technology may allow assays to be performed at significantly reduced costs on unprecedented scales. Nucleic acid amplification methods are likely to be married to microarray platforms for the identification of amplified DNA by hybridization. For instance, the pattern of hybridization of labeled and amplified ITS 1 rDNA to a chip containing thousands of ITS sequences from all known fungal pathogens may be useful for identifying fungi in clinical samples or mixed communities. Interpreting the results of microarray assays will likely require a great deal of experience derived from empirical observations using known amounts of fungal DNA from different species as input. Cross-hybridization of rDNA species to unintended spots on the microarray is one potential problem with this approach. Detection of fungal nucleic acid sequences by microarray alone is not likely to detect fungi with sufficient sensitivity in human infections, thus necessitating use of an amplification step prior to hybridization. Considering the challenges evident with the introduction of relatively simple molecular diagnostics in mycology, such as PCR, it is unlikely that more advanced technology platforms will be adopted in the immediate future.

CONCLUSIONS

Advances in molecular mycology have made our lives more complicated by identifying new fungal genera and cryptic species, and by creating new taxonomic groups for existing fungal pathogens. The same advances allow us to better resolve differences between fungal species, creating new opportunities for understanding the epidemiology of infection and microbe-disease associations. Molecular sequence data will be instrumental in improving the diagnosis of fungal infections, filling a significant gap in our ability to provide optimal care to patients. As the diversity of fungal pathogens that cause human disease continues to expand, so does our ability to detect them.

REFERENCES

1. Yeo SF, Wong B. Current status of nonculture methods for diagnosis of invasive fungal infections. Clin Microbiol Rev 2002; 15(3):465–84.
2. Stevens DA. Diagnosis of fungal infections: current status. J Antimicrob Chemother 2002; 49(Suppl. 1):11–9.
3. Mahfouz T, Anaissie E. Prevention of fungal infections in the immunocompromised host. Curr Opin Investig Drugs 2003; 4(8):974–90.
4. Taylor JW, Fisher MC. Fungal multilocus sequence typing—it's not just for bacteria. Curr Opin Microbiol 2003; 6(4):351–6.
5. Kwon-Chung KJ, Bennett JE. Rhinosporidiosis. Medical Mycology. Philadelphia, PA: Lea & Febiger, 1992:695–706.
6. Levy MG, Meuten DJ, Breitschwerdt EB. Cultivation of *Rhinosporidium seeberi* in vitro: interaction with epithelial cells. Science 1986; 234(4775):474–6.
7. Fredricks DN, et al. *Rhinosporidium seeberi*: a human pathogen from a novel group of aquatic protistan parasites. Emerg Infect Dis 2000; 6(3):273–82.
8. Herr RA, et al. Phylogenetic analysis of *Rhinosporidium seeberi*'s 18S small-subunit ribosomal DNA groups this pathogen among members of the protoctistan *Mesomycetozoa* clade. J Clin Microbiol 1999; 37(9):2750–4.

9. Ragan MA, Murphy CA, Rand TG. Are Ichthyosporea animals or fungi? Bayesian phylogenetic analysis of elongation factor 1alpha of *Ichthyophonus irregularis* Mol Phylogenet Evol 2003; 29(3):550–62.

10. Ragan MA, et al. A novel clade of protistan parasites near the animal-fungal divergence. Proc Natl Acad Sci USA 1996; 93(21):11907–12.

11. Mendoza L, Taylor JW, Ajello L. The class *mesomycetozoea*: a heterogeneous group of microorganisms at the animal-fungal boundary. Annu Rev Microbiol 2002; 56:315–44.

12. Taborda PR, Taborda VA, McGinnis MR. *Lacazia loboi* gen. nov., comb. nov., the etiologic agent of lobomycosis. J Clin Microbiol 1999; 37(6):2031–3.

13. Kwon-Chung KJ, Bennett JE. Lobomycosis. Medical Mycology. Philadelphia, PA: Lea & Febiger, 1992:514–23.

14. Belone AF, et al. Experimental reproduction of the Jorge Lobo's disease in BAlb/c mice inoculated with *Lacazia loboi* obtained from a previously infected mouse. Mycopathologia 2002; 155(4):191–4.

15. Fischer M, et al. Sucessful treatment with clofazimine and itraconazole in a 46 year old patient after 32 years duration of disease. Hautarzt 2002; 53(10):677–81.

16. Herr RA, et al. Phylogenetic analysis of *Lacazia loboi* places this previously uncharacterized pathogen within the dimorphic Onygenales. J Clin Microbiol 2001; 39(1):309–14.

17. Hughes WT. *Pneumocystis carinii*: taxing taxonomy. Eur J Epidemiol 1989; 5(3):265–9.

18. Bedrossian CW. Ultrastructure of *Pneumocystis carinii*: a review of internal and surface characteristics. Semin Diagn Pathol 1989; 6(3):212–37.

19. ul Haque A, et al. *Pneumocystis carinii*. Taxonomy as viewed by electron microscopy. Am J Clin Pathol 1987; 87(4):504–10.

20. Pixley FJ, et al. Mitochondrial gene sequences show fungal homology for *Pneumocystis carinii*. Mol Microbiol 1991; 5(6):1347–51.

21. Stringer SL, et al. *Pneumocystis carinii*: sequence from ribosomal RNA implies a close relationship with fungi. Exp Parasitol 1989; 68(4):450–61.

22. Edman JC, et al. Ribosomal RNA sequence shows *Pneumocystis carinii* to be a member of the fungi. Nature 1988; 334(6182):519–22.

23. Liu YJ, Whelen S, Hall BD. Phylogenetic relationships among ascomycetes: evidence from an RNA polymerse II subunit. Mol Biol Evol 1999; 16(12):1799–808.

24. Stringer JR, et al. Molecular genetic distinction of *Pneumocystis carinii* from rats and humans. J Eukaryot Microbiol 1993; 40(6):733–41.

25. Stringer JR, et al. A new name (*Pneumocystis jiroveci*) for *Pneumocystis* from humans. Emerg Infect Dis 2002; 8(9):891–6.

26. Stringer JR. Pneumocystis. Int J Med Microbiol 2002; 292(5–6):391–404.

27. Kwon-Chung KJ, Bennett JE. Infections caused by *Malassezia* species. Medical Mycology. Philadelphia, PA: Lea & Febiger, 1992:170–82.

28. Marcon MJ, Powell DA. Human infections due to *Malassezia* spp. Clin Microbiol Rev 1992; 5(2):101–19.

29. Gueho E, Midgley G, Guillot J. The genus *Malassezia* with description of four new species. Antonie Van Leeuwenhoek 1996; 69(4):337–55.

30. Sugita T, et al. A new yeast, *Malassezia yamatoensis*, isolated from a patient with seborrheic dermatitis, and its distribution in patients and healthy subjects. Microbiol Immunol 2004; 48(8):579–83.

31. Sugita T, et al. Description of a new yeast species, *Malassezia japonica*, and its detection in patients with atopic dermatitis and healthy subjects. J Clin Microbiol 2003; 41(10):4695–9.

32. Sugita T, et al. New yeast species, *Malassezia dermatis*, isolated from patients with atopic dermatitis. J Clin Microbiol 2002; 40(4):1363–7.

33. Hirai A, et al. *Malassezia nana* sp. nov., a novel lipid-dependent yeast species isolated from animals. Int J Syst Evol Microbiol 2004; 54(Pt 2):623–7.

34. Yamada Y, et al. DNA base alignment and taxonomic study of genus *Malassezia* based upon partial sequences of mitochondrial large subunit ribosomal RNA gene. Microbiol Immunol 2003; 47(6):475–8.

35. Makimura K, et al. Species identification and strain typing of *Malassezia* species stock strains and clinical isolates based on the DNA sequences of nuclear ribosomal internal transcribed spacer 1 regions. J Med Microbiol 2000; 49(1):29–35.

36. Kano R, et al. Chitin synthase 2 gene sequence of *Malassezia* species. Microbiol Immunol 1999; 43(8):813–5.

37. Aspiroz C, et al. Differentiation of three biotypes of *Malassezia* species on human normal skin correspondence with *M. globosa*, *M. sympodialis* and *M. restricta*. Mycopathologia 1999; 145(2):69–74.

38. Sugita T, et al. Molecular analysis of *Malassezia* microflora on the skin of atopic dermatitis patients and healthy subjects. J Clin Microbiol 2001; 39(10):3486–90.

39. Gemmer CM, et al. Fast, noninvasive method for molecular detection and differentiation of *Malassezia* yeast species on human skin and application of the method to dandruff microbiology. J Clin Microbiol 2002; 40(9):3350–7.

40. Koufopanou V, Burt A, Taylor JW. Concordance of gene genealogies reveals reproductive isolation in the pathogenic fungus *Coccidioides immitis*. Proc Natl Acad Sci USA 1997; 94(10):5478–82.

41. Koufopanou V, et al. Gene genealogies, cryptic species, and molecular evolution in the human pathogen *Coccidioides immitis* and relatives (*Ascomycota, Onygenales*). Mol Biol Evol 2001; 18(7):1246–58.

42. Pan S, Sigler L, Cole GT. Evidence for a phylogenetic connection between *Coccidioides immitis* and *Uncinocarpus reesii* (*Onygenaceae*). Microbiology 1994; 140(Pt 6):1481–94.

43. Kasuga T, Taylor JW, White TJ. Phylogenetic relationships of varieties and geographical groups of the human pathogenic fungus *Histoplasma capsulatum* darling. J Clin Microbiol 1999; 37(3):653–63.

44. Kasuga T, et al. Phylogeography of the fungal pathogen *Histoplasma capsulatum*. Mol Ecol 2003; 12(12):3383–401.

45. Franzot SP, Salkin IF, Casadevall A. *Cryptococcus neoformans* var. *grubii*: separate varietal status for *Cryptococcus neoformans* serotype A isolates. J Clin Microbiol 1999; 37(3):838–40.

46. Sugita T, Ikeda R, Shinoda T. Diversity among strains of *Cryptococcus neoformans* var. *gattii* as revealed by a sequence analysis of multiple genes and a chemotype analysis of capsular polysaccharide. Microbiol Immunol 2001; 45(11):757–68.

47. Guarro J, Gene J, Stchigel AM. Developments in fungal taxonomy. Clin Microbiol Rev 1999; 12(3):454–500.
48. Taylor JW, et al. The evolutionary biology and population genetics underlying fungal strain typing. Clin Microbiol Rev 1999; 12(1):126–46.
49. Taylor JW, et al. Phylogenetic species recognition and species concepts in fungi. Fungal Genet Biol 2000; 31(1):21–32.
50. Balajee SA, et al. *Aspergillus fumigatus* variant with decreased susceptibility to multiple antifungals. Antimicrob Agents Chemother 2004; 48(4):1197–203.
51. Balajee SA, et al. *Aspergillus lentulus* sp. nov., a new sibling species of *A. fumigatus*. Eukaryot Cell 2005; 4(3):625–32.
52. Hong SB, et al. Polyphasic taxonomy of *Aspergillus fumigatus* and related species. Mycologia 2005; 97(6):1316–29.
53. Tarrand JJ, et al. *Aspergillus* hyphae in infected tissue: evidence of physiologic adaptation and effect on culture recovery. J Clin Microbiol 2005; 43(1):382–6.
54. Hugenholtz P, Goebel BM, Pace NR. Impact of culture-independent studies on the emerging phylogenetic view of bacterial diversity. J Bacteriol 1998; 180(18):4765–74.
55. Anderson IC, Cairney JW. Diversity and ecology of soil fungal communities: increased understanding through the application of molecular techniques. Environ Microbiol 2004; 6(8):769–79.
56. Vandenkoornhuyse P, et al. Extensive fungal diversity in plant roots. Science 2002; 295(5562):2051.
57. Fredricks DN, Relman DA. Sequence-based identification of microbial pathogens: a reconsideration of Koch's postulates. Clin Microbiol Rev 1996; 9(1):18–33.
58. Jahagirdar BN, Morrison VA. Emerging fungal pathogens in patients with hematologic malignancies and marrow/stem-cell transplant recipients. Semin Respir Infect 2002; 17(2):113–20.
59. Nucci M, Marr KA. Emerging fungal diseases. Clin Infect Dis 2005; 41(4):521–6.
60. Marr KA, et al. Invasive aspergillosis in allogeneic stem cell transplant recipients: changes in epidemiology and risk factors. Blood 2002; 100(13):4358–66.
61. Hazen KC. New and emerging yeast pathogens. Clin Microbiol Rev 1995; 8(4):462–78.
62. Perfect JR, Schell WA. The new fungal opportunists are coming. Clin Infect Dis 1996; 22(Suppl. 2):S112–8.
63. Walsh TJ, et al. Infections due to emerging and uncommon medically important fungal pathogens. Clin Microbiol Infect 2004; 10(Suppl. 1):48–66.
64. Husain S, et al. Opportunistic mycelial fungal infections in organ transplant recipients: emerging importance of non-*Aspergillus* mycelial fungi. Clin Infect Dis 2003; 37(2):221–9.
65. Imhof A, et al. Breakthrough fungal infections in stem cell transplant recipients receiving voriconazole. Clin Infect Dis 2004; 39(5):743–6.
66. Marty FM, Cosimi LA, Baden LR. Breakthrough zygomycosis after voriconazole treatment in recipients of hematopoietic stem-cell transplants. N Engl J Med 2004; 350(9):950–2.
67. Siwek GT, et al. Invasive zygomycosis in hematopoietic stem cell transplant recipients receiving voriconazole prophylaxis. Clin Infect Dis 2004; 39(4):584–7.

68. Kontoyiannis DP, et al. Zygomycosis in the 1990s in a tertiary-care cancer center. Clin Infect Dis 2000; 30(6):851–6.

69. Kontoyiannis DP, et al. Zygomycosis in a tertiary-care cancer center in the era of *Aspergillus*-active antifungal therapy: a case-control observational study of 27 recent cases. J Infect Dis 2005; 191(8):1350–60.

70. Fredricks DN, Relman DA. Application of polymerase chain reaction to the diagnosis of infectious diseases. Clin Infect Dis 1999; 29(3):475–86 (Quiz 487–8).

Index

About the Editors

Johan A. Maertens is Associate Professor of Hematology, Department of Hematology, Universitaire Ziekenhuizen Leuven, Belgium, campus Gasthuisberg. Dr. Maertens is a member of the Immunocompromised Host Society, the International Society of Human and Animal Mycology, the Belgian Infectious Diseases Advisory Board, the Multinational Association of Supportive Care in Cancer, the American Society of Hematology, the European Blood and Marrow Transplantation, and the European Organization for Research and Treatment of Cancer (EORTC)-Infectious Diseases Group (of which he is the current chair person), among other organizations. He is one of the steering committee members of the European Conference on Infections in Leukaemia (ECIL)-meetings. Dr. Maertens has published articles on management and diagnosis of fungal infections in several esteemed journals, including the *New England Journal of Medicine*. Dr. Maertens received the M.D. degree from the Catholic University of Leuven, Belgium. He completed an internal medicine residency and clinical hematology fellowship at the University Hospital, Leuven, Belgium.

Kieren A. Marr is a Professor of Medicine, Division of Infectious Diseases, at Oregon Health and Science University, Portland, Oregon, U.S.A., where she serves as Director of the Transplant Infectious Diseases Program and the Infectious Diseases Clinical Research Center. She is also an Affiliate Investigator at the Fred Hutchinson Cancer Research Center, Seattle, Washington, U.S.A. Her research is focused on *Aspergillus* pathogenesis, and the prevention and early diagnosis of invasive infections in immunocompromised patients. Dr. Marr is the recipient of numerous awards, including the Cancer Federation Award, the American Medical Women's Association Citation, and a Medical Mycology Fellowship from the National Federation of Infectious Diseases. She has served on the program committee of the Infectious Diseases Society of America, the council of the Immunocompromised Host Society, and multiple editorial boards. Dr. Marr received the M.D. degree at Hahnemann University, Philadelphia, Pennsylvania, U.S.A., and completed an internship and residency in internal medicine at Duke University, Durham, North Carolina, U.S.A. She completed infectious diseases training at the University of Washington, Seattle, Washington, U.S.A.